Nutrition in Gynecologic Disease

Nutrition in Gynecologic Disease

Editor

Pasquapina Ciarmela

MDPI • Basel • Beijing • Wuhan • Barcelona • Belgrade • Manchester • Tokyo • Cluj • Tianjin

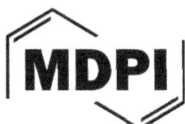

Editor
Pasquapina Ciarmela
Università Politecnica delle Marche
Italy

Editorial Office
MDPI
St. Alban-Anlage 66
4052 Basel, Switzerland

This is a reprint of articles from the Special Issue published online in the open access journal *Nutrients* (ISSN 2072-6643) (available at: https://www.mdpi.com/journal/nutrients/special_issues/Nutrition_Gynecologic_Disease).

For citation purposes, cite each article independently as indicated on the article page online and as indicated below:

LastName, A.A.; LastName, B.B.; LastName, C.C. Article Title. *Journal Name* **Year**, *Volume Number*, Page Range.

ISBN 978-3-0365-3280-6 (Hbk)
ISBN 978-3-0365-3281-3 (PDF)

© 2022 by the authors. Articles in this book are Open Access and distributed under the Creative Commons Attribution (CC BY) license, which allows users to download, copy and build upon published articles, as long as the author and publisher are properly credited, which ensures maximum dissemination and a wider impact of our publications.

The book as a whole is distributed by MDPI under the terms and conditions of the Creative Commons license CC BY-NC-ND.

Contents

About the Editor vii

Pasquapina Ciarmela
Nutrition in Gynecologic Disease
Reprinted from: *Nutrients* **2022**, *14*, 707, doi:10.3390/nu14030707 1

Yung-Jiun Chien, Chun-Yu Chang, Meng-Yu Wu, Chih-Hao Chen, Yi-Shiung Horng and Hsin-Chi Wu
Effects of Curcumin on Glycemic Control and Lipid Profile in Polycystic Ovary Syndrome: Systematic Review with Meta-Analysis and Trial Sequential Analysis
Reprinted from: *Nutrients* **2021**, *13*, 684, doi:10.3390/nu13020684 3

Michał Ciebiera, Sahar Esfandyari, Hiba Siblini, Lillian Prince, Hoda Elkafas, Cezary Wojtyła, Ayman Al-Hendy and Mohamed Ali
Nutrition in Gynecological Diseases: Current Perspectives
Reprinted from: *Nutrients* **2021**, *13*, 1178, doi:10.3390/nu13041178 17

Thais R. Silva, Karen Oppermann, Fernando M. Reis and Poli Mara Spritzer
Nutrition in Menopausal Women: A Narrative Review
Reprinted from: *Nutrients* **2021**, *13*, 2149, doi:10.3390/nu13072149 51

Małgorzata Szczuko, Justyna Kikut, Urszula Szczuko, Iwona Szydłowska, Jolanta Nawrocka-Rutkowska, Maciej Ziętek, Donatella Verbanac and Luciano Saso
Nutrition Strategy and Life Style in Polycystic Ovary Syndrome—Narrative Review
Reprinted from: *Nutrients* **2021**, *13*, 2452, doi:10.3390/nu13072452 65

Ludovica Bartiromo, Matteo Schimberni, Roberta Villanacci, Jessica Ottolina, Carolina Dolci, Noemi Salmeri, Paola Viganò and Massimo Candiani
Endometriosis and Phytoestrogens: Friends or Foes? A Systematic Review
Reprinted from: *Nutrients* **2021**, *13*, 2532, doi:10.3390/nu13082532 83

Enrrico Bloise, Jair R. S. Braga, Cherley B. V. Andrade, Guinever E. Imperio, Lilian M. Martinelli, Roberto A. Antunes, Karina R. Silva, Cristiana B. Nunes, Luigi Cobellis, Flavia F. Bloise, Stephen G. Matthews, Kristin L. Connor and Tania M. Ortiga-Carvalho
Altered Umbilical Cord Blood Nutrient Levels, Placental Cell Turnover and Transporter Expression in Human Term Pregnancies Conceived by Intracytoplasmic Sperm Injection (ICSI)
Reprinted from: *Nutrients* **2021**, *13*, 2587, doi:10.3390/ nu13082587 113

Karina Ryterska, Agnieszka Kordek and Patrycja Załęska
Has Menstruation Disappeared? Functional Hypothalamic Amenorrhea—What Is This Story about?
Reprinted from: *Nutrients* **2021**, *13*, 2827, doi:10.3390/nu13082827 131

Linda Yu, Eddy Rios, Lysandra Castro, Jingli Liu, Yitang Yan and Darlene Dixon
Genistein: Dual Role in Women's Health
Reprinted from: *Nutrients* **2021**, *13*, 3048, doi:10.3390/nu13093048 147

Yi-Fen Chiang, Hsin-Yuan Chen, Mohamed Ali, Tzong-Ming Shieh, Yun-Ju Huang,
Kai-Lee Wang, Hsin-Yi Chang, Tsui-Chin Huang, Yong-Han Hong and Shih-Min Hsia
The Role of Cell Proliferation and Extracellular Matrix Accumulation Induced by Food Additive
Butylated Hydroxytoluene in Uterine Leiomyoma
Reprinted from: *Nutrients* **2021**, *13*, 3074, doi:10.3390/nu13093074 . . . . **171**

Paula Benvindo Ferreira, Anderson Fellyp Avelino Diniz, Francisco Fernandes Lacerda Júnior,
Maria da Conceição Correia Silva, Glêbia Alexa Cardoso, Alexandre Sérgio Silva and
Bagnólia Araújo da Silva
Supplementation with *Spirulina platensis* Prevents Uterine Diseases Related to Muscle Reactivity and
Oxidative Stress in Rats Undergoing Strength Training
Reprinted from: *Nutrients* **2021**, *13*, 3763, doi:10.3390/nu13113763 . . . . **185**

Stefania Greco, Pamela Pellegrino, Alessandro Zannotti, Giovanni Delli Carpini,
Andrea Ciavattini, Fernando M. Reis and Pasquapina Ciarmela
Phytoprogestins: Unexplored Food Compounds with Potential Preventive and Therapeutic
Effects in Female Diseases
Reprinted from: *Nutrients* **2021**, *13*, 4326, doi:10.3390/nu13124326 . . . . **199**

About the Editor

Pasquapina Ciarmela is an Associate Professor of Human Anatomy at Università Politecnica delle Marche, Italy. Her research focuses on uterine physiology and pathophysiology and explores the role of growth factors and the extracellular matrix. Her investigation aims at understanding the pathogenesis of uterine fibroids and developing potential therapeutic agents, including nutritional components.

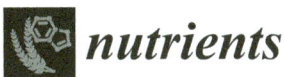

Editorial

Nutrition in Gynecologic Disease

Pasquapina Ciarmela

Department of Experimental and Clinical Medicine, Università Politecnica delle Marche, 60126 Ancona, Italy; p.ciarmela@univpm.it; Tel.: +39-071-220-6270

The pathologies concerning the gynecological organs are very varied and range from tumoral pathologies to hormonal dysfunctions. The frequency of benign and malignant disease affecting women's health is very high.

Epidemiological studies show that lifestyle can be an important risk factor for gynecological diseases. One such modifiable lifestyle factor is the diet. The father of medicine, Hippocrates, proclaimed "Let food be the medicine and medicine be the food" almost 25 centuries ago. The relationship between diet and health is yet to be fully explored. The human diet contains a wide variety of plant-based foods that provide essential nutrients for the body. Besides, plant-based foods possess a huge variety of non-nutritive components that offer beneficial health effects.

This book, based on a Special Issue of Nutrients, contains a total of 11 papers (four original research, six reviews and one systematic review) focusing on nutrition in gynecologic disease.

The original articles include studies on uterine and ovarian dysfunctions and placental development.

The first study of this book is in vivo and it focuses on the effect of food supplementation in preventing uterine dysfunction. In detail, it demonstrated that *Spirulina platensis*, an antioxidant blue algae, prevents changes in reactivity and oxidative stress induced by strength training in rat uteri [1]. The second article describe an in vitro study on leiomyoma, the most common benign uterine tumor in reproductive-age women. The commonly used food additive butylated hydroxytoluene (BHT) has a proliferative and fibrotic effect on the ELT-3 leiomyoma cell line. BHT exposure may therefore have a harmful effect on leiomyoma progression and the mechanism may be related to PI_3K modulation [2].

Following this, an article is included that reports on the possible mechanism that may increase the risk for abnormal placental development in assisted reproductive technologies, studied through tissual evaluation of human placenta and fasting blood nutrient levels from term pregnancy conceived naturally or by intracytoplasmic sperm injection. Hence, in term pregnancy, intracytoplasmic sperm injection impairs placental amino acids transporter expression, cell turnover, and altern umbilical vein levels of specific nutrients [3].

Finally, there is an article on the effect of curcumin on glycemic control and lipid profile in patients with polycystic ovary syndrome (PCOS). Systemic review with meta-analysis and trial sequential analysis suggest that curcumin may improve glycemic control, lipid metabolism, and metabolic abnormality in patients with PCOS [4].

Regarding the reviews, two papers on the effect of phytosteroids (phytoprogestins and phytoestrogens) have been included [5,6]. First, there is a review on possible terapeutic phytoprogestins for female disease studied so far, such as kaempferol, apigenin, luteolin, and naringenin. Although limited data are available, it seems that phytoprogestins could be a promising tool for preventing and treating hormone-dependent diseases [5]. Among the extensively studied phytoestrogens, the second review focuses on genistein, an isoflavone which structurally resembles endogenous estrogen often consumed via soya products [6].

Next, there are two reviews on nutritional aspects in pathological situations, such as functional hypothalamic amenorrhea (FHA) [7], and PCOS [8]. Furthermore, there is a further review on the importance of the nutritional habits for health promotion and lifestyle adaptation to the menopausal period [9].

Citation: Ciarmela, P. Nutrition in Gynecologic Disease. *Nutrients* 2022, 14, 707. https://doi.org/10.3390/nu14030707

Received: 18 January 2022
Accepted: 28 January 2022
Published: 8 February 2022

Publisher's Note: MDPI stays neutral with regard to jurisdictional claims in published maps and institutional affiliations.

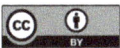

Copyright: © 2022 by the author. Licensee MDPI, Basel, Switzerland. This article is an open access article distributed under the terms and conditions of the Creative Commons Attribution (CC BY) license (https://creativecommons.org/licenses/by/4.0/).

The last review is a comprehensive general paper that summarizes and furnishes the current perspectives on the importance of nutrition in gynecological disease [10].

The book ends with a systematic review that provides comprehensive and available data on the possible role of phytoestrogens for the treatment of endometriosis [11].

I believe that this collection includes important current studies on the benefits of nutrients in prevention, therapy, and management of female dysfunctions.

Conflicts of Interest: The author declares no conflict of interest.

References

1. Ferreira, P.B.; Diniz, A.F.A.; Lacerda Júnior, F.F.; Silva, M.d.C.C.; Cardoso, G.A.; Silva, A.S.; da Silva, B.A. Supplementation with Spirulina platensis Prevents Uterine Diseases Related to Muscle Reactivity and Oxidative Stress in Rats Undergoing Strength Training. *Nutrients* **2021**, *13*, 3763. [CrossRef]
2. Chiang, Y.-F.; Chen, H.-Y.; Ali, M.; Shieh, T.-M.; Huang, Y.-J.; Wang, K.-L.; Chang, H.-Y.; Huang, T.-C.; Hong, Y.-H.; Hsia, S.-M. The Role of Cell Proliferation and Extracellular Matrix Accumulation Induced by Food Additive Butylated Hydroxytoluene in Uterine Leiomyoma. *Nutrients* **2021**, *13*, 3074. [CrossRef]
3. Bloise, E.; Braga, J.R.S.; Andrade, C.B.V.; Imperio, G.E.; Martinelli, L.M.; Antunes, R.A.; Silva, K.R.; Nunes, C.B.; Cobellis, L.; Bloise, F.F.; et al. Altered Umbilical Cord Blood Nutrient Levels, Placental Cell Turnover and Transporter Expression in Human Term Pregnancies Conceived by Intracytoplasmic Sperm Injection (ICSI). *Nutrients* **2021**, *13*, 2587. [CrossRef] [PubMed]
4. Chien, Y.-J.; Chang, C.-Y.; Wu, M.-Y.; Chen, C.-H.; Horng, Y.-S.; Wu, H.-C. Effects of Curcumin on Glycemic Control and Lipid Profile in Polycystic Ovary Syndrome: Systematic Review with Meta-Analysis and Trial Sequential Analysis. *Nutrients* **2021**, *13*, 684. [CrossRef] [PubMed]
5. Greco, S.; Pellegrino, P.; Zannotti, A.; Delli Carpini, G.; Ciavattini, A.; Reis, F.M.; Ciarmela, P. Phytoprogestins: Unexplored Food Compounds with Potential Preventive and Therapeutic Effects in Female Diseases. *Nutrients* **2021**, *13*, 4326. [CrossRef] [PubMed]
6. Yu, L.; Rios, E.; Castro, L.; Liu, J.; Yan, Y.; Dixon, D. Genistein: Dual Role in Women's Health. *Nutrients* **2021**, *13*, 3048. [CrossRef] [PubMed]
7. Ryterska, K.; Kordek, A.; Załęska, P. Has Menstruation Disappeared? Functional Hypothalamic Amenorrhea—What Is This Story about? *Nutrients* **2021**, *13*, 2827. [CrossRef] [PubMed]
8. Szczuko, M.; Kikut, J.; Szczuko, U.; Szydłowska, I.; Nawrocka-Rutkowska, J.; Ziętek, M.; Verbanac, D.; Saso, L. Nutrition Strategy and Life Style in Polycystic Ovary Syndrome—Narrative Review. *Nutrients* **2021**, *13*, 2452. [CrossRef] [PubMed]
9. Silva, T.R.; Oppermann, K.; Reis, F.M.; Spritzer, P.M. Nutrition in Menopausal Women: A Narrative Review. *Nutrients* **2021**, *13*, 2149. [CrossRef] [PubMed]
10. Ciebiera, M.; Esfandyari, S.; Siblini, H.; Prince, L.; Elkafas, H.; Wojtyła, C.; Al-Hendy, A.; Ali, M. Nutrition in Gynecological Diseases: Current Perspectives. *Nutrients* **2021**, *13*, 1178. [CrossRef] [PubMed]
11. Bartiromo, L.; Schimberni, M.; Villanacci, R.; Ottolina, J.; Dolci, C.; Salmeri, N.; Viganò, P.; Candiani, M. Endometriosis and Phytoestrogens: Friends or Foes? A Systematic Review. *Nutrients* **2021**, *13*, 2532. [CrossRef] [PubMed]

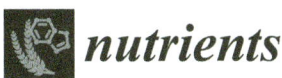

Article

Effects of Curcumin on Glycemic Control and Lipid Profile in Polycystic Ovary Syndrome: Systematic Review with Meta-Analysis and Trial Sequential Analysis

Yung-Jiun Chien [1,2], Chun-Yu Chang [2,3], Meng-Yu Wu [2,4], Chih-Hao Chen [5], Yi-Shiung Horng [1,2,*] and Hsin-Chi Wu [1,2,*]

1. Department of Physical Medicine and Rehabilitation, Taipei Tzu Chi Hospital, Buddhist Tzu Chi Medical Foundation, New Taipei City 231, Taiwan; jessica.kan.48@gmail.com
2. School of Medicine, Tzu Chi University, Hualien 970, Taiwan; paulchang1231@gmail.com (C.-Y.C.); skyshangrila@gmail.com (M.-Y.W.)
3. Department of Anesthesiology, Taipei Tzu Chi Hospital, Buddhist Tzu Chi Medical Foundation, New Taipei City 231, Taiwan
4. Department of Emergency Medicine, Taipei Tzu Chi Hospital, Buddhist Tzu Chi Medical Foundation, New Taipei City 231, Taiwan
5. Department of Otolaryngology-Head and Neck Surgery, Taipei Veterans General Hospital, Taipei 112, Taiwan; michaelchen808@gmail.com
* Correspondence: yshorng2015@gmail.com (Y.-S.H.); taipeitzuchi2021@gmail.com (H.-C.W.)

Abstract: The therapeutic effects of curcumin for polycystic ovary syndrome (PCOS) remain inconclusive. The present study aims to evaluate the effects of curcumin on glycemic control and lipid profile in patients with PCOS. PubMed, Embase, Scopus, Web of Science, and Cochrane Library were searched from the inception through 28 November 2020. Randomized control trials (RCTs), which enrolled adult patients with PCOS, compared curcumin with placebo regarding the glycemic control and lipid profile, and reported sufficient information for performing meta-analysis, were included. Three RCTs were included. Curcumin significantly improves fasting glucose (mean difference (MD): −2.77, 95% confidence interval (CI): −4.16 to −1.38), fasting insulin (MD: −1.33, 95% CI: −2.18 to −0.49), Homeostasis Model Assessment of Insulin Resistance (HOMA-IR) (MD: −0.32, 95% CI: −0.52 to −0.12), and quantitative insulin sensitivity check index (QUICKI) (MD: 0.010, 95% CI: 0.003–0.018). It also significantly improves high-density lipoprotein (MD: 1.92, 95% CI: 0.33–3.51) and total cholesterol (MD: −12.45, 95% CI: −22.05 to −2.85). In contrast, there is no statistically significant difference in the improvement in low-density lipoprotein (MD: −6.02, 95% CI: −26.66 to 14.62) and triglyceride (MD: 8.22, 95% CI: −26.10 to 42.53) between curcumin and placebo. The results of the fasting glucose, fasting insulin, HOMA-IR, QUICKI, and total cholesterol are conclusive as indicated by the trial sequential analysis. Curcumin may improve glycemic control and lipid metabolism in patients with PCOS and metabolic abnormality without significant adverse effects. Further studies are advocated to investigate the potential effects of curcumin on hyperandrogenism.

Keywords: cholesterol; curcumin; insulin resistance; meta-analysis; polycystic ovary syndrome; trial sequential analysis

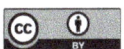

1. Introduction

Polycystic ovary syndrome (PCOS) is the most common endocrine disorder in women of reproductive age, with prevalence up to 10% to 16% [1,2]. It is characterized by hyperandrogenism, ovulatory dysfunction, and polycystic ovaries [3]. In addition, nearly half of adult patients with PCOS develop metabolic syndrome and insulin resistance [4,5], and are associated with considerably higher risks of type 2 diabetes mellitus, cardiovascular disease, and even cancer [6,7].

The pathophysiology of PCOS is complex and is believed to involve functional ovarian hyperandrogenism caused by hyperresponsiveness to the stimulation of luteinizing hormone and failed downregulation of thecal androgen production [8,9]. A distinctive feature of PCOS is insulin-resistant hyperinsulinemia. It aggravates hyperandrogenism by counteracting the luteinizing hormone-induced homologous desensitization via upregulation of the activity of cytochrome P450c17 and luteinizing hormone receptor binding sites [10,11]. Moreover, the excessive insulin synergizes with androgen to prematurely luteinize granulosa cells, leading to follicle maturation arrest and anovulation [12]. Furthermore, proinflammatory cytokines have also been demonstrated to upregulate the activity of cytochrome P450c17 [13]. The goals of therapy for patients with PCOS include improving hyperandrogenic features, managing metabolic abnormalities, and ovulation induction or contraception depending on whether a pregnancy is pursued.

More than a third of women with PCOS suffered from metabolic syndrome [14]. The severity of metabolic syndrome and the phenotype of PCOS are strongly associated with the degree of hyperandrogenism and hyperinsulinemia [15,16]. Decreasing plasma insulin level and improving insulin resistance in patients with PCOS not only benefit hyperandrogenism and ovulation but also reduce cardiovascular risks [1,12,17]. Besides lifestyle modification, metformin is commonly used as an insulin sensitive agent that reduces fasting glucose, improving insulin resistance in patients with PCOS [18]. Combination therapy with metformin and clomiphene also showed positive results for ovulation in patients with PCOS [19]. However, emerging studies on phytomedicine as well as complementary medicine had shown promising results in the treatment of PCOS.

Curcumin, also known as turmeric, is a polyphenol derived from curcumin longa, and is traditionally used in various Asian cuisine [20]. Recently, curcumin has been studied to adjunctly treat broad spectrum of disease from type 2 diabetes mellitus to telogen effluvium [21]. Curcumin elicits antidiabetic effects via several mechanisms, including the increase in glycolysis and glycogen synthesis and the decrease in gluconeogenesis in the liver, as well as the increase in glucose uptake, glycolysis, and glycogen synthesis in the skeletal muscle [22]. Curcumin has also been known to reduce plasma cholesterol and triglyceride by increasing the activity of lipoprotein lipase and through mechanisms which alter lipid and cholesterol gene expression [23,24]. In addition, the anti-inflammatory effects of curcumin have been demonstrated to reduce the oxidative stress in patients with PCOS [25,26]. Previous literature reveals that curcumin significantly improves fasting blood glucose and triglyceride in patients with metabolic syndrome [27]. In vivo study further demonstrates similar effects in the PCOS model [28]. However, the effects of curcumin on metabolic abnormalities in patients with PCOS are not conclusive. The present study aims to evaluate the effects of curcumin on glycemic control and lipid profile in patients with PCOS.

2. Materials and Methods

2.1. Study Design

The present study is a systematic review and meta-analysis of randomized control trials. The primary aim is to investigate the effects of curcumin on glycemic control in patients with PCOS, which is assessed by fasting glucose, fasting insulin, Homeostasis Model Assessment of Insulin Resistance (HOMA-IR), and quantitative insulin sensitivity check index (QUICKI). The secondary aim is to investigate the effects of curcumin on lipid profile, which is assessed by plasma high-density lipoprotein (HDL), low-density lipoprotein (LDL), triglyceride, and total cholesterol. This study was registered with the International Prospective Register of Systematic Reviews (PROSPERO registration number CRD42021223898) and abides the Preferred Reporting Items for Systematic Review and Meta-Analysis (PRISMA) statement [29].

2.2. Search Strategy

Two authors (Y.-J. Chien and C.-Y. Chang) searched five electronic databases from the inception through 18 November 2020, including PubMed, Embase, Scopus, Web of Science, and Cochrane Library. Subject headings (MeSH terms in PubMed and Cochrane Library, and Emtree terms in Embase) and search field tags of title, abstracts and keywords were used to facilitate searching. Terms used for searching relevant records included: "polycystic ovary syndrome", "polycystic ovarian syndrome", "Stein-Leventhal syndrome", "sclerocystic ovarian degeneration", "sclerocystic ovary syndrome", "sclerocystic ovary", "sclerocystic ovaries", "curcumin", "curcumins", "curcuminoid", "curcuminoids", "curcuma longa", "tumeric", "turmeric", "curqfen", "theracurmin", "nanocurcumin", "turmeric yellow", and "diferuloylmethane". Supplementary Table S1 presents the detailed search strategy. The records identified from the databases were screened by titles, abstracts, and keywords. A full-text review was then carried out on those with potential eligibility. The authors also manually searched the references that were cited in the included studies to retrieve potentially eligible studies.

2.3. Eligibility Criteria

Studies were considered eligible if they met the following criteria: (a) the study was a randomized control trial enrolling patients with PCOS; (b) the study compared curcumin with placebo with regard to the outcomes of interest; (c) the study presented information that could be used to calculate the effect estimates for meta-analysis. Studies were not excluded according to publication date, country or language. All studies were selected against the eligibility criteria by two authors (Y.-J. Chien and C.-Y. Chang). Disagreements in the study selection were resolved through discussion and consensus with the third author (M.-Y. Wu)

2.4. Risk of Bias Assessment

The revised Cochrane Risk of Bias Tool 2 was used to assess the methodological quality of the included studies [30]. Disagreements were resolved by discussion or consensus with a third reviewer (M.-Y. Wu).

2.5. Data Extraction

Data extraction was performed by two reviewers (Y.-J. Chien and C.-Y. Chang) from the included studies. The required information included the author's name, year of publication, country, number and mean age of patients, dosing regimen and duration of curcumin therapy, diagnostic criteria of PCOS, and the effect estimates of curcumin on the outcomes of interest.

2.6. Statistical Analysis

The effects of curcumin on the continuous outcome variables were estimated by comparing the mean difference (MD) and standard deviation of changes before and after the therapy in the curcumin group with those in the placebo group (i.e., curcumin–placebo). The MD and 95% confidence interval (CI) were then calculated for each study using the aforementioned information. Alternatively, the MD and 95% CI were directly extracted if they were reported in the study. The pooled MD was synthesized using the inverse variance method with the random-effects model (DerSimonian–Laird estimator) [31,32]. Statistical heterogeneity was assessed by the Cochran's Q statistic and quantified by the I^2 statistic. In addition, an a priori meta-regression was planned to explore the influence of daily dose of curcumin and duration of therapy on the pooled effect estimates that are pooled from ≥ 10 studies [33].

In order to evaluate whether the results of the conventional meta-analysis were subject to type I or type II error due to sparse data and lack of power, trial sequential analysis (TSA) was applied to calculate the diversity-adjusted required information size (RIS) and trial sequential monitoring boundaries [34]. The models were set at an alpha of 5% and a power of 80% for all outcomes. Influence analysis was carried out as a sensitivity analysis by omitting one study at a time and recalculating the pooled results from each subset of the studies. Finally, if the pooled results were synthesized from greater than 10 studies, a contour-enhanced funnel plot and Egger's test were conducted to evaluate whether the publication bias existed [33,35,36]. In the case of significant asymmetry indicated by Egger's test, the trim-and-fill method was performed to identify the missing studies [37]. The statistical analyses were carried out using R software version 3.6.1 (R Foundation for Statistical Computing, Vienna, Austria) [38] with "dmetar", "meta", and "metafor" packages. TSA was performed with TSA software version 0.9.5.10 Beta (Copenhagen Trial Unit, Copenhagen, Denmark) [39]. A p-value < 0.05 was considered statistically significant.

3. Results

3.1. Study Identification and Selection

A total of 177 studies were identified from five databases, including PubMed (n = 10), EMBASE (n = 36), Cochrane Library (n = 14), SCOPUS (n = 112), and Web of Science (n = 5). After removing 51 duplicates, the remaining studies were screened for eligibility. A total of 117 records were excluded due to irrelevant topics by screening titles and abstracts. Therefore, nine studies were assessed for full-text review. Six studies were excluded due to ongoing trials and not having outcomes of interest. Finally, three studies involving 168 patients were included. The detailed PRISMA flow diagram is presented in Figure 1.

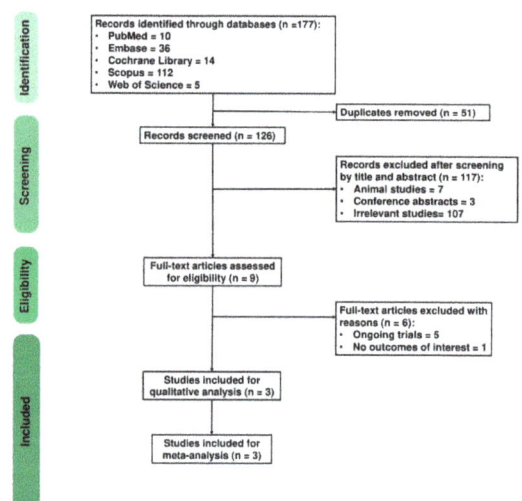

Figure 1. PRISMA flow diagram.

3.2. Study Characteristics and Risk of Bias Assessment

The characteristics of the included studies are presented in Table 1. All studies are randomized control trials. The dosing regimen of curcumin ranges from 500 mg once per day [40] to 500 mg three times per day [41]. Maltodextrin is used as placebo in one study [41], starch is used in another [40], and the other does not specify what consists of placebo [42]. The duration of therapy ranges from 6 weeks [42] to 12 weeks [40,41]. The diagnosis of PCOS is based on Rotterdam criteria in all the included studies [3]. In addition, the datasets extracted from each included study with regard to the outcomes of interest are presented in Table 2. Moreover, all the included studies are of low risk of overall bias despite some concerns raised from the randomization process, measurement of the outcome, and deviation from intended interventions. Notably, despite the measures taken to ensure the patient's adherence (e.g., returning the medication containers, and the reminders of taking medication by cell phone), deviation from intended interventions may, though unlikely, have occurred. The detailed risk of bias assessment for each included study is presented in Supplementary Figure S1.

Table 1. Study characteristics.

Scheme	Country	Study Design	Duration (Weeks)	Sample Size		Mean Age [†]		Regimen		Diagnostic Criteria
				Intervention	Control	Intervention	Control	Intervention	Control	
Sohaei et al. 2019 [42]	Iran	Double-blind RCT	6	27	24	29.4 (5.3)	29.6 (5.0)	Curcumin 500 mg BID	Placebo BID	Rotterdam criteria
Heshmati et al. 2020 [41]	Iran	Double-blind RCT	12	34	33	31.0 (5.2)	30.8 (8.0)	Curcumin 500 mg TID	Placebo (maltodextrin) TID	Rotterdam criteria
Jamilian et al. 2020 [40]	Iran	Double-blind RCT	12	26	24	28.6 (4.7)	27.2 (3.4)	Curcumin 500 mg QD	Placebo (starch) QD	Rotterdam criteria

[†] Mean age is presented as mean (standard deviation). BID: twice per day; QD: once per day; RCT: randomized control trial; TID: three times per day.

Table 2. Measurement of glycemic control and lipid profile in the curcumin and placebo group.

Study	Mean Difference (Standard Deviation) [†]		Mean Difference (95% Confidence Interval) [‡]
	Curcumin	Placebo	Curcumin−Placebo
	Fasting glucose (mg/dL)		
Sohaei et al. 2019 [42]	2.62 (9.48)	4.50 (10.80)	-
Heshmati et al. 2020 [41]	−5.09 (7.29)	−0.98 (9.11)	-
Jamilian et al. 2020 [40]	-	-	−2.63 (−4.21, −1.05)
	Fasting insulin (µIU/mL)		
Sohaei et al. 2019 [42]	−3.06 (6.44)	−0.88 (5.93)	-
Heshmati et al. 2020 [41]	−1.35 (4.90)	0.63 (4.77)	-
Jamilian et al. 2020 [40]	-	-	−1.16 (−2.12, −0.19)
	HOMA-IR		
Sohaei et al. 2019 [42]	−0.69 (1.87)	−0.07 (1.65)	-
Heshmati et al. 2020 [41]	−0.47 (1.22)	0.16 (1.17)	-
Jamilian et al. 2020 [40]	-	-	−0.26 (−0.48, −0.03)
	QUICKI		
Sohaei et al. 2019 [42]	0.010 (0.010)	0.000 (0.010)	-
Heshmati et al. 2020 [41]	0.020 (0.040)	−0.010 (0.040)	-
Jamilian et al. 2020 [40]	-	-	0.006 (0.001, 0.010)
	HDL (mg/dL)		
Sohaei et al. 2019 [42]	1.82 (6.30)	1.03 (7.99)	-
Jamilian et al. 2020 [40]	-	-	2.14 (0.36, 3.92)
	LDL (mg/dL)		
Sohaei et al. 2019 [42]	3.20 (21.82)	−1.79 (23.34)	-
Jamilian et al. 2020 [40]	-	-	−16.09 (−25.11, −7.06)
	Triglyceride (mg/dL)		
Sohaei et al. 2019 [42]	8.81 (70.73)	−21.62 (53.96)	-
Jamilian et al. 2020 [40]	-	-	−5.58 (−12.93, 1.77)
	Total cholesterol (mg/dL)		
Sohaei et al. 2019 [42]	−3.33 (18.58)	2.08 (33.67)	-
Jamilian et al. 2020 [40]	-	-	−15.86 (−24.48, −7.24)

[†] The mean difference refers to the changes before and after the therapy in the curcumin and placebo group. [‡] The mean difference refers to the difference in changes before and after the therapy between the curcumin and placebo group. HDL: high-density lipoprotein; HOMA-IR: Homeostasis Model Assessment of Insulin Resistance; LDL: low-density lipoprotein; QUICKI: quantitative insulin sensitivity check index.

3.3. Outcomes

3.3.1. Glycemic Control

The forest plot of glycemic control is presented in Figure 2. Fasting glucose, fasting insulin, HOMA-IR, and QUICKI were reported in all the included studies. The improvement in fasting glucose (MD: −2.77, 95% CI: −4.16 to −1.38; $p < 0.001$; $I^2 = 0\%$), fasting insulin (MD: −1.33, 95% CI: −2.18 to −0.49; P = 0.002; $I^2 = 0\%$), HOMA-IR (MD: −0.32, 95% CI: −0.52 to −0.12; P = 0.002; $I^2 = 0\%$), and QUICKI (MD: 0.010, 95% CI: 0.003–0.018; P = 0.005; $I^2 = 69\%$) are significantly greater in patients taking curcumin than those taking placebo.

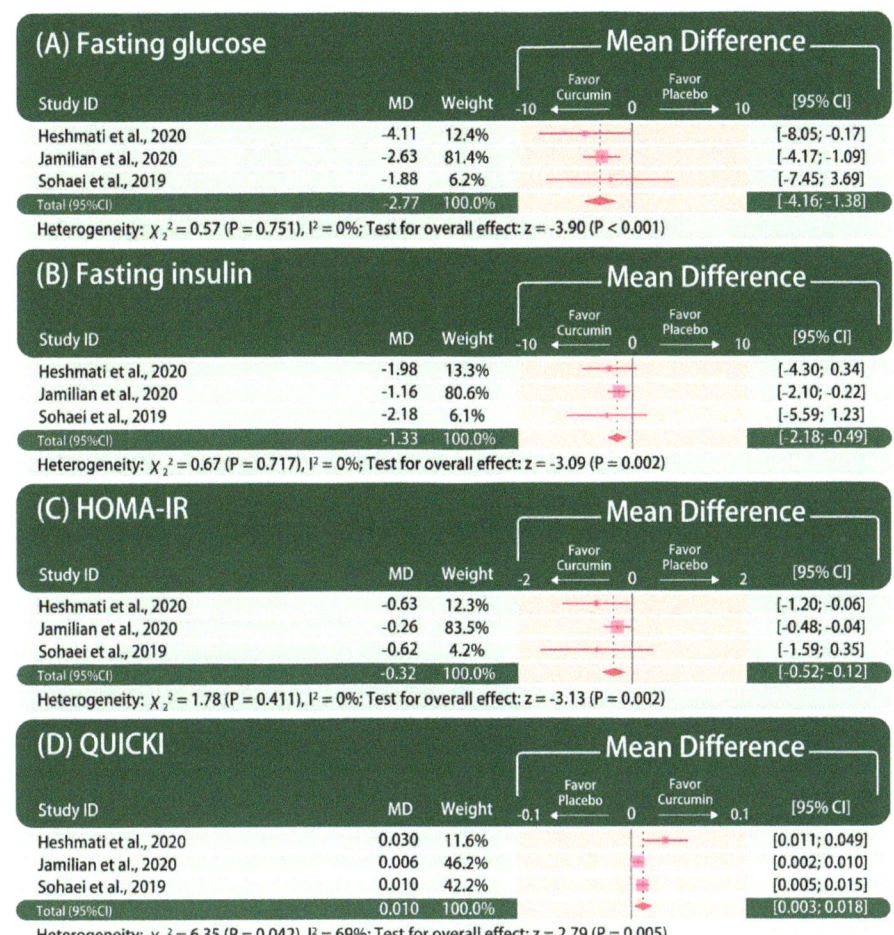

Figure 2. Forest plot of glycemic control. The mean difference between curcumin and placebo is calculated as the value in the curcumin group subtracted by that in the placebo group (curcumin–placebo). CI: confidence interval. MD: mean difference.

3.3.2. Lipid Profile

The forest plot of the lipid profile is presented in Figure 3. HDL, LDL, triglyceride, and total cholesterol were reported in only two studies [40,42]. The improvement in HDL (MD: 1.92, 95% CI: 0.33–3.51; P = 0.018; I^2 = 0%) and total cholesterol (MD: −12.45, 95% CI: −22.05 to −2.85; P = 0.011; I^2 = 32%) are significantly greater in patients taking curcumin than those taking placebo. In contrast, there is no statistically significant difference in the improvement in LDL (MD: −6.02, 95% CI: −26.66 to 14.62; P = 0.567; I^2 = 86%) and triglyceride (MD: 8.22, 95% CI: −26.10 to 42.53; P = 0.639; I^2 = 75%) between patients taking curcumin and those taking placebo.

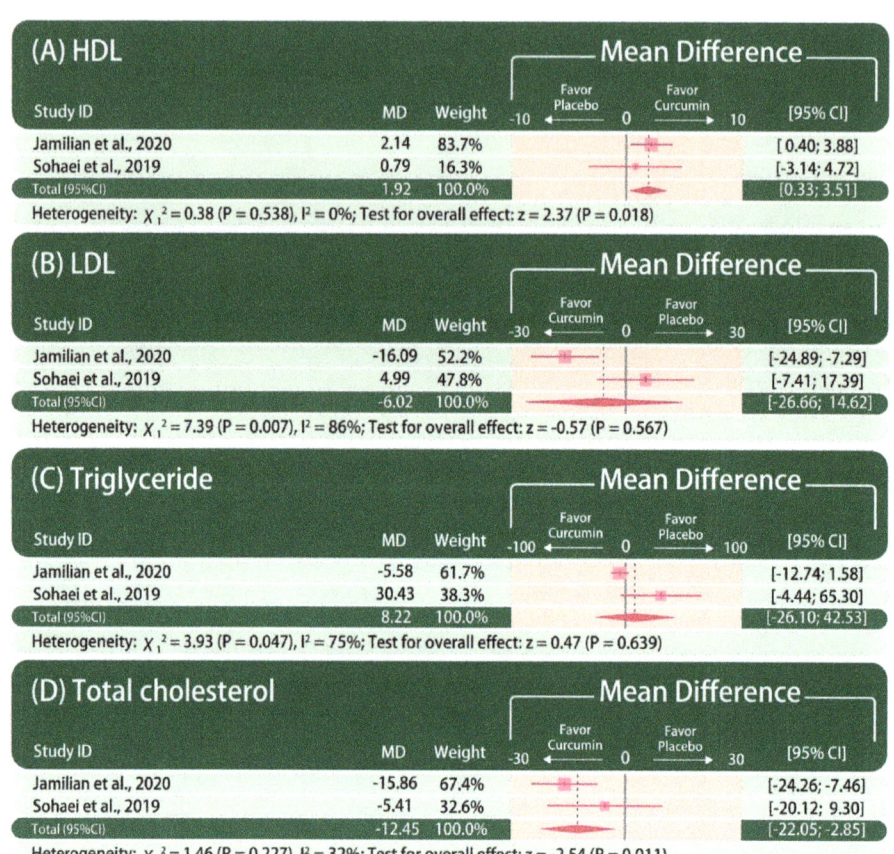

Figure 3. Forest plot of lipid profile. The mean difference between curcumin and placebo is calculated as the value in the curcumin group subtracted by that in the placebo group (curcumin–placebo). CI: confidence interval. MD: mean difference.

3.3.3. Influence Analysis

The influence analysis is presented in Supplementary Figure S2. For the fasting glucose, fasting insulin and QUICKI, the influence analysis reveals that the pooled point estimates after omitting each included study one at a time lie within the 95% CI of the overall pooled results for these outcomes. In contrast, the influence analysis of HOMA-IR reveals that the pooled point estimate after omitting the study by Jamilian et al. lies outside of the 95% CI of the overall pooled result. The influence analysis of the lipid profile was not performed due to limited number of studies in each outcome.

3.3.4. Trial Sequential Analysis

The cumulative Z-curve has reached the estimated RIS and has passed the traditional significance boundary in favor of curcumin in the TSA of fasting glucose, fasting insulin, HOMA-IR, and QUICKI (Supplementary Figures S3–S6). In the TSA of total cholesterol, although the cumulative Z-curve has not yet reached the estimated RIS, it passes the adjusted significance boundary in favor of curcumin (Supplementary Figure S7). In contrast, in the TSA of HDL, although the cumulative Z-curve passes the traditional significance boundary, it has not yet reached the estimated RIS, and has not passed the adjusted significance boundary in favor of curcumin (Supplementary Figure S8). In the TSA of LDL and triglyceride, the cumulative Z-curves have not reached the estimated RIS (2432 for

LDL and 3609 for triglyceride), and the sequential monitoring boundaries are ignored due to too few patients relative to the estimated RIS (Supplementary Figures S9 and S10).

3.3.5. Meta-Regression and Publication Bias

Despite the pre-planned attempts to evaluate the effects of daily dose of curcumin and duration of therapy on the pooled effect estimates, a meta-regression is not performed due to limited number of studies eligible for inclusion. Similarly, publication bias is not assessed by a funnel plot and performing Egger's test due to few numbers of included studies.

4. Discussion

The principal finding of the present study is that patients with PCOS taking curcumin have significantly greater improvement in glycemic control than those taking placebo, reflected by the fasting glucose, fasting insulin, HOMA-IR and QUICKI. In addition, curcumin also shows beneficial effects in improving lipid profile, including HDL and total cholesterol. In contrast, there is no statistically significant difference in LDL and triglyceride between patients taking curcumin and placebo. The TSA shows that the results of the current meta-analysis with regard to the fasting glucose, fasting insulin, HOMA-IR, QUICKI, and total cholesterol are conclusive. In contrast, the TSA indicates that the effects of curcumin on HDL, LDL, and triglyceride are not yet conclusive, and thus more large-scaled trials to determine these results are required. A visual summary abstract is presented in Figure 4.

Among the included studies, the curcumin dosage ranged from 500 mg to 1500 mg per day and the treatment period ranged from 6 weeks to 12 weeks. All of the patients were diagnosed with Rotterdam criteria and were studied in Iran. One study by Sohaei et al. mentioned the concentration and detailed manufacturing of curcumin with 95% of standardized turmeric powder. One study took place in infertility center but none of the included studies discuss the effects of curcumin in ovulation or reproduction.

The effects of curcumin on glycemic control and lipid metabolism are complex and involve several mechanisms that underlie the observation in the present study. Curcumin stimulates insulin-mediated glucose uptake by the phosphatidylinositol 3-kinase (PI3K)/Akt pathway, which in turn upregulates the translocation of glucose transporter 4 (GLUT4) to the membrane of adipocyte and skeletal muscle, leading to an increase in glucose uptake [43,44]. Curcumin also activates adenosine monophosphate-activated protein kinase, which not only suppresses gluconeogenesis in hepatocyte via inhibiting glucose-6-phosphatase and phosphoenolpyruvate carboxykinase [45,46], but also enhances GLUT4 translocation and glucose uptake in adipocytes [47]. Moreover, curcumin improves glucose homeostasis by activating glucose transporter 2 and glucokinases in liver via increasing the transcription of peroxisome proliferator-activated receptor-gamma (PPAR-γ) [48,49]. In the study by Jamilian et al., significant upregulation of PPAR-γ has been observed after taking curcumin for 12 weeks [40]. With regard to lipid metabolism, curcumin upregulates LDL receptors and inhibits the synthesis of cholesterol and triglyceride in hepatocyte [50,51]. It also promotes cholesterol catabolism and fecal excretion of bile acids [52].

The anti-inflammatory property of curcumin may also play a role in glucose and lipid metabolisms and may mitigate hyperandrogenism. Proinflammatory cytokines, such as tumor necrosis factor-α (TNF-α), are found to be significantly higher in patients with PCOS [53]. TNF-α has been known to stimulate serine phosphorylation of insulin receptor substrate 1, resulting in insulin resistance [54]. Moreover, serine phosphorylation of cytochrome P450c17 enhances the activity of 17,20-lyase and promotes thecal production of androgen [55]. Curcumin inhibits PI3K/Akt/mechanistic target of rapamycin (mTOR) signaling pathway, resulting in the degradation of nuclear factor kappa-light-chain-enhancer of activated B cells (NF-κB) and downregulation of TNF-α and other proinflammatory cytokines [56,57]. Curcumin has been demonstrated to significantly reduce the plasma levels of TNF-α and interleukin (IL)-6 [58,59] and, subsequently, improves insulin sensitivity and decreases obesity-induced insulin resistance [60,61]. In addition, patients with PCOS are associated with higher oxidative stress [62]. A recent study has demonstrated beneficial effects of curcumin on upregulating the gene expression of peroxisome proliferator-activated receptor-gamma coactivator 1 alpha (PGC-1α), which in turn increases the activity of glutathione peroxidase, reducing the oxidative stress expression [25].

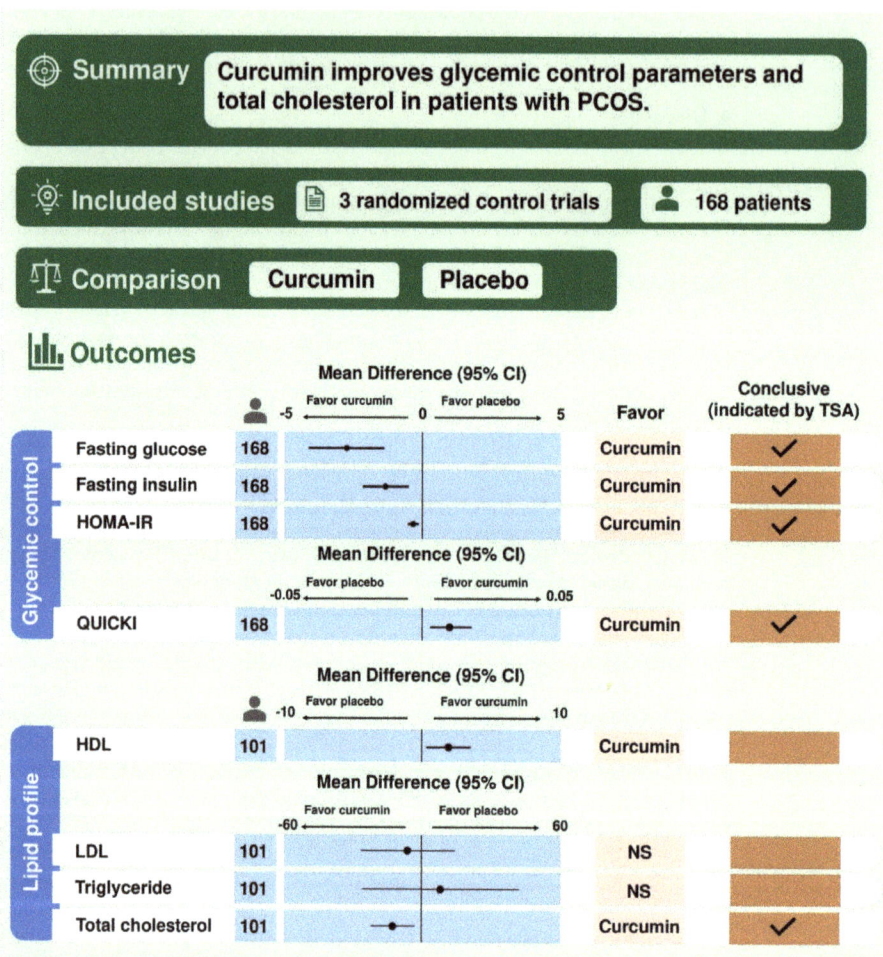

Figure 4. Visual summary abstract. CI: confidence interval. HDL: high-density lipoprotein. HOMA-IR: Homeostasis Model Assessment of Insulin Resistance. LDL: low-density lipoprotein. NS: non-significant. PCOS: polycystic ovary syndrome. QUICKI: quantitative insulin sensitivity check index. TSA: trial sequential analysis.

Curcumin may have promising effects in improving hyperandrogenism, though this is not demonstrated in the present study because meta-analysis, which evaluates and reports the influence of curcumin on thecal androgen production, is not performed due to the limited number of studies. In the study by Heshmati et al., the plasma levels of dehydroepiandrosterone (DHEA) are significantly reduced in patients taking curcumin compared to those taking placebo for 12 weeks [41]. This observation is likely attributed to the downregulation of the activity of cytochrome P450c17. Curcumin has been demonstrated to reduce the activity of cytochrome P450c17 in a dose-dependent manner in vitro [63]. In an animal model, the expression of cytochrome P450c17 in the ovaries of the curcumin-treated mice is reduced to the same level as in those of the wild-type ones [64]. Together with the anti-inflammatory property of curcumin, these results collectively support the notion that curcumin inhibits the activity of cytochrome P450c17, and thereby reduces the synthesis of DHEA.

There are several limitations of the present study. First, the number of studies that are eligible for inclusion is limited. Nevertheless, a TSA is performed to evaluate the robustness of the results. While some of the outcomes remain inconclusive and require more investigation, most of the results in the present study are conclusive as indicated by the TSA. However, all of the included studies were from Iran. The results of our meta-analysis should be carefully interpreted with populations other than Middle Eastern ethnicity. Second, the dosing regimen and duration of curcumin therapy varied across studies. The daily dosage of curcumin in the included studies ranged from 500 mg to 1500 mg. However, the duration of curcumin was relatively short from 6 weeks up to 12 weeks. Despite the pre-planned meta-regression to assess the effects of these covariates on the pooled effect estimates, it was not performed due to limited number of studies. Third, the detailed information regarding the preparation of the capsule and concentration of curcumin is not mentioned in the included studies. It is well documented that curcumin has poor bio-availability due to low absorption in intestines [65]. The difference in capsule design may affect the plasma concentration and the duration of the effects of curcumin. Finally, the effects of curcumin on sex hormone abnormalities in patients with PCOS are not assessed in the present study due to a lack of investigation in the included studies. Although the comprehensive therapy for PCOS is beyond the scope of the present study, the potential of curcumin in lowering plasma levels of androgen, as demonstrated in the study by Heshmati et al., is promising. Further investigation to confirm this result is advocated.

5. Conclusions

Curcumin may improve glycemic control and lipid metabolism in patients with PCOS and metabolic abnormality without significant adverse effects. Further studies are advocated to investigate the potential effects of curcumin on hyperandrogenism.

Supplementary Materials: The following are available online at https://www.mdpi.com/2072-6643/13/2/684/s1, Figure S1: Risk of bias summary and graph, Figure S2: Influence analysis of fasting glucose, fasting insulin, Homeostasis Model Assessment of Insulin Resistance (HOMA-IR) and quantitative insulin sensitivity check index (QUICKI), Figure S3: Trial sequential analysis of fasting glucose, Figure S4: Trial sequential analysis of fasting insulin, Figure S5: Trial sequential analysis of HOMA-IR, Figure S6: Trial sequential analysis of QUICKI, Figure S7: Trial sequential analysis of total cholesterol, Figure S8: Trial sequential analysis of HDL, Figure S9: Trial sequential analysis of LDL, Figure S10: Trial sequential analysis of triglyceride, Table S1: Detailed search strategy.

Author Contributions: Conceptualization, Y.-J.C. and C.-Y.C.; methodology, Y.-J.C., C.-Y.C. and M.-Y.W.; software, Y.-J.C. and C.-Y.C.; writing—original draft preparation, Y.-J.C. and C.-Y.C.; writing—review and editing, Y.-J.C., C.-Y.C., C.-H.C., Y.-S.H., and H.-C.W.; visualization, C.-Y.C. and M.-Y.W. All authors have read and agreed to the published version of the manuscript.

Funding: This study was supported by a grant from the Taipei Tzu Chi Hospital, Buddhist Tzu Chi Medical Foundation (TCRD-TPE-109-RT-6).

Conflicts of Interest: The authors declare no conflict of interest.

References

1. McCartney, C.R.; Marshall, J.C. Polycystic ovary syndrome. *N. Engl. J. Med.* **2016**, *375*, 54–64. [CrossRef]
2. Lauritsen, M.P.; Bentzen, J.G.; Pinborg, A.; Loft, A.; Forman, J.L.; Thuesen, L.L.; Cohen, A.; Hougaard, D.M.; Nyboe Andersen, A. The prevalence of polycystic ovary syndrome in a normal population according to the Rotterdam criteria versus revised criteria including anti-Mullerian hormone. *Hum. Reprod.* **2014**, *29*, 791–801. [CrossRef]
3. Chang, J.; Azziz, R.; Legro, R.; Dewailly, D.; Franks, S.; Tarlatzis, R.; Fauser, B.; Balen, A.; Bouchard, P.; Dalgien, E.; et al. Revised 2003 consensus on diagnostic criteria and long-term health risks related to polycystic ovary syndrome. *Fertil. Steril.* **2004**, *81*, 19–25. [CrossRef]

4. Apridonidze, T.; Essah, P.A.; Iuorno, M.J.; Nestler, J.E. Prevalence and characteristics of the metabolic syndrome in women with polycystic ovary syndrome. *J. Clin. Endocrinol. Metab.* **2005**, *90*, 1929–1935. [CrossRef] [PubMed]
5. Ciaraldi, T.P.; Aroda, V.; Mudaliar, S.; Chang, R.J.; Henry, R.R. Polycystic ovary syndrome is associated with tissue-specific differences in insulin resistance. *J. Clin. Endocrinol. Metab.* **2009**, *94*, 157–163. [CrossRef]
6. Wekker, V.; Van Dammen, L.; Koning, A.; Heida, K.Y.; Painter, R.C.; Limpens, J.; Laven, J.S.E.; Roeters van Lennep, J.E.; Roseboom, T.J.; Hoek, A. Long-term cardiometabolic disease risk in women with PCOS: A systematic review and meta-analysis. *Hum. Reprod. Update* **2020**, *26*, 942–960. [CrossRef] [PubMed]
7. Chandrasekaran, S.; Sagili, H. Metabolic syndrome in women with polycystic ovary syndrome. *Obstet. Gynaecol.* **2018**, *20*, 245–252. [CrossRef]
8. Gilling-Smith, C.; Story, H.; Rogers, V.; Franks, S. Evidence for a primary abnormality of thecal cell steroidogenesis in the polycystic ovary syndrome. *Clin. Endocrinol.* **1997**, *47*, 93–99. [CrossRef] [PubMed]
9. Rosenfield, R.L.; Barnes, R.B.; Ehrmann, D.A. Studies of the nature of 17-hydroxyprogesterone hyperresonsiveness to gonadotropin-releasing hormone agonist challenge in functional ovarian hyperandrogenism. *J. Clin. Endocrinol. Metab.* **1994**, *79*, 1686–1692. [CrossRef]
10. Cara, J.F.; Rosenfield, R.L. Insulin-like growth factor I and insulin potentiate luteinizing hormone-induced androgen synthesis by rat ovarian thecal-interstitial cells. *Endocrinology* **1988**, *123*, 733–739. [CrossRef] [PubMed]
11. McAllister, J.M.; Byrd, W.; Simpson, E.R. The effects of growth factors and phorbol esters on steroid biosynthesis in isolated human theca interna and granulosa-lutein cells in long term culture. *J. Clin. Endocrinol. Metab.* **1994**, *79*, 106–112. [CrossRef]
12. Rosenfield, R.L.; Ehrmann, D.A. The Pathogenesis of Polycystic Ovary Syndrome (PCOS): The hypothesis of PCOS as functional ovarian hyperandrogenism revisited. *Endocr. Rev.* **2016**, *37*, 467–520. [CrossRef]
13. Fox, C.W.; Zhang, L.; Sohni, A.; Doblado, M.; Wilkinson, M.F.; Chang, R.J.; Duleba, A.J. Inflammatory stimuli trigger increased androgen production and shifts in gene expression in theca-interstitial cells. *Endocrinology* **2019**, *160*, 2946–2958. [CrossRef] [PubMed]
14. Mandrelle, K.; Kamath, M.S.; Bondu, D.J.; Chandy, A.; Aleyamma, T.; George, K. Prevalence of metabolic syndrome in women with polycystic ovary syndrome attending an infertility clinic in a tertiary care hospital in South India. *J. Hum. Reprod. Sci.* **2012**, *5*, 26–31. [CrossRef]
15. Garruti, G.; Depalo, R.; Vita, M.G.; Lorusso, F.; Giampetruzzi, F.; Damato, A.B.; Giorgino, F. Adipose tissue, metabolic syndrome and polycystic ovary syndrome: From pathophysiology to treatment. *Reprod. Biomed. Online* **2009**, *19*, 552–563. [CrossRef] [PubMed]
16. Yang, R.; Yang, S.; Li, R.; Liu, P.; Qiao, J.; Zhang, Y. Effects of hyperandrogenism on metabolic abnormalities in patients with polycystic ovary syndrome: A meta-analysis. *Reprod. Biol. Endocrinol.* **2016**, *14*, 67. [CrossRef] [PubMed]
17. Nestler, J.E.; Jakubowicz, D.J. Decreases in ovarian cytochrome P450c17 alpha activity and serum free testosterone after reduction of insulin secretion in polycystic ovary syndrome. *N. Engl. J. Med.* **1996**, *335*, 617–623. [CrossRef] [PubMed]
18. Baillargeon, J.P.; Jakubowicz, D.J.; Iuorno, M.J.; Jakubowicz, S.; Nestler, J.E. Effects of metformin and rosiglitazone, alone and in combination, in nonobese women with polycystic ovary syndrome and normal indices of insulin sensitivity. *Fertil. Steril.* **2004**, *82*, 893–902. [CrossRef]
19. Legro, R.S.; Barnhart, H.X.; Schlaff, W.D.; Carr, B.R.; Diamond, M.P.; Carson, S.A.; Steinkampf, M.P.; Coutifaris, C.; McGovern, P.G.; Cataldo, N.A.; et al. Clomiphene, metformin, or both for infertility in the polycystic ovary syndrome. *N. Engl. J. Med.* **2007**, *356*, 551–566. [CrossRef]
20. Hewlings, S.J.; Kalman, D.S. Curcumin: A review of its effects on human health. *Foods* **2017**, *6*, 92. [CrossRef]
21. Nistico, S.; Tamburi, F.; Bennardo, L.; Dastoli, S.; Schipani, G.; Caro, G.; Fortuna, M.C.; Rossi, A. Treatment of telogen effluvium using a dietary supplement containing Boswellia serrata, Curcuma longa, and Vitis vinifera: Results of an observational study. *Dermatol. Ther.* **2019**, *32*, e12842. [CrossRef] [PubMed]
22. Wojcik, M.; Krawczyk, M.; Wojcik, P.; Cypryk, K.; Wozniak, L.A. Molecular mechanisms underlying curcumin-mediated therapeutic effects in type 2 diabetes and cancer. *Oxid. Med. Cell. Longev.* **2018**, *2018*, 9698258. [CrossRef]
23. Jimenez-Osorio, A.S.; Monroy, A.; Alavez, S. Curcumin and insulin resistance-molecular targets and clinical evidences. *Biofactors* **2016**, *42*, 561–580. [CrossRef] [PubMed]
24. Shin, S.K.; Ha, T.Y.; McGregor, R.A.; Choi, M.S. Long-term curcumin administration protects against atherosclerosis via hepatic regulation of lipoprotein cholesterol metabolism. *Mol. Nutr. Food Res.* **2011**, *55*, 1829–1840. [CrossRef]
25. Heshmati, J.; Golab, F.; Morvaridzadeh, M.; Potter, E.; Akbari-Fakhrabadi, M.; Farsi, F.; Tanbakooei, S.; Shidfar, F. The effects of curcumin supplementation on oxidative stress, Sirtuin-1 and peroxisome proliferator activated receptor gamma coactivator 1alpha gene expression in polycystic ovarian syndrome (PCOS) patients: A randomized placebo-controlled clinical trial. *Diabetes Metab. Syndr.* **2020**, *14*, 77–82. [CrossRef]
26. Shishodia, S.; Singh, T.; Chaturvedi, M.M. Modulation of transcription factors by curcumin. *Adv. Exp. Med. Biol.* **2007**, *595*, 127–148. [CrossRef]
27. Azhdari, M.; Karandish, M.; Mansoori, A. Metabolic benefits of curcumin supplementation in patients with metabolic syndrome: A systematic review and meta-analysis of randomized controlled trials. *Phytother. Res.* **2019**, *33*, 1289–1301. [CrossRef] [PubMed]
28. Reddy, P.S.; Begum, N.; Mutha, S.; Bakshi, V. Beneficial effect of Curcumin in Letrozole induced polycystic ovary syndrome. *Asian Pac. J. Reprod.* **2016**, *5*, 116–122. [CrossRef]

29. Moher, D.; Liberati, A.; Tetzlaff, J.; Altman, D.G.; Group, P. Preferred reporting items for systematic reviews and meta-analyses: The PRISMA statement. *Int. J. Surg.* **2009**, *339*, b2535. [CrossRef]
30. Sterne, J.A.C.; Savovic, J.; Page, M.J.; Elbers, R.G.; Blencowe, N.S.; Boutron, I.; Cates, C.J.; Cheng, H.Y.; Corbett, M.S.; Eldridge, S.M.; et al. RoB 2: A revised tool for assessing risk of bias in randomised trials. *BMJ* **2019**, *366*, l4898. [CrossRef]
31. Borenstein, M.; Hedges, L.; Rothstein, H. Meta-Analysis: Fixed Effect vs. Random Effects. Available online: https://www.meta-analysis.com/downloads/M-a_f_e_v_r_e_sv.pdf (accessed on 20 April 2020).
32. DerSimonian, R.; Laird, N. Meta-analysis in clinical trials. *Control. Clin. Trials* **1986**, *7*, 177–188. [CrossRef]
33. Higgins, J.P.T.; Thomas, J.; Chandler, J.; Cumpston, M.; Li, T.; Page, M.J.; Welch, V.A. *Cochrane Handbook for Systematic Reviews of Interventions version 6.0 (updated July 2019)*; Cochrane: London, UK, 2019.
34. Wetterslev, J.; Jakobsen, J.C.; Gluud, C. Trial sequential analysis in systematic reviews with meta-analysis. *BMC Med. Res. Methodol.* **2017**, *17*, 39. [CrossRef]
35. Peters, J.L.; Sutton, A.J.; Jones, D.R.; Abrams, K.R.; Rushton, L. Contour-enhanced meta-analysis funnel plots help distinguish publication bias from other causes of asymmetry. *J. Clin. Epidemiol.* **2008**, *61*, 991–996. [CrossRef]
36. Egger, M.; Davey Smith, G.; Schneider, M.; Minder, C. Bias in meta-analysis detected by a simple, graphical test. *BMJ* **1997**, *315*, 629–634. [CrossRef] [PubMed]
37. Duval, S.; Tweedie, R. Trim and fill: A simple funnel-plot-based method of testing and adjusting for publication bias in meta-analysis. *Biometrics* **2000**, *56*, 455–463. [CrossRef]
38. R Core Team. *R: A Language and Environment for Statistical Computing*; R Foundation for Statistical Computing: Vienna, Austria, 2019; Available online: https://www.R-project.org/ (accessed on 10 December 2020).
39. Centre for Clinical Intervention Research Copenhagen Trial Unit, Rigshospitalet. Trial Sequential Analysis Software Copenhagen. 2016. Available online: http://www.ctu.dk/tsa/ (accessed on 10 December 2020).
40. Jamilian, M.; Foroozanfard, F.; Kavossian, E.; Aghadavod, E.; Shafabakhsh, R.; Hoseini, A.; Asemi, Z. Effects of curcumin on body weight, glycemic control and serum lipids in women with polycystic ovary syndrome: A randomized, double-blind, placebo-controlled trial. *Clin. Nutr. ESPEN* **2020**. [CrossRef] [PubMed]
41. Heshmati, J.; Moini, A.; Sepidarkish, M.; Morvaridzadeh, M.; Salehi, M.; Palmowski, A.; Mojtahedi, M.F.; Shidfar, F. Effects of curcumin supplementation on blood glucose, insulin resistance and androgens in patients with polycystic ovary syndrome: A randomized double-blind placebo-controlled clinical trial. *Phytomedicine* **2020**, *80*, 153395. [CrossRef]
42. Sohaei, S.; Amani, R.; Tarrahi, M.J.; Ghasemi-Tehrani, H. The effects of curcumin supplementation on glycemic status, lipid profile and hs-CRP levels in overweight/obese women with polycystic ovary syndrome: A randomized, double-blind, placebo-controlled clinical trial. *Complementary Ther. Med.* **2019**, *47*, 102201. [CrossRef] [PubMed]
43. Lin, J.; Zheng, S.; Chen, A. Curcumin attenuates the effects of insulin on stimulating hepatic stellate cell activation by interrupting insulin signaling and attenuating oxidative stress. *Lab. Investig.* **2009**, *89*, 1397–1409. [CrossRef]
44. Den Hartogh, D.J.; Gabriel, A.; Tsiani, E. Antidiabetic properties of curcumin I: Evidence from in vitro studies. *Nutrients* **2020**, *12*, 118. [CrossRef] [PubMed]
45. Srivastava, R.A.; Pinkosky, S.L.; Filippov, S.; Hanselman, J.C.; Cramer, C.T.; Newton, R.S. AMP-activated protein kinase: An emerging drug target to regulate imbalances in lipid and carbohydrate metabolism to treat cardio-metabolic diseases. *J. Lipid Res.* **2012**, *53*, 2490–2514. [CrossRef] [PubMed]
46. Fujiwara, H.; Hosokawa, M.; Zhou, X.; Fujimoto, S.; Fukuda, K.; Toyoda, K.; Nishi, Y.; Fujita, Y.; Yamada, K.; Yamada, Y.; et al. Curcumin inhibits glucose production in isolated mice hepatocytes. *Diabetes Res. Clin. Pract.* **2008**, *80*, 185–191. [CrossRef]
47. Yamaguchi, S.; Katahira, H.; Ozawa, S.; Nakamichi, Y.; Tanaka, T.; Shimoyama, T.; Takahashi, K.; Yoshimoto, K.; Imaizumi, M.O.; Nagamatsu, S.; et al. Activators of AMP-activated protein kinase enhance GLUT4 translocation and its glucose transport activity in 3T3-L1 adipocytes. *Am. J. Physiol. Endocrinol. Metab.* **2005**, *289*, E643–E649. [CrossRef] [PubMed]
48. Jacob, A.; Wu, R.; Zhou, M.; Wang, P. Mechanism of the anti-inflammatory effect of curcumin: PPAR-gamma activation. *PPAR Res.* **2007**, *2007*, 89369. [CrossRef] [PubMed]
49. Kim, H.I.; Ahn, Y.H. Role of peroxisome proliferator-activated receptor-gamma in the glucose-sensing apparatus of liver and beta-cells. *Diabetes* **2004**, *53*, S60–S65. [CrossRef] [PubMed]
50. Kim, M.; Kim, Y. Hypocholesterolemic effects of curcumin via up-regulation of cholesterol 7a-hydroxylase in rats fed a high fat diet. *Nutr. Res. Pract.* **2010**, *4*, 191–195. [CrossRef]
51. Peschel, D.; Koerting, R.; Nass, N. Curcumin induces changes in expression of genes involved in cholesterol homeostasis. *J. Nutr. Biochem.* **2007**, *18*, 113–119. [CrossRef] [PubMed]
52. Rao, D.S.; Sekhara, N.C.; Satyanarayana, M.N.; Srinivasan, M. Effect of curcumin on serum and liver cholesterol levels in the rat. *J. Nutr.* **1970**, *100*, 1307–1315. [CrossRef]
53. Gao, L.; Gu, Y.; Yin, X. High serum tumor necrosis factor-alpha levels in women with polycystic ovary syndrome: A meta-analysis. *PLoS ONE* **2016**, *11*, e0164021. [CrossRef]
54. Rui, L.; Aguirre, V.; Kim, J.K.; Shulman, G.I.; Lee, A.; Corbould, A.; Dunaif, A.; White, M.F. Insulin/IGF-1 and TNF-alpha stimulate phosphorylation of IRS-1 at inhibitory Ser307 via distinct pathways. *J. Clin. Investig.* **2001**, *107*, 181–189. [CrossRef] [PubMed]
55. Miller, W.L.; Tee, M.K. The post-translational regulation of 17,20 lyase activity. *Mol. Cell. Endocrinol.* **2015**, *408*, 99–106. [CrossRef]

56. Zhang, C.; Hao, Y.; Wu, L.; Dong, X.; Jiang, N.; Cong, B.; Liu, J.; Zhang, W.; Tang, D.; De Perrot, M.; et al. Curcumin induces apoptosis and inhibits angiogenesis in murine malignant mesothelioma. *Int. J. Oncol.* **2018**, *53*, 2531–2541. [CrossRef] [PubMed]
57. Jobin, C.; Bradham, C.A.; Russo, M.P.; Juma, B.; Narula, A.S.; Brenner, D.A.; Sartor, R.B. Curcumin blocks cytokine-mediated NF-kappa B activation and proinflammatory gene expression by inhibiting inhibitory factor I-kappa B kinase activity. *J. Immunol.* **1999**, *163*, 3474–3483.
58. Sahebkar, A.; Cicero, A.F.G.; Simental-Mendia, L.E.; Aggarwal, B.B.; Gupta, S.C. Curcumin downregulates human tumor necrosis factor-alpha levels: A systematic review and meta-analysis of randomized controlled trials. *Pharmacol. Res.* **2016**, *107*, 234–242. [CrossRef]
59. Derosa, G.; Maffioli, P.; Simental-Mendia, L.E.; Bo, S.; Sahebkar, A. Effect of curcumin on circulating interleukin-6 concentrations: A systematic review and meta-analysis of randomized controlled trials. *Pharmacol. Res.* **2016**, *111*, 394–404. [CrossRef] [PubMed]
60. Akash, M.S.H.; Rehman, K.; Liaqat, A. Tumor necrosis factor-alpha: Role in development of insulin resistance and pathogenesis of type 2 diabetes mellitus. *J. Cell. Biochem.* **2018**, *119*, 105–110. [CrossRef]
61. Moller, D.E. Potential role of TNF-alpha in the pathogenesis of insulin resistance and type 2 diabetes. *Trends Endocrinol. Metab.* **2000**, *11*, 212–217. [CrossRef]
62. Sabuncu, T.; Vural, H.; Harma, M.; Harma, M. Oxidative stress in polycystic ovary syndrome and its contribution to the risk of cardiovascular disease. *Clin. Biochem.* **2001**, *34*, 407–413. [CrossRef]
63. Rodriguez Castano, P.; Parween, S.; Pandey, A.V. Bioactivity of curcumin on the cytochrome P450 enzymes of the steroidogenic pathway. *Int. J. Mol. Sci.* **2019**, *20*, 4606. [CrossRef] [PubMed]
64. Tiwari-Pandey, R.; Ram Sairam, M. Modulation of ovarian structure and abdominal obesity in curcumin- and flutamide-treated aging FSH-R haploinsufficient mice. *Reprod. Sci.* **2009**, *16*, 539–550. [CrossRef]
65. Dei Cas, M.; Ghidoni, R. Dietary curcumin: Correlation between bioavailability and health potential. *Nutrients* **2019**, *11*, 2147. [CrossRef] [PubMed]

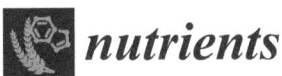

Review

Nutrition in Gynecological Diseases: Current Perspectives

Michał Ciebiera [1], Sahar Esfandyari [2], Hiba Siblini [3], Lillian Prince [4], Hoda Elkafas [2,5], Cezary Wojtyła [6], Ayman Al-Hendy [3] and Mohamed Ali [7,*]

1. Second Department of Obstetrics and Gynecology, Center of Postgraduate Medical Education, 01-809 Warsaw, Poland; michal.ciebiera@cmkp.edu.pl
2. Department of Surgery, University of Illinois at Chicago, Chicago, IL 60612, USA; sesfan2@uic.edu (S.E.); helkaf2@uic.edu (H.E.)
3. Department of Obstetrics and Gynecology, University of Chicago, Chicago, IL 60637, USA; hsiblini@bsd.uchicago.edu (H.S.); aalhendy@bsd.uchicago.edu (A.A.-H.)
4. Biological Sciences Division, Public Health Sciences, University of Chicago, Chicago, IL 60637, USA; lprince@uchicago.edu
5. Department of Pharmacology and Toxicology, Egyptian Drug Authority (EDA), Cairo 15301, Egypt
6. International Prevention Research Institute-Collaborating Centre, Calisia University, 62-800 Kalisz, Poland; cezary.wojtyla@gmail.com
7. Clinical Pharmacy Department, Faculty of Pharmacy, Ain Shams University, Cairo 11566, Egypt
* Correspondence: mohamed.aboouf@pharma.asu.edu.eg

Abstract: Diet and nutrition are fundamental in maintaining the general health of populations, including women's health. Health status can be affected by nutrient deficiency and vice versa. Gene–nutrient interactions are important contributors to health management and disease prevention. Nutrition can alter gene expression, as well as the susceptibility to diseases, including cancer, through several mechanisms. Gynecological diseases in general are diseases involving the female reproductive system and include benign and malignant tumors, infections, and endocrine diseases. Benign diseases such as uterine fibroids and endometriosis are common, with a negative impact on women's quality of life, while malignant tumors are among the most common cause of death in the recent years. In this comprehensive review article, a bibliographic search was performed for retrieving information about nutrients and how their deficiencies can be associated with gynecological diseases, namely polycystic ovary syndrome, infertility, uterine fibroids, endometriosis, dysmenorrhea, and infections, as well as cervical, endometrial, and ovarian cancers. Moreover, we discussed the potential beneficial impact of promising natural compounds and dietary supplements on alleviating these significant diseases.

Keywords: nutrition; gynecological diseases; infertility; PCOS; uterine fibroids; endometriosis; microbiome; infection; cervical cancer; endometrial cancer; ovarian cancer; dysmenorrhea; diet; nutrients; complementary and alternative medicine

1. Introduction

Gynecological diseases are diseases of the female reproductive organs; these diseases are considered a public health and social problem. These diseases include benign and malignant tumors, infections, and endocrine disorders. All these diseases significantly impact women's quality of life, and many of them, unfortunately, are still lacking efficient treatment plans. Promoting both primary and secondary prevention is essential for the sake of these afflicted women and their reproductive health [1]. Sometimes, applying such preventive approaches is as or even more important than curative procedures. Educating patients about the significance of a healthy lifestyle and explaining hygienic and dietary measures are among these imperative procedures.

Gene–nutrient interactions are central contributors to health management and disease prevention. Nutrigenomics and nutrigenetics are defined as sciences that investigate the relationship between genetic variations and nutrient requirements [2]. Interestingly, it

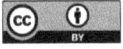

was recently reported that nutrients can drive epigenetic changes that can influence such requirements. Nutrition can alter gene expression, as well as the susceptibility to several diseases, including cancer, through genetic and epigenetic changes [3]. During the past decade, it has become clearer that nutrition can exert imprinting effects on the human genome, with many studies indicating that early life nutrition could influence the risk of developing chronic diseases in adulthood [4,5]. For example, with regard to the role of nutrition in cancer development, existing evidence suggests that dietary components can impact disease pathogenesis via the activation of tumor suppressor genes, cellular apoptosis, protein translation, and noncoding microRNAs (miRNAs) with roles in messenger RNA (mRNA) stability and translation [6,7]. In this article, we summarized published research in the public domain regarding the existing correlation between nutrients and dietary supplements with common gynecological diseases, highlighting the essential role of nutrients and dietary supplements in halting disease progression.

2. Infertility

Infertility is estimated to affect 8–16% of reproductive-age couples worldwide [8]. Lifestyle and nutritional factors have been shown to be important elements of normal reproductive function [9,10]. The literature exploring the relationship between diet and infertility has expanded over the past decade. Studies agree that the intake of folic acid is recommended for the prevention of neural tube defects and has been shown to be related to a lower frequency of infertility and a lower risk of pregnancy loss [11,12]. Further nutritional components or types of diet have been studied in relation to female infertility, including the Mediterranean diet, fats, vitamins, caffeine, smoking, alcohol, and, more recently, probiotics [11].

2.1. Mediterranean Diet

The Mediterranean diet is a diet rich in vegetables, fruits, whole grains, legumes, nuts, and olive oil and low in red meat. It has proven to be beneficial in several aspects of human health in general [13] and has also been studied in relation to fertility [14]. Previously, Vujkovic et al. studied the association between a preconception diet and in vitro fertilization (IVF) in a cohort of subfertile couples in the Netherlands and showed that adherence to the Mediterranean diet is associated with a higher chance of pregnancy [15]. A similar effect was later confirmed in a Dutch cohort of couples undergoing first-time in vitro fertilization (IVF), and the authors explained that the high fat content of vegetable oil as part of this diet could be the driving force behind this association. Subsequently, a prospective cohort study of 244 non-obese women who underwent their first IVF in Athens showed that adherence to the Mediterranean diet is associated with an increased chance of clinical pregnancy and live birth [16]. Results from the Nurses' Health Study cohort, which included 438 reported infertilities related to ovulation disorders, showed a significant association between female fertility and consumption of low-glycemic carbohydrates, monounsaturated fatty acids, proteins of plant origin, and supplements with iron, folate, and vitamins [17]. The authors concluded that adherence to such components, which are essentially present in the Mediterranean diet, is associated with a lower risk of ovulatory infertility [17].

2.2. Fats

Long-chain omega-3 fatty acids seem to improve female infertility, although it is unclear whether environmental toxins in such food sources, such as fish, can reduce this benefit [18]. In a prospective study of a cohort of 1228 women attempting pregnancy followed for up to six menstrual cycles, the preconception plasma phospholipid fatty acid level was measured at baseline [18]. The authors concluded that monounsaturated fatty acids (MUFAs) are associated with increased fecundability or a shorter time to pregnancy, whereas polyunsaturated fatty acids show the opposite effect. The role of polyunsaturated fatty acids (PUFAs) to decrease fecundability may be due to their effect on androgen synthesis, and androgens have been associated with ovulatory disorders such as polycystic ovary syndrome. Fatty acids are also thought to effect fecundability through changes in insulin sensitivity and inflammation, as these pathways also influence ovulatory function [19].

2.3. Vitamins

Despite promising evidence from preclinical animal model studies, vitamin D deficiency does not appear to influence human fertility [20,21]. Among women attempting pregnancy in the Nurses' Health Study II (NHSII) cohort, higher intake of vitamin D was not associated with a risk of ovulatory infertility [22]. Similarly, among another large cohorts of women with no history of infertility but with one to two prior pregnancy losses, no association was found between baseline vitamin D levels or vitamin D deficiency and fecundability [23].

A more recent topic of interest is the role of antioxidant consumption based on evidence from experimental association between low antioxidant status and infertility [24]. In one study, increased intake of beta carotene, vitamin C, and vitamin E was associated with a shorter time to pregnancy (TTP), but the effects varied with the body mass index (BMI) and age. A shorter TTP was observed among women with a body mass index (BMI) of <25 kg/m^2 with increasing vitamin C, among women with a BMI of $\geq$25 kg/m^2 with increasing beta carotene, among women aged <35 years with increasing beta carotene and vitamin C, and among women aged $\geq$35 years with increasing vitamin E [25].

2.4. Probiotics

Considerable attention is lately being given toward probiotics and the effect of the gut microbiome on diseases [26]. Nevertheless, the role of the microbiome in infertility and the role of probiotics in infertility management have not been extensively studied. Lactobacilli are the most studied probiotic bacteria, and they show several mechanisms in protecting the vaginal environment, including production of lactic acid that deters pathogens by lowering the pH and yielding an acidic environment to the cervico-vaginal mucus [27]; production of bacteriocins, which are antimicrobial peptides and proteins that protect against microbial invasion; and enhancement of immunomodulation by producing H_2O_2 and stimulating anti-inflammatory action [28]. In a recent review article, Younis et al. drew attention to the importance of further exploring in future clinical research the role of probiotics in managing infertility [29]. Bhandari et al. demonstrated that Lactobacillis plantarum works to competitively exclude sperm-agglutinating Escherichia coli (E. coli) bacteria. They treated a mice model with E. coli for 10 days intravaginally and then administered L. plantarum to find out that the fertility of this group was comparable to that of the control group, which reinforces the hypothesis that Lactobacillus probiotics may be used as an infertility therapeutic agent [30]. However, further research at the clinical level is needed to confirm these findings.

3. Polycystic Ovary Syndrome

Polycystic ovary syndrome (PCOS) is a complex and common hormonal condition in women of reproductive age, characterized by ovulatory dysfunction, chronic anovulation, altered menstruation, and ovarian small cysts on one or both ovaries, which may affect fertility [31]. It is found in approximately 5% to 10% of women aged between 18 and 44 years, making it among the most widespread diseases of reproductive-age women. Based on the previous literature, PCOS is associated with other common disorders, such as insulin resistance, obesity, type 2 diabetes, hypertension, endometrial cancer, and hyperandrogenemia. Indeed, most women with PCOS have insulin resistance [32–34].

Although the actual cause of PCOS remains unclear, evidence points to the role of environmental factors, including lifestyle and dietary habits, in the prevention and treatment of PCOS. Therefore, considering these factors may propose new therapeutic strategies for PCOS patients [35,36]. One of the most prominent approaches in treating PCOS is diet therapy for the sake of reducing insulin resistance and reproductive dysfunction. Considering the association of PCOS with obesity and insulin resistance, it should be noted that approximately a 5% to 10% decrease in weight may increase reproductive activity. This might be achieved by weight loss, a decrease in the intake of foods with a high glycemic index and foods rich in fatty acids, and intake of sufficient omega-3, vitamin D, and chromium [35]. There are several studies considering the effects of these nutritional components on the control of PCOS, which we will discuss in this review.

First, foods rich in fat, mainly saturated fatty acids, increase the risk of insulin resistance and its related complications, while diets rich in unsaturated fatty acids decrease the risk of these diseases [35,37]. In this manner, the intake of omega-3 unsaturated fatty acids reduces the risk of PCOS in women with insulin resistance [35]. Moreover, another study indicated that the intake of unsaturated fatty acids affects the levels of pregnanediol 3-glucuronide in cases with PCOS, although the levels of sex hormones do not alter [38].

Current evidence has revealed the role of vitamin D in different metabolic pathways, including the insulin signaling pathway [39]. Previous studies have shown that the vitamin D signaling pathway directly contributes to the activation of the insulin receptor gene [39]. Hence, sub-optimal vitamin D levels may be associated with the pathogenesis of insulin resistance and PCOS [39,40]. In this context, a recent systematic review and meta-analysis demonstrated the association between vitamin D levels and the metabolic profile, including high-density lipoprotein (HDL-C), fasting blood glucose, and insulin, in PCOS women. Furthermore, vitamin D levels had a positive relationship with sexual hormone binding globulin (SHBG). These findings suggested an important role of vitamin D supplementation in infertile women with PCOS who undergo ovarian stimulation [41].

Recently, attention has shifted toward the effect of vitamin D on ovarian function in PCOS. However, the underlying mechanism of vitamin D on ovarian function is still not fully determined. One possible mechanism is the role of vitamin D in alleviating the inflammatory pathways causing insulin resistance [35]. Previous studies have also indicated the existence of a vitamin D receptor in the granulosa cells of ovaries [42,43]. Moreover, another study showed that the anti-Müllerian hormone (AMH) promoter is under vitamin D down-regulation. AMH is produced by growing follicles, and its excess excretion is linked to PCOS. Therefore, it seems likely that vitamin D supplementation can affect ovarian function and alleviate PCOS [44]. A clinical trial reported that vitamin D supplementation in PCOS women with vitamin D deficiency was related to lower levels of AMH [45]. Consequently, it is tempting to speculate that vitamin D supplementation may be effective in PCOS patients.

Many natural anti-androgen foods have driven scientists' attention to their effects on PCOS therapy. Considering the effect of high insulin levels on the production of testosterone and the high levels of this androgen in PCOS women, improving insulin sensitivity by changing the diet and lifestyle may be regarded as the first-line treatment in this disorder [46,47]. According to previous studies, a low-carbohydrate diet is correlated with a lower risk of metabolic diseases, including insulin resistance, type 2 diabetes, and obesity, along with a lower risk of reproductive disorders [48–50]. However, other studies have shown that a low-carbohydrate diet does not affect the metabolic profile and levels of sex hormones in PCOS women [36,51].

Here, we mention some of the most notable natural anti-androgen foods used in PCOS studies. Soybean comprises isoflavone and phytoestrogens, which are critical in modulating many androgens in the human body [52]. A study showed that soybean phytoestrogen decreased the level of testosterone after three months [53]. Green tea with a high amount of antioxidants was used in a study on PCOS women and promoted insulin sensitivity and lowered the levels of testosterone [54]. Licorice is another phytoestrogen that alleviates the symptoms of PCOS patients and reduces the levels of testosterone [55]. Collectively, natural anti-androgen foods can be considered in the lifestyle to lower testosterone levels and alleviate PCOS.

Flavonoids are polyphenolic compounds of plants that have antioxidant, antiestrogenic, and antidiabetic properties [56]. These natural compounds are emerging as important mediators in the pathogenesis of many reproductive disorders, such as PCOS. Among them, quercetin as a bioflavonoid with antioxidant activity is effective in PCOS therapy [57]. It is reported that quercetin may reduce many androgens in rats [58]. Quercetin also reduced insulin resistance in an animal model of PCOS [59].

A clinical trial showed that quercetin improves insulin resistance and hormonal profile in PCOS women [60]. Another study demonstrated that a daily dose of 1000 mg of quercetin for 12 weeks was effective in alleviating PCOS features [61]. Moreover, previous studies have also indicated the potential effects of other flavonoids, such as resveratrol and soy isoflavones, in the treatment of PCOS through the regulation of steroidogenesis, metabolic parameters, ovarian cysts, and follicular development [62–64].

Several studies have suggested the role of minerals in the pathogenesis of PCOS [65]. In this regard, chromium is one of the most important minerals playing a role in carbohydrate and lipid metabolism, whose deficiency is observed in patients with type 2 diabetes. Subsequently, it seems plausible that chromium deficiency increases the risk of insulin resistance [66]. Furthermore, it is evident that PCOS patients have a lower level of chromium, which is associated with insulin resistance [67]. Interestingly, chromium supplementation with a dose of 200 µg for three months improved glucose tolerance in PCOS patients. However, it did not change the reproductive function [68]. Another study demonstrated that chromium supplementation with a daily dose of 200 µg for eight weeks improved insulin resistance and other metabolic parameters in PCOS women compared to the placebo [69]. It is also reported that chromium picolinate might decrease hirsutism and improve the symptoms of PCOS [70].

Other minerals that participate in reproductive function and are important in the pathogenesis of PCOS are calcium, selenium, zinc, and magnesium [65]. Calcium is a key mineral involved in follicular development and oocyte maturation [71]. It is demonstrated that calcium plays an important role in the insulin signaling pathway. Thus, calcium deficiency may be correlated with insulin resistance and the following PCOS. Obese women with PCOS have lower levels of calcium compared with healthy individuals. Interestingly, vitamin D receptor (VDR) is associated with calcium homeostasis [66,71,72]. A study reported that supplementation of calcium in combination with vitamin D and metformin 1500 mg for six months decreases the body mass index of PCOS patients. The authors also observed that this supplementation improves follicular development and the fertility rate, although the results were not statistically significant [73].

Selenium is an antioxidant mineral important for the development and activity of reproductive tissues [74]. Lower levels of selenium as well as a higher amount of free radicals have been reported in PCOS patients, which cause a higher production of androgens, luteinizing hormone (LH), and testosterone [75]. Interestingly, selenium also has insulin-like activities [76]. Therefore, it may affect carbohydrate and lipid metabolism. A clinical trial showed that selenium supplementation at a daily dose of 200 µg for eight weeks alleviates insulin resistance in PCOS patients [77]. Hence, selenium supplementation seems to have potential in the adjustment and improvement of insulin resistance and PCOS.

Another mineral, zinc, is a cofactor for many enzymes in carbohydrate and lipid metabolism [78]. Therefore, it also plays a key role in insulin resistance and PCOS. It is reported that women with PCOS represent lower levels of zinc [79,80]. Collectively, zinc supplementation may provide an adjunctive nutritional treatment for inducing insulin sensitivity in women with PCOS. Magnesium as a regulator of ATP use is also an important trace element for the metabolism of insulin [81]. A low level of magnesium was observed in women with insulin resistance and high levels of testosterone [82]. It should be noted that only limited studies have investigated the association between magnesium levels and the pathogenesis of PCOS. Hence, their relationship remains unrecognized [65].

4. Uterine Fibroids

Uterine fibroids (UFs) are the most common gynecological tumors and a major cause of gynecological morbidity in reproductive-age women [83,84]. They are also the leading cause of hysterectomies in the United States, with more than 200,000 hysterectomies yearly [85]. The annual costs attributed to UFs range between $5.9 and $34.4 billion per year in the United States alone and hundreds of billions worldwide [86]. Although UFs are benign tumors, they can cause a myriad of symptoms and outcomes, including pelvic pain, abnormal uterine bleeding, bladder dysfunction, and even infertility [87]. Despite the high morbidity and cost associated with UFs, the exact pathophysiology is not completely delineated [88], yet there are theories and reports of associated risk factors. Some of these risk factors include an increased body mass index, early age at menarche, nulliparity, vitamin D deficiency, and African American ethnicity [89]. A growing body of research has shed light on increasing evidence that dietary factors may play a role in UF etiology and growth [90]. This is hypothesized to be due to their ability to modify endogenous hormones as well as their inflammatory or anti-inflammatory effects.

4.1. Fats

Fats have been extensively studied in relation to UFs, seeing their effect on the inflammatory milieu. For example, trans fats are reported to influence levels of interleukin 6 (IL-6) and other inflammatory markers [91]. Fats also have an effect on hormone levels, as a meta-analysis of 13 intervention studies reported that reducing fat consumption results in lower serum estradiol levels [92].

As previously mentioned, the African American race is considered a risk factor for UFs, and the time of onset is estimated to be 10 to 15 years earlier for this race cohort [93]. In addition, the source of dietary fat intake is shown to be generally different between black and white women in the United States, with black women consuming more fat from meat and fish and less from dairy products as compared to white women [94]. The Black Women's Healthy Study (BWHS) [95] was the first prospective study comprising solely a black women cohort to study the association between dietary fat and UF risk. More than 12,000 African American women were followed for eight years, with 2695 having fibroids that were self-reported, ultrasound detected, or detected during hysterectomy or other surgery. Wise et al. studied data from the BWHS and reported an increased risk of fibroids with the intake of specific ω-3 polyunsaturated fatty acids (PUFAs) but no consistent association with total fat or other fat subtypes, with the exception of total monounsaturated fatty acid (MUFA) intake, for which a positive association was identified [96]. Nevertheless, fish consumption was the main source of PUFAs in this population, so results may have been confounded by environmental contaminants in fish intake. Biomarker measurements of exposure to pollutants in future studies could help differentiate the extent to which the association is explained by pollutants or fatty acids themselves.

Moreover, the BWHS did not measure circulating fatty acids (FAs) that reflect dietary intake and FA metabolism and reflect the internal dose more precisely than estimations based on diet assessment questionnaires, and UF case identification has been based on self-reporting. To expand on the literature, Wise et al. studied this association in the Study of Environment, Lifestyle, and Fibroids (SELF), in which a prospective cohort of African American women underwent serial ultrasound screening for UF incidence during a five-year period [97]. Findings were consistent with those from the BWHS, in which higher intake of marine ω-3 PUFAs are associated with a 13–21% increased risk of UFs.

A more recent prospective study done by Harris et al. examined a cohort aged 25–42 in the NHS II and studied the erythrocyte membrane FA levels of a subset of women [98]. This allowed considering dietary intake and endogenous synthesis and transformation of FAs instead of serum FA levels alone, since erythrocytes reflect long-term intake better than plasma. This study showed an inverse association between total ω-3 PUFAs and a positive association of trans FAs and the onset of uterine fibroids. Moreover, it has been shown that there is an estrogenic or inflammatory effect of dietary fat reflected by the reduction in women's quality of life [92] and by an increase in T helper cytokines associated with fat intake, which is hypothesized to promote chronic inflammation and fibroid tissue growth [99]. However, total trans FAs were associated with higher odds of fibroids. In contrast, an Italian case–control study of 843 histologically confirmed UF cases and 1557 controls reported no association between butter, margarine, or oil intake during the year prior to the study and fibroid risk [100]. Also consistent with these null results was a cross-sectional study of Japanese women including 54 UF cases and 234 controls that reported no association between all fat subtypes and fibroid risk [101]. Islam et al. stated that the myometrium has a higher amount of arachidonic acid than UFs, with alpha-linolenic acid (ALA) being higher in UFs. Treatment with eicosapentaenoic acid (EPA) and docosahexaenoic acid (DHA) reduced the monounsaturated fatty acid content in UFs and controls. However, these did not reflect changes in the mRNA expression of extracellular matrix (ECM) components. Omega-3 fatty acids reduced the levels of sterol regulatory molecules (e.g., ATP-binding cassette sub-family G member 1 (ABCG1) or ATP-binding cassette transporter member 1 (ABCA1)) in both cell types. It also reduced a cytochrome 450 family member CYP11A1, the mitochondrial enzyme that catalyzes the conversion of cholesterol to pregnenolone. The authors concluded that omega-3 fatty acids modulate the lipid profile, mechanical signaling, and cellular lipid accumulation in UFs [102].

4.2. Vegetables, Meat, and Phytochemicals

National surveys have shown that African Americans have a lower intake of vegetables and fruits [103,104]. Several studies have demonstrated that diets rich in vegetables, fruits, and dairy foods play a positive and sometimes protective role in UFs [105] and, conversely, that substantial intake of red meat might increase the risk of fibroids. Fruits and vegetables are good sources of vitamins, antioxidants, and phytochemicals, and numerous studies have shown that they may decease fibroid risk. Wise et al. evaluated the association between fruit and vegetable intake and UF risk in the BWHS [105]. They studied specific components such as carotenoids, folate, fiber, and vitamins A, C, and E. Results suggested that fruit intake is inversely associated with UF risk, with the highest reduction observed for citrus fruit intake. It has been hypothesized that citrus fruit may reduce UF risk through pathways mediated by sex hormones or by inhibition of sex hormones receptors.

In a case–control study in China, He and co-authors confirmed the reduced UF risk with fruits and vegetables but found no association with meat intake [106]. The authors hypothesized that the protective role of a high intake of vegetables and fruits may be related to fibers and lycopene. Fibers can influence sex hormone and bile acid metabolism by interrupting the enterohepatic circulation. Lycopene, which makes up the red pigment in tomatoes, has been proven to decrease fibroid size in a Japanese quail study, but these results are yet to be proven in humans [107]. Phytoestrogens, which are bioactive nutrients found in plants such as soy, have been found to have moderate estrogen and antiestrogen activity [108]. Because of the presence of the phenol ring, soy isoflavone, a type of phytoestrogen, can bind to the estrogen receptor and compete with estradiol. Recently, an in vitro study explored the effects of quercetin and indole-3-carbinol (I3C) on ECM expression, cell migration, and proliferation in human myometrial and UF cells [109]. Quercetin is a flavonoid with known antifibrotic effects found in most edible fruits and vegetables, such as tea, lemon, tomato, onion leaves, and strawberry, while I3C is a naturally occurring glucosinolate in cruciferous vegetables. Results showed that both treatments significantly reduce the expression of ECM markers collagen type I and fibronectin but not versican. Moreover, the treatments inhibited UF cell migration [109].

Anthocyanins are water-soluble flavonoid pigments that are abundant in blueberries, raspberries, and strawberries [110]. Strawberries have anti-inflammatory, anti-oxidative, anti-proliferative, and genomic-protective effects [111,112]. Islam et al. explored the effect of different strawberry Alba cultivar extracts on apoptosis, fibrosis, and oxidation in the myometrium and UF cells. Results showed that anthocyanin-rich strawberries induce apoptosis but suppress glycolysis and fibrosis in UF cells. Following strawberry treatment, the authors observed an increase in reactive oxygen species levels in UFs. Additionally, the anthocyanin-rich extract significantly reduced fibronectin, collagen, and versican mRNA expression in UF cells [113]. In addition, a recent study tested five different strawberry cultivars to identify the one with the best anti-UF effects. The authors found that Alba and Romina cultivars presented the best results: they decreased collagen 1A1, fibronectin, versican, and activin A mRNA expression in UF cells [112]. In vitro studies have shown that curcumin, which is abundantly found in turmeric, prevents fibroid growth as it inhibits UF cell proliferation by regulating the apoptotic pathway [87]. Isoliquiritigenin, which is abundantly found in liquorice, and soybean have been reported to induce growth inhibition and apoptosis of UF cells [114]. On the other hand, studies have also shown both stimulatory and inhibitory effects of genistein, which is abundantly found in soybeans and fava beans, on fibroid cell proliferation [115,116]. Lower concentrations (≤ 1 μg/mL) stimulated proliferation, whereas higher concentrations (≥ 10 μg/mL) significantly inhibited proliferation, decreased proliferating cell nuclear antigen (PCNA), and increased apoptosis of both myometrial and leiomyoma cells. Finally, resveratrol, found in mulberries, peanuts, and grapes, is shown to be inversely associated with the proliferation of fibroids also via inducing apoptosis of UF cells in vitro [87].

Al Hendy et al. showed that intake of epigallocatechin gallate (EGCG), a green tea extract, reduces fibroid size [87]. Thirty-nine reproductive-age women with symptomatic UFs were studied, and although the placebo group was found to have an increase in fibroid size, those randomized to the green tea extract treatment showed an average of 32.6% ($p = 0.0001$) reduction in UF volume. This was attributed to EGCG's inhibitory effect on the proliferation of leiomyoma cells and induction of apoptosis, as was proven by Al Hendy et al. preclinically.

4.3. Dairy Foods and Vitamins

National surveys have shown that African Americans consume less dairy food than white Americans do, and they are less likely to take vitamin supplements as well [117]. Dairy foods have antitumorigenic constituents, including calcium, vitamin D, butyric acid, and milk proteins [118]. Yet, milk may contain estrogen and progesterone that may increase the risk of hormone-dependent tumors [119]. In the BWHS cohort, Wise et al. prospectively studied the effect of dairy food on UF risk and found that women who had four of more dairy servings per day had a 30% reduction in the incidence of fibroids [120]. Calcium, phosphorus, and the calcium-to-phosphorus ratio (as an indicator of calcium bioavailability) were inversely associated with UF risk. It is hypothesized that calcium may reduce fat-induced cell proliferation. In this study, Wise et al. did not find an effect of dietary vitamin D, and this was attributed to the fact that the largest bioavailable sources of vitamin D are derived from sun exposure and supplements. In a later study, Wise identified single-nucleotide polymorphisms in genes involved in vitamin D metabolism that were significantly associated with UFs [121]. It has also been shown African American women have lower serum vitamin D levels than white Americans, which could explain the increased risk of UFs [122]. Al Hendy et al. observed that vitamin D could be a potent antiestrogenic agent that reduces the expression of sex steroid receptors and consequently the risk of UFs [123]. Vitamin D has been shown to be a potent antitumor agent inhibiting UF cell proliferation and decreasing UF size in in vivo animal models as well as several clinical trials [122,124,125]. Mechanistically, vitamin D might exert its anti-UF effects via induction of DNA repair genes and amelioration of DNA damage both in UF cells and in myometrial cells at risk of developing UFs [126–128]. More recently, Sheng et al. published a protocol for the first open-label randomized controlled trial to evaluate whether supplementation with vitamin D can reduce the risk of UFs in reproductive-age women, and future results of this study could provide new evidence of the benefit of vitamin D intake [129].

4.4. Pollutants and Metaloestrogens

As explained previously, fibroid development is mostly mediated by estrogen and progesterone receptors. Many pollutants resemble these steroid hormones and affect these receptors as endocrine-disrupting chemicals (EDCs). As described in a recent review, these include phthalates, parabens, environmental phenols, alternate plasticizers, diethylstilbestrol, organophosphate esters, and tributyltin. The US National Institute of

Environmental Health Sciences (NIEHS) defines EDCs as "chemicals that interfere with the body's endocrine system and produce adverse developmental, reproductive, neurological and immune effects." EDCs have been described to bind to nuclear receptors, such as estrogen receptors, and alter hormone functions by mimicking endogenous hormones and/or blocking them from interacting with their receptors. EDCs may also induce genomic and nongenomic signaling. For example, bisphenol A and diethylstilbesterol have been shown to activate nongenomic signaling through estrogen receptors [130]. Epidemiologic studies have shown that exposure to certain EDCs is associated with increased fibroid risk and severity [131].

Some heavy metals, which are mostly present in tobacco smoke, polluted air, seafood, and leafy green vegetables, are also associated with increased fibroid risk. The Endometriosis: Natural History, Diagnosis, and Outcomes (ENDO) study demonstrated a direct link between fibroids and increased serum levels of cadmium and lead and urinary cobalt levels [132]. Heavy metals as metaloestrogens activate the estrogen receptor in the absence of estradiol and affect the hypothalamic–pituitary–ovarian axis as do endocrine-disrupting compounds [133].

5. Endometriosis

Endometriosis is an inflammatory and estrogen-dependent gynecological disorder characterized by the proliferation of endometrial cells outside the uterine cavity [134]. Indeed, endometrial cells migrate from their original site, the uterus, to other organs and produce endometrial-like tissues in various anatomical sites outside the uterine cavity, particularly the ovaries and the peritoneum [134,135]. Although the symptoms of endometriosis are not specific and most of them are similar to symptoms of other gynecological diseases, it may cause pelvic pain and infertility. Exosomes act as biomarkers for female reproductive disease diagnosis and therapy [136]. Moreover, it should be noted that endometriosis creates a significant burden in terms of health expenditure and quality of life all over the world [136]. It is a disorder with approximately 3 to 11 years of diagnostic delay, resulting in the dysfunction of the reproductive cycle in reproductive-age women. The exact prevalence of endometriosis is not determined due to a lack of proper non-invasive diagnostic techniques, but it is estimated that about 10% of women of reproductive age suffer from endometriosis. Furthermore, its prevalence rises to approximately 20% to 50% in women with pelvic pain or infertility [136–138].

Endometriosis is a multifactorial disorder that involves genetic and immunologic pathways, contraction of the smooth muscle, and inflammation, as well as environmental factors, including dietary habits and nutrition components. According to previous studies, the development of endometriosis requires alterations in several biological pathways for disease establishment [139,140]. The present work aimed to summarize the biological effects of nutrition components, including omega-3, omega-6, vitamin D, N-acetylcysteine, flavonoids, and L-carnitine, on the prevention and treatment of endometriosis.

Foods rich in omega-6 fatty acids, such as red meat, are correlated with higher levels of estradiol and estrone sulfate, which is linked to higher concentrations of steroids, inflammation, and the development of endometriosis [141]. Instead, supplementation with omega-3 may decrease the growth of endometrial implants and the production of inflammatory factors, particularly in patients with stage III or IV endometriosis [142].

Vitamin D is a classic regulator of inflammatory pathways and has been widely studied in the field of endometriosis. Macrophages, lymphocytes, and dendritic cells (DCs) express enzymes that use this vitamin [143]. It has been shown that these cells express CYP27B1, while DCs also express CYP2R1, which are both key enzymes in vitamin D metabolism. All these cell types can convert hydroxy vitamin D3 (25(OH)D3) into bioactive dihydroxy vitamin D3 (1,25(OH)2D3), enabling them to respond not only to the active vitamin D metabolite but also to its precursors]. Vitamin D boosts the shift away from Th1-type responses to a Th2-type immunity by repressing the secretion of IL-12, IL-2, tumor necrosis factor (TNF), and γ-interferon by macrophages, T cells, and DCs [143]. Therefore, the active form of vitamin D may act in the endometriosis lesion by lowering the production of prostaglandins and inflammatory cytokines [143]. A clinical trial demonstrated that patients with dysmenorrhea treated with a dose of 300,000 IU of vitamin D had lower pain along with lower use of nonsteroidal anti-inflammatory drugs (NSAIDs) [144]. However, another clinical trial reported that vitamin D supplementation at a dose of 50,000 IU weekly for 12 weeks did not affect endometriosis-related pain [145]. Hence, further studies are required in this area of research.

N-acetylcysteine, also known as acetylcysteine, can effectively reduce inflammation and alleviate endometriosis. Interestingly, foods with N-acetylcysteine, including onions, garlic, wheat germ, broccoli, and Brussels sprouts, are reported to have the ability to control cell proliferation and oxidative stress in endometriotic cells [146]. A study observed that the size of the endometrioma in patients supplemented with N-acetylcysteine at a dose of 1800 mg reduced significantly [147].

Studies have shown that quercetin acts as a natural flavonoid in endometriosis therapy [148]. A study reported that quercetin affected the hypothalamic–pituitary–gonadal (HPGA) axis in an animal model of endometriosis. Therefore, quercetin decreased the levels of Luteinizing hormone (LH) and follicle-stimulating hormone (FSH). Furthermore, it reduced the levels of estrogen and progesterone receptors [149]. Resveratrol is a polyphenol ingredient found in grapes, peanuts, and cocoa with anti-inflammatory and antioxidant activities. A study reported that resveratrol supplementation reduced the size of endometriomas in an animal model. Moreover, it reduced the levels of vascular endothelial growth factor (VEGF) in endometrial tissue, which is efficient for endometriosis therapy [150]. A randomized exploratory trial in infertile patients with endometriosis (stage III–IV) within the window of implantation revealed that receiving resveratrol (400 mg) for 12–14 weeks significantly attenuated the levels of VEGF and TNF-α genes and protein in the ectopic endometrium compared with the placebo group [151]. Several studies have reported that sulforaphane (SFN), an isothiocyanate in cruciferous vegetables such as cauliflower, cabbage, and broccoli, has antioxidative, antitumor, anti-inflammatory, and immune-enhancing effects [152,153]. Zhou et al. reported that administrating SFN in an endometriosis rat model for three weeks dose-dependently attenuated the volumes of the adhesion score and endometriotic foci. Further, post-treatment of SFN repressed levels of VEGF, interferon gamma (IFN-γ), TNF-α, IL-6 and IL-10 in plasma and peritoneal fluid and regulated the expression of cleaved caspase-3, bcl-2, Bax, and VEGF in endometrial tissue by repression of the PI3K/Akt pathway [152]. These studies suggest that flavonoids may inhibit ectopic endometrium growth.

L-carnitine is an amino acid analogue involved in fatty acid oxidation and energy metabolism [154]. Studies have shown that L-carnitine supplementation acts as a double-edged sword in the progression of endometriosis. For instance, it was reported that L-carnitine intensified an already presented endometriotic lesion when cells expressed estrogen receptors, while it improved this situation when cells did not express estrogen receptors. Clearly, the underlying mechanism is linked to the cellular features of cells arising from the endometrium [155].

Altogether, there are many studies on the role of different nutrients in endometriosis, which provide promising approaches to disease control. It seems that foods rich in omega-3, N-acetylcysteine, and polyphenol, in addition to decreased consumption of omega-6 fatty acids, may lower the plausible risk of endometriosis. Therefore, dietary education appears to be a promising strategy for the control of the disease.

6. Vaginal Microbiome, Nutrients, and Female Reproductive Tract Infections

The worldwide burden of reproductive tract infections (RTIs) is a vast and major public health concern, particularly in developing countries where RTIs are widespread [156]. RTIs, except for human immunodeficiency virus (HIV), are considered the next major cause of disease burden (after maternity-related causes) in young women in developing countries. RTIs involve three sets of infections [156,157]: sexually transmitted infections

(STIs), infections that arise from the overgrowth of organisms usually present in the reproductive tract, and, finally, infections connected with therapeutic plans, including abortion and insertion of intrauterine devices.

Female RTIs usually start in the lower genital tract as vaginitis or cervicitis and may exhibit irregular vaginal discharge, genital discomfort, itching, and burning sensation with urination. RTIs causes a heavy burden on women if untreated, and they can cause serious infertility, cervical cancer, ectopic pregnancy, menstrual disturbances, pregnancy wastage, and low-birth-weight babies [158].

An environment's microbiota consists of resident bacteria, viruses, fungi, protists, and archaea. Either culture-based or sequence-based techniques can distinguish the bacterial microbiome. Both methods have been used to define various sites within the women's reproductive tract, including the vagina, cervix, and uterus. While sequence-based techniques are not routinely used to recognize bacteria in the female reproductive tract, this is an emerging research interest field. Bacterial infections of the female reproductive tract, including vaginitis, cervicitis, and endometritis, have been described [159], as this pathogenic environment may cause inflammation and immune activation in the endometrium, impairing embryo implantation and the onset of a successful pregnancy [159,160].

The interplay between nutrition and infectious diseases has been identified. In the era before antibiotics, the diet was a vital part of controlling infections [161]. Malnutrition, including undernutrition and overnutrition, can increase sensitivity to infectious diseases and magnify the infection severity, which can worsen by malnutrition; the gut microbiota has been attracting interest as an essential mediator in the complex relationships linking food, the human body, and infectious diseases [162].

An optimal vaginal microbiota is controlled by Lactobacillus species, which produce the metabolite lactic acid. Lactic acid decreases the pH of the vaginal microenvironment [163] and, throughout immunomodulatory and direct inhibitory effects, may defend against the acquisition of STIs, including Chlamydia trachomatis (CT) and HIV [164,165]. Women with a non-optimal microbiota, as epitomized by the clinical condition of bacterial vaginosis (BV), have vaginal microbial communities low in Lactobacillus spp. and are instead colonized by a variety of anaerobes that generally produce little or no lactic acid. Some of these bacteria produce metabolites such as biogenic amines and short-chain fatty acids that may be pro-inflammatory and linked with symptoms such as vaginal malodor and discomfort. These metabolites may also increase susceptibility to STIs. Moreover, women with a low-Lactobacillus non-optimal vaginal microbiota have an increased risk of being infected with STIs and ascending infection, including pelvic inflammatory disease (PID) and increased risk of preterm birth (PTB) [166].

Bacterial vaginosis (BV) is the most common reason for vaginal complaints amongst reproductive-age women. The prevalence of BV in infertile women is high (19%), and an abnormal microflora occurs in 39% of infertile patients [167,168]. BV is a clinical case marked by a transformation from a Lactobacillus-dominant bacterial community to higher diversity and a greater abundance of anaerobes and a subsequent rise in vaginal pH (>4.5) [169,170].

BV is considered a risk factor for several common sexual transmitted infections [171], including those induced by the bacteria Neisseria gonorrhea, CT, and Mycoplasma genitalium; the protozoan Trichomonas vaginalis; and viruses such as HIV, human papillomavirus (HPV), and herpes simplex virus type 2 (HSV-2) [158,169,170]. Many data have reported the relationship between diet and nutritional status in BV, but the mechanism is still unclear [162,172]. Many studies have found associations between BV and low micronutrient status, including vitamins A, C, E, and D and β-carotene, and low dietary intake of folate and calcium [162,170,172–174].

6.1. Bacterial Vaginosis and Vitamin D Deficiency

Many records describe higher frequencies of BV among women with low vitamin D concentrations (often marked as <20 nmol/L or <30 nmol/L) [175,176]. In addition, vitamin

D supplementation is effective in eliminating BV [177]. Race/ethnicity has significant population-level impacts on vitamin D status, BV status, and pregnancy outcomes. Women of African heritage are also doubly as likely to receive a clinical diagnosis of BV, and analyses of the vaginal microbiota reveal that it is more likely to be colonized by specific BV-associated bacteria.

6.2. Role of a High-Fat Diet and a High-Sugar-Diet on Altering the Vaginal Microbiome

In specific subsets of women, a correlation between a high-saturated-fat diet, a higher glycemic load, and lower nutritional density with BV has been found, in addition to a contrary relationship between BV and higher folate, vitamin E, and calcium consumption [170,172,178]. BV has also been epidemiologically combined with obesity [169]. Subsequently, shifts in the vaginal microbiota balance due to infection with BV alters the composition referred to as polybacterial dysbiosis and to disease such as vaginal HPV [179]. In addition, BV has been associated with acquiring and transmitting HIV and other sexually transmitted pathogens [180,181].

Lactobacillus dominance is that the high starch content of human diets leads to high glycogen levels in the vaginal tract, creating a suitable Lactobacillus environment. Lactobacilli and other fermentative bacteria and vaginal epithelial cells produce lactic acid and are responsible for acidifying the vaginal microenvironment pH to <4.5, which gives the vaginal microbiota a certain level of balance and ability to withstand some infections. This microbiota is shown by a low degree of diversity and the high dynamics of its structure changes under the control of various exogenous and endogenous factors. Nutrients play an important role in altering the vaginal microbiome diversity. A diet deficient in vitamin A, C, D, and E, calcium, folate, and beta-carotene but rich in fats and sugar, causes vaginal infections such as BV, which are linked to preterm birth, increased risk of HIV transmission, increased risk of HPV infection, and cervical, endometrial, and ovarian cancers (Figure 1).

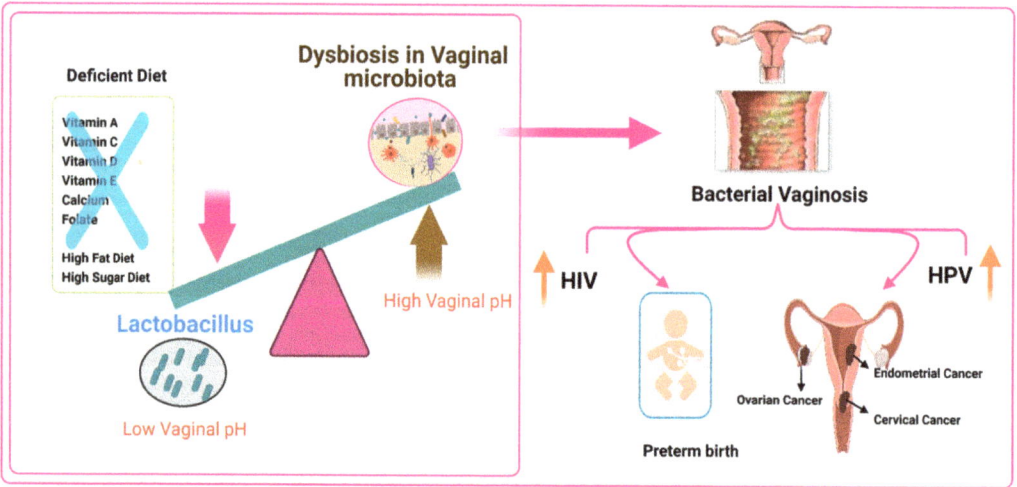

Figure 1. Impact of diet on the vaginal microbiome. A diet deficient in vitamins A, C, D, and E, calcium, folate, and beta-carotene but loaded with fats and sugar leads to altering the vaginal microbiota and increase susceptibility to infections causing bacterial vaginosis, which are associated with preterm birth, raising the risk of human immunodeficiency virus (HIV) transmission, human papillomavirus (HPV) infection, and cervical, endometrial, and ovarian cancers.

7. Gynecological Cancers

Neoplastic diseases are a growing public health problem, considering their incidence and subsequent health care burden [182,183]. Interdisciplinary oncological care is extremely important for the sake of successful cancer cure. Adequate prophylaxis, diagnostic work-up, and therapeutic plan are essential in order to either achieve a curative goal in the case of curable diseases or prolong patient survival and quality of life in the case of an incurable disease. In gynecological oncology, the utility of prophylaxis and health-promoting behavior strategies can result in three outcomes: effective, leading to poor effects, or ineffective. Examples of the first outcome are vaccination and the application of effective screening tools in cervical cancer, with subsequent reduced morbidity and mortality [184]. Intermediate effective outcomes are achieved in endometrial cancer, where behaviors such as avoiding aggravating factors and following their effective treatment in co-morbid conditions (diabetes, hypertension, and obesity) reduced morbidity in some groups [185]. Unfortunately, following the same measures in the case of ovarian cancer resulted in practically ineffective outcomes [186].

Diet and nutritional intervention plans in oncology should be individualized and focused on adjusting nutrient needs for cancer patients [187]. The literature estimates that diet and nutritional compounds may contribute to approximately 20–60% of cancers worldwide [188]. Collectively, more investment should be made in research detailing the role diet/nutrition plays both in the occurrence of cancer and in its cure, such as tolerance to radiation and chemotherapy. The current literature relatively ignores this important angle, while focusing on exploring new chemotherapeutics, immunological therapies, and new operative techniques, including those only for women [189]. Recent findings have shown that neither fruits nor vegetables might be convincingly or possibly associated with the risk of any cancer. Moreover, vitamins and mineral compounds do not reduce cancer risk in populations that are well nourished. Therefore, they should not be used for standard cancer prevention. However, specific components of certain fruits and vegetables might present protective properties [189]. Seemingly, even if studies in this area are scarce, it is worth collecting at least some available data to draw conclusions for future research.

7.1. Cervical Cancer

Cervical cancer has been studied for many years. Unlike other cancers, cervical cancer is caused by sexually transmitted infections (STIs) with certain types of HPV. A persistent viral infection in high-risk groups was recognized as necessary for the development, maintenance, and progression of cervical intraepithelial neoplasia (CIN) and cervical cancer [190]. Some environmental and lifestyle co-factors were found to influence such disease progression, including inappropriate diet, cigarette smoking, coexistence of STIs, combined oral contraceptive (COC) use, high parity, low socioeconomic status, early sexual activity, or multiple sexual partners.

Available studies have demonstrated that reactive oxygen species (ROS), either independently or orchestrated with HPV, may play a role in cervical cancer pathogenesis. Therefore, consumption of dietary antioxidants, such as carotenes, ascorbic acid, and vitamin D, might offer a protective role via neutralizing such harmful ROS [188]. Moreover, antioxidants may modulate the immune system in favor of a better response to the cancer microenvironment [191].

Likewise, natural antioxidants may slow down or protect against persistent HPV infection and thus later cervical cancer development [192,193]. For example, Tomita et al. highlighted an existing correlation between both low intake of fruits and vegetables and smoking habits with an increasing risk of developing high-grade CIN [192]. In addition, in 2012, Jia et al. published data suggesting that eating higher amounts of fresh vegetables and drinking green tea may reduce the overall risk of cervical cancer [194]. Interestingly, vitamins such as C and E can serve as efficient antioxidants, with studies linking higher serum antioxidant vitamin levels with a lower risk of cervical cancer, especially in passive smokers [195]. It was also demonstrated that the dietary intake of carotenoids or retinols, lutein, different xanthines, and ascorbic acid was associated with a reduced incidence of HPV persistence in infected women [196]. Furthermore, low serum levels of lycopene, retinol, and tocopherols are suspected to increase the risk of high-grade CIN, while higher serum levels of carotenoids and gamma tocopherol could even reduce the overall risk of this kind of dysplasia [192].

A summarized review by Ono et al. in 2020 concluded that various nutritional antioxidants may affect HPV infection-derived cervical diseases. They suggested that the intake of vitamin A, carotenoids, and vitamin D may inhibit cervical cancer development at early stages. Conversely, the intake of vitamin C and E may be useful in the inhibition of the cervical cancer development process [197], while vitamin A's main effect is inhibition of HPV infection and CIN development [188]. In 2000, Yeo. et al. found that women with low serum retinol levels were at an increased risk of low-degree CIN compared with women who had higher levels of retinol [198]. Interestingly, Huang et al. (2020) found that the dietary intake of vitamin A, equal to or higher than 1448.155 mcg, increased the risk of HPV infection by 70% [199]. Vitamin E is a group of fat-soluble compounds including tocopherols and tocotrienols with antioxidant effects protecting cell membranes from ROS [200]. Studies have confirmed the same findings that high circulating levels or a greater intake of vitamin E might reduce the risk of CIN or cervical cancer [201]. Concerning other nutrients such as vitamin D and folic acid, a recent randomized controlled trial by Vahedpoor et al. (2017) performed in 58 women diagnosed with low-grade CIN revealed that after six months of vitamin D administration, the regression of lesions was observed more commonly in women who consumed vitamin D compared with controls [202]. Folic acid has not been extensively studied recently, and the available data are relatively old. Hernandez et al. (2003) reported that the total folate serum level presented an inverse, dose-responsive correlation with low-grade cervical squamous intraepithelial lesions and high-grade squamous intraepithelial lesions [203].

Natural compounds with chemopreventive/chemotherapeutic potential and antioxidant features have received increased attention in the past few years. Some natural compounds extracted from plants, such as curcumin and EGCG, have been found to exhibit anticancer properties, e.g., increasing tumor cell sensitization to different forms of therapy [204,205]. Seemingly, curcumin requires special attention. This compound (also known as diferuloylmethane) is present in the turmeric rhizome and shows different anti-inflammatory and antioxidant properties [205]. Briefly, curcumin contributes to the inhibition of nuclear factor kappa B-regulated gene factors that control apoptosis, proliferation, invasion, or angiogenesis, in addition to inhibition of nuclear factor kappa B activation through the modulation of different kinases [205], which contributes to the resistance of human cervical cancer cells and results in increased cell death [206]. EGCG is another interesting compound with anticancer properties. It is a polyphenol with proven antiproliferative, antiangiogenic, antimetastatic, and proapoptotic properties in several tumor models [207]. EGCG is a potent inhibitor of several kinases as well as the mammalian target of rapamycin (mTOR) signaling, besides acting as a modulator in inflammatory processes [208]. EGCG modulates ROS production, which might be linked to its antitumorigenic effects. The EGCG-derived modulation/inhibition of nuclear factor kappa B signaling is responsible for its effect against angiogenesis, cell movement, and viability [208]. Finally, resveratrol, which is a phytoalexin found in fruits like grapes, blueberries, or peanuts, exhibits anticancer effects via interacting with several important molecules involved in tumor development, such as activators, kinases, or nuclear factor kappa B. Moreover, resveratrol shows antiproliferative effects on cervical cancer cell lines through cell cycle modulation with accumulation of the cells in the S phase [204].

To conclude, several nutrients with antioxidant effects may present potent abilities to intervene in the natural history of cervical cancer tumorigenesis connected with HPV infection [197]. Selected vitamins (such as vitamins A and D) and natural compounds (e.g., EGCG) demonstrate a positive effect in halting the cervical cancer disease process.

Obviously, the available data are inconclusive, and their quality may be undermined. Therefore, more well-designed, large randomized clinical studies are needed.

7.2. Endometrial Cancer

Endometrial cancer (EC) is currently one of the most common malignant neoplasms affecting women worldwide. Unfortunately, the direct underlying etiology has not been clearly described and understood. EC is known to occur mainly in postmenopausal women [209]. Contributing risk factors are older age, nulliparity, diabetes, estrogen-only hormone replacement therapy, and obesity [210]. Fortunately, the survival rate ranges from about 75% to 90% in patients diagnosed at early stages [211]. Differences in histological patterns and clinical outcomes divide EC into two types. Type I cancers present as endometrioid adenocarcinomas, and this kind of tumor is often preceded by endometrial hyperplasia. Importantly, the development of this kind of tumor is mostly influenced by the long-lasting stimulation of estrogens on the endometrium [210,212]. Type II tumors are mostly represented by serous cancers, and they are rather estrogen independent. We may observe them arising from the atrophic endometrium [210,212].

Regarding the potential preventive effects of diet intake on EC risk, limited data are available with conclusions of negligible correlation. In their review, Bandera et al. (2009) found an inverse relationship of EC risk with the dietary intake of carotenes, ascorbic acid, and tocopherols. They highlighted that additional larger studies are necessary to confirm this association [213]. Later, a Nurses' Health Study denied such association between EC risk and the consumption of dietary carotenoids and vitamins A, C, or E [214].

The incidence of precancerous changes was found to be higher in overweight and obese patients. Interestingly, higher fat energy intake was found to be associated with increased EC risk, but the energy from carbohydrates and proteins did not increase that risk [215]. Therefore, it was interesting for researchers to explore the role of diet in the pathophysiology of EC in the context of inflammation. Studies have suggested that elevated levels of prostaglandins might underlie the transformation of a normal endometrium into neoplastic tissue, which might be attributed to inflammation-induced cell division with subsequent possibility of ineffective DNA repair and mutations. Interestingly, polyunsaturated fatty acids (e.g., available in seafood) are thought to be anti-inflammatory, and one might think play a possible beneficial role against EC. For example, Brasky et al. (2014) showed that high consumption of dietary eicosapentaenoic acid and docosahexaenoic acid increased the risk of EC by 80% compared to a lower consumption rate [216]. Alcohol was thought to increase EC risk via increasing the circulating serum sex steroids. Rinaldi et al. (2006) showed that sex-hormone-binding globulin levels are approximately 15% lower in alcohol consumers (25 g of alcohol daily) compared with non-consumers [217]. Interestingly, recent data from a prospective study performed in 301,051 European women showed that alcohol consumption is not associated with EC risk [218].

The effect of some plant-derived compounds on EC is attributed to their hormonal effect, for example, phytoestrogens, which have low estrogenic activity, while others might possess antioxidant and antimutagenic properties [219]. Flavonoids are a class of polyphenolic metabolites that have antioxidant and anti-mutagenic properties, so it is believed that they may reduce cancer risk, e.g., in EC [220]. Unfortunately, it has not been confirmed in further studies. A randomized controlled trial by Wang et al. (2009) revealed no association between selected flavones and flavonols and EC risk [221]. Similarly, Bandera et al. (2009) showed no association between isoflavones and EC [222]. However, slightly different data were presented by Ollberding et al. (2012), who demonstrated that a greater consumption of isoflavone-containing foods was associated with a reduced risk of EC in postmenopausal women [223]. This might be explained by the fact that isoflavones possess some selective estrogen receptor modulator activity, with varying estrogenic and antiestrogenic potential, depending on the receptor characteristics of the target tissue. Isoflavones are abundant in soy, whose consumption has been studied in numerous publications. A review by Zhang et al. (2015) revealed that soy intake might be associated with lower EC risk; however, the authors highlighted that the exact mechanisms are still unknown [224]. Furthermore, a meta-analysis by Zhong et al. (2018) revealed that the consumption of larger amounts of dietary isoflavones from soy products and legumes weakly decreased the risk of EC in the selected population [225]. Remarkably, some authors indicated a negative effect of high soy isoflavone consumption that resulted in a relatively high incidence of endometrial hyperplasia [226]. Therefore, the protective effect of soy isoflavones on EC should be interpreted with caution, and their introduction into cancer therapy might be rather challenging now.

If it is about other compounds, the data are scarce. An inverse association between ultraviolet irradiance and EC incidence was demonstrated, suggesting a possible beneficial effect of vitamin D, considering its multitargeted effects [227]. However, available meta-analyses have revealed no significant relationship between the intake of vitamin D and the incidence of EC [228]. In a study by Bandera et al. (2009), increased intake of quercetin (a bitter plant flavonol found in different fruits and vegetables) was associated with a decreased risk of EC [222]. Similarly, kaempferol, a natural dietary flavonoid, was explored against EC cells, considering its anticancer, anti-inflammatory, and antioxidant properties, and studies have shown that it suppresses cellular proliferation through various mechanisms [229,230].

Some research was conducted on the association between tea consumption and the risk of EC. In 2015, Yang et al. demonstrated little or no association between tea consumption and the risk of EC [231], while a meta-analysis published later highlighted that a higher dietary intake of green tea might be connected with a reduced risk of EC. Notably, such correlation was not demonstrated in the case of black tea. The authors suggested that the reduced risk might be due to the markedly higher content of catechins in green tea in comparison with black tea. Catechins, such as EGCG, may modulate the estrogen-induced activation of endometrial cells and also induce the apoptosis of neoplastic cells as well as cell cycle arrest [232].

Taking all together, available data on the effect of nutritional compounds on EC pathophysiology are of poor quality and insufficient. Nevertheless, exploring new natural dietary compounds in the prophylaxis or treatment of this disease is encouraged.

7.3. Ovarian Cancer

Ovarian cancer is a malignant tumor of the ovaries, occurring mainly in peri- or postmenopausal women. Unfortunately, it is associated with the poorest prognosis and the highest mortality rate among all gynecological cancers [233]. Research shows that the number and frequency of ovulations in a woman's lifetime are linked to the risk of her developing ovarian cancer [234], since it is associated with the rupture of the ovarian epithelium and the sensitizing effect of the follicular fluid with a high content of estrogens [235]. Ovarian cancers are histologically and clinically divided into two different types. Type I cancers are low-grade endometrioid, mucinous, and clear-cell cancers, whereas type II cancers are of a higher histological grade in which tumors may develop de novo from the tubal and/or ovarian surface epithelium and include serous cancers [234]. Surgery is the critical modality in the treatment of ovarian cancer, as well as chemotherapy [234]. Regrettably, due to the unclear etiology of ovarian cancer, it may not always be prevented. However, some factors have been shown to limit the risk of its development, e.g., lactation or the use of combined oral contraception. Therefore, exploring the potential role of nutritional compounds in prophylaxis or supportive treatment is valid.

The available literature suggests a possible link between ovarian cancer and inappropriate dietary habits. For instance, chronic inflammation was implied as an underlying mechanism contributing to ovarian carcinogenesis [236]. A study by Shivappa et al. (2016) showed that ovarian cancer risk increases in women who consume higher amounts of pro-inflammatory products [237]. On the contrary, Dolecek et al. (2010) and Playdon et al. (2017) demonstrated the influence of a healthy diet on the clinical course of ovarian cancer [238,239]. The former study showed that only yellow and cruciferous vegetables significantly favored the survival rate, whereas a negative correlation was shown for meat [238]. Playdon et al. (2017) demonstrated a trend toward lower mortality with higher fruit intake. Moreover, a higher intake of green leafy vegetables was inversely associated with mortality. Compared to the previously discussed study, the authors did not show such a strong influence of cruciferous vegetables [239]. An important meta-analysis published by Qiu et al. revealed that a high consumption of total, saturated, and trans fats increased ovarian cancer risk. The authors emphasized that different histological subtypes had different susceptibilities to dietary fat, and provided an example of saturated fats that might increase the overall risk of serous and endometrioid ovarian cancers [240].

A variety of studies are available considering phytoestrogens, including the beneficial effect of isoflavones on ovarian cancer, with nonconclusive findings. In a study by Bandera et al. (2011), phytoestrogen presented a trend for a reduction in ovarian cancer risk. However, no significant associations were found. However, an inverse association with total phytoestrogen consumption was found after adjusting for age, race, education, body mass index, and total energy [241]. Moreover, an analysis by Neill et al. (2014) showed a pattern of inverse associations between the increasing intake of phytoestrogens, isoflavones, or lignans and the risk of ovarian cancer, but it should be emphasized that significance was only proved for two lignans—matairesinol and lariciresinol [242]. Isoflavones were found to have a protective effect against ovarian cancer, which may be attributed to the inhibition of the growth and proliferation of ovarian cell lines. Furthermore, they may regulate cancer inflammation pathways [188]. Conversely, Hedelin et al. (2010) found no association between phytoestrogens, fiber intake, and ovarian cancer risk. The authors found that fiber and coumestrol intake was inversely associated with borderline tumors but not with invasive types [243]. Finally, in 2016, Hua et al. showed in their meta-analysis that the intake of dietary flavonoids might decrease ovarian cancer risk. According to this analysis, ovarian cancer risk decreases with isoflavones and flavonols, but there was no evidence that the dietary intake of flavones was protective in the case of ovarian cancer [244].

Herein, we present some examples of such flavonoids that might offer beneficial effects against ovarian cancer. Quercetin, a plant flavonol, inhibits oxidation and acts as a free-radical scavenger with estrogenic activities on both types of estrogen receptors (α and β) [87]. Quercetin presented antitumor and anti-inflammatory properties with a cytotoxic influence on ovarian cancer, which Shafabakhsh et al. attributed to its anti-inflammatory, pro-oxidative, antiproliferation, and apoptosis induction activities [245]. A different already described flavonoid, kaempferol, was also found to be a good inhibitor of angiogenesis [246]. Finally, a flavonol named galangin was found to be selective against cancer cells where it induced apoptosis. It was suggested that future research might prove its usability in platinum-resistant ovarian cancers [247].

Curcumin is a well-known natural compound found in turmeric. It is a diarylheptanoid and belongs to the group of curcuminoids, which are natural phenols. Curcumin exhibited a wide range of effects, e.g., anticancer, anti-inflammatory, and antioxidant capabilities. In 2007, Lin et al. showed that curcumin might inhibit nuclear factor kappa B activation and suppress both proliferation and angiogenesis in ovarian cancer cells [248]. Since curcumin has been extensively studied in cancer treatment, data might suggest additional efficacy due to sensitization of the resistance of cancer cells to current therapies [249]. For example, a study conducted by Wahl et al. (2007) demonstrated that curcumin used in a combination with a special anticancer ligand (Apo2L) results in reduced chemoresistance to conventional chemotherapeutic agents [250]. More recently, He et al. (2016) found that curcumin significantly increases epithelial ovarian cancer sensitivity to cisplatin and abolishes the sphere-forming ability [251]. An earlier study by Yallapu et al. in 2010 showed that this compound reduces the dose of both radiation and cisplatin needed for cell growth suppression in cisplatin-resistant ovarian cancer cells [252]. Berberine is a plant-based alkaloid with a tetracyclic skeleton with anti-inflammatory, antiproliferative, pro-apoptotic, and antimetastatic actions [253]. A recent study by Liu et al. (2019) proposed that the co-use of berberine and cisplatin enhances ovarian cancer cell death by inducing apoptosis and necroptosis. Tissue samples revealed the typical apoptotic and necrotic cell death morphology with the inhibition of proliferating cell nuclear antigen and Ki67 and a higher expression of selected caspases [254].

Finally, we highlight new agents that might be of interest for future research on ovarian cancer therapy. The first is honokiol, a natural biphenolic lignan extracted from different parts of magnolia. Regarding the possible effects on ovarian cancer, honokiol regulates the nuclear factor kappa B activation pathway and VEGF expression [255]. Recently, a study showed that the anticancer activities of honokiol in ovarian cancer cells are mediated through the activation of adenosine 5′ phosphate-activated protein kinase. Honokiol induced apoptosis with the activation of various caspases. Moreover, honokiol inhibited the migration and invasion of ovarian cancer cells [256]. The second new compound is bufalin, which is a steroid isolated from toad venom. According to available studies, bufalin presents antitumor effects against various malignancies, including lung cancer [257]. A study by Su et al. published in 2020 demonstrated its usefulness in ovarian cancer, where it acted as a potent inhibitor of cell growth and migration in ovarian cancer cells through the suppression of mTOR activation and hypoxia-inducible factor 1-alpha (HIF1α) induction. The authors concluded that bufalin might be used as an additive to cisplatin in ovarian cancer therapy [258]. Lastly, tetramethylpyrazine (also named ligustrazine) is a chemical compound classified as an alkylpyrazine found in fermented soybeans and cocoa beans [259]. It is a natural compound reported to present anticancer activity. In 2020, Zhang et al. found that tetramethylpyrazine inhibits the viability, proliferation, migration, and invasion ability of selected ovarian cancer cell lines in a dose-dependent manner [260].

Vitamin D may be significant in reproductive organ tumors [261]. A systematic review of the literature has not identified any human studies regarding the effect of vitamin D or its analogues on ovarian cancer patients, and such supplementation or treatment cannot be recommended [262]. Regardless of vitamin D, calcium seems to be significant in the pathophysiology and therapy of ovarian cancer. An available meta-analysis by Song et al. published in 2017 supported the hypothesis that increased calcium intake might reduce ovarian cancer risk. In the analysis, dietary calcium was significantly associated with a reduced risk of ovarian cancer among cohort and case–control studies. However, the authors concluded that further studies, mostly those on larger groups, might lead to more decisive conclusions [263].

Although the discussed data indicated some influence of nutritional compounds on the development and course of ovarian cancer, there is a paucity of valuable clinical data that may be translated into evidence-based medicine. Flavonoids seem to play the most significant role. However, more research is encouraged in order to explore novel compounds.

8. Menstrual Disorders

8.1. Menorrhagia

Menorrhagia is described as excessive uterine bleeding, in terms of flow and duration, during regular cyclical intervals. Its clinical definition includes blood loss greater than 80 mL per cycle or menses lasting longer than 7 days [264]. Diet should be considered when managing menorrhagia. Ideally, the diet should be low in animal fat and rich in fish oils and linolenic and linoleic acids. Therefore, flaxseeds and soy protein have been frequently suggested due to their ability to regulate the menstrual cycle [265]. Here, we briefly discuss supplements and nutrients that have been explored for their potential role in managing menorrhagia.

8.1.1. Iron

Blood loss is one of the major causes of iron deficiency anemia. However, it is less well known that chronic iron deficiency can be a contributor to menorrhagia, in turn. Therefore, women experiencing heavy blood loss should consume iron-rich foods such as Brewer's yeast, wheat germ, blackstrap molasses, organic liver and kidneys, apricots, eggs, ground beef, raisins, beans, cooked spinach, and chicken. In addition, yogurt, sour fruits, and citrus juices can aid in the absorption of iron [266].

8.1.2. Vitamin A

Adult women experiencing menorrhagia may have low levels of vitamin A. One study in which vitamin A was used to treat women with menorrhagia showed that those who received 60,000 IU of vitamin A for 35 days experienced both a return to normal and a reduction in blood loss compared to the placebo group [264,267].

8.1.3. Vitamin B Complex

Vitamin B deficiency may be related to menorrhagia. Studies have shown that vitamin B complex deficiencies result in failure of the liver to inactivate estrogen. Thus, the excess estrogen's effect on the endometrium ends up with more bleeding, while vitamin B complex may help normalize estrogen metabolism and thus reduce bleeding [268].

8.1.4. Vitamin C and Bioflavonoids

Vitamin C and bioflavonoids improve heavy bleeding via making the capillary walls less fragile. Livdans-Forret noted that 16 of 18 women who took vitamin C and bioflavonoids for heavy menstrual bleeding reported an improvement [264]. Moreover, vitamin C can benefit women with iron deficiency due to menorrhagia by increasing iron absorbency [269].

Some herbal and nutritional supplements have shown beneficial effects against menorrhagia, including the chaste tree or chasteberry (Vitex agnus castus), which is a well-known herb in Europe for the treatment of hormonal imbalances and abnormal bleeding in women. In addition, astringent herbs such as shepherd's purse have a long history of use for inhibiting gynecological hemorrhage. Tonic herbs such as life root, also known as ragwort, have been used for conditions such as menstrual cramps, menorrhagia, and subdued menstruation. Traditional herbs such as yarrow have been used since medieval times to treat bleeding wounds. Yarrow is a uterine stimulant that increases muscular tone, stimulates reproductive activity, and effectively treats menstrual problems [264].

8.2. Dysmenorrhea

Dysmenorrhea is commonly described as painful menstruation in the form of lower abdominal pain, which has a range of severity and associated symptoms. These include nausea, vomiting and loss of appetite, fatigue, diarrhea, headache, restlessness, insomnia, and fainting [270]. Primary dysmenorrhea has been primarily associated with the extra production of prostaglandins and leukotrienes. Prostaglandins (PGF2-α) temporarily limit or stop the blood supply to the uterus by stimulating its contraction, which reduces the amount of blood perfusing the uterus through myometrial compression of the blood vessels. This deprives the uterus of oxygen, which results in cramping and abdominal pain. Higher concentrations of PGF2-α and leukotrienes in menstrual blood and in uterine smears were observed in women with signs of painful menstruation. Several studies have explored the efficacy of supplements and nutrients against dysmenorrhea [271–273], which we discuss next in the article.

8.2.1. Calcium and Magnesium

Dietary calcium and magnesium intake has a protective effect against dysmenorrhea. Following absorption from the upper intestine, they can manage the muscle cells' response to nerve stimuli through numerous functions [274]. Even though the tocolytic effect of magnesium has already been proven in vivo and in vitro, the best dosage for treating or preventing dysmenorrhea is not yet clear [275].

8.2.2. Olive Oil

The polyphenolic compound oleocanthal in extra virgin olive oil has been shown to have anti-inflammatory and antioxidant effects. A study examining its inhibitory effect on prostaglandin-induced uterine hypercontraction showed that oleocanthal, dose-dependently, inhibited the PGF2α-induced contraction amplitude [276]. Thus, the authors concluded that extra virgin olive oil and oleocanthal can reduce oxidative stress and uterine hypercontraction.

8.2.3. Fennel

Fennel, or Foeniculum vulgare, is a herbal therapy proposed to alleviate menstrual pain by lowering the prostaglandin levels in blood. A meta-analysis showed the equivalent effects of fennel on pain reduction compared with drug therapy, and the pooled results showed favorable effects of fennel on pain reduction compared to the placebo [277]. Fennel in the form of capsules, pill, or oils (excluding massage oil) was used in the 12 studies included in the meta-analysis.

8.2.4. Dietary Fiber

Since dietary fat and fiber alter estrogen levels, they may be related to dysmenorrhea by affecting hormones. Fiber intake reduces blood estrogen levels, whereas fat has been associated with increased estrogen levels. Nagata et al. found that intake of dietary fiber is significantly inversely correlated with the menstrual pain scale after adjusting for age, smoking status, age at menarche, and total energy intake [278].

8.2.5. Omega-3 and Omega-6 Fatty Acids

Western diets are rich in omega-6 fatty acids (e.g., vegetable oil, eggs, and margarine) but poor in omega-3 fatty acids (e.g., fish, canola oil, and wheat germ). Omega-6 fatty acids contribute to the formation of pro-inflammatory eicosanoids, such as Prostaglandin E2 (PGE2), thromboxane A2, and leukotriene B4, whereas omega-3 fatty acids, specifically eicosapentanoic and docosahexanoic acids, lead to the formation of less inflammatory eicosanoids (e.g., PGE3, thromboxane A3, and leukotriene B5). There is some epidemiologic evidence that a diet rich in omega-3 fatty acids can decrease painful menses. Several studies have shown a significant decrease in menstrual pain in those using fish oil [279,280].

8.2.6. Vitamin D

Vitamin D receptors are located in the human uterus, and vitamin D inhibits the synthesis of prostaglandins [144]. Calcitriol (1,25[OH]2D) decreases, in vitro, the level of pro-inflammatory cytokines such as interleukin 6 and tumor necrosis factor and regulates the expression of several key genes involved in the prostaglandin pathway, causing decreased biological activity of prostaglandins [144]. Thus, vitamin D has been suggested to halt the extra prostaglandin production found in primary dysmenorrhea. One study showed an inverse correlation of 25(OH)D levels with the pain score as well as a significant reduction in pain in women taking vitamin D, with the greatest reduction found in women who reported severe pain at baseline [281]. Studies in Iran and Italy have shown that the use of a single dose of oral cholecalciferol (300,000 IU) for five days before the beginning of menstrual bleeding significantly decreased the pain of severe primary dysmenorrhea, while another trial found that the administration of 50,000 IU of vitamin D for eight weeks significantly reduced pain severity [282]. Another study found that low levels of vitamin D are inversely related to the severity of primary dysmenorrhea and that vitamin D and calcium intake could reduce its severity [283].

8.2.7. Vitamin E

Vitamin E is thought to reduce prostaglandin formation by inhibiting arachidonic acid release. A review article about the positive effects of vitamin E on the alleviation of primary dysmenorrhea pain showed a significant reduction in pain severity in women treated with this vitamin [264]. Two studies have shown a significant reduction in pain when 150 to 500 IU/day of vitamin E was administered a few days before and during menses compared with the placebo for two to three cycles [264].

8.2.8. Qixuehe

Formulations of Chinese herbs may be beneficial but lack rigorous testing to evaluate their mechanistic action. One study found that QiXueHe Capsule (QXHC) can alleviate pathological changes in menstrual disorders. Researchers identified 1022 targets of 15 herbs in QXHC to investigate its pharmacological mechanisms on menstrual disorders. Results showed that targets in the treatment of menstrual disorders are significantly associated with several biological pathways, such as VEGF and chemokine signaling pathways and alanine, aspartate, and glutamate metabolism, which are involved in the major pathological processes of menstrual disorders. The authors also found 20 pairs of QXHC candidate targets, and the corresponding chemical components had the strong binding free energy. These results showed that the pharmacological mechanisms of QXHC in the treatment of menstrual disorders may be associated with its involvement in hemopoiesis, analgesia, nutrient absorption and metabolism, mood regulation, as well as immune modulation [284].

8.2.9. Zinc

Zinc has been found to reduce the synthesis of prostaglandins via its action as an endogenous antioxidant catalyst and as an anti-inflammatory agent that can improve microcirculation of endometrial tissue. This was shown in a study that found that zinc significantly lowered the pain duration and severity in women compared to the control group and improved the patients' quality of life [285]. One study suggested that daily intake of 30 mg of zinc one to four days prior to menstruation can prevent menstrual cramping pain, without harmful side effects, while another showed evidence that zinc can treat primary dysmenorrhea in adolescent girls [286].

8.2.10. Vitamin K

A few studies have investigated vitamin K (phylloquinone) injection to treat primary dysmenorrhea. Treatment with vitamin K may shorten the length of the extended menstrual flow due to its action on prothrombin, which is a coagulation protein produced in the liver and is dependent on vitamin K [287]. Chao et al. reported that women indicated a significant decrease in pain after vitamin K injection in both legs and increased plasma phylloquinone levels [287]. Wade et al. noted that both women given vitamin K3 using an acupuncture point injection or deep muscle injection experienced a decrease in average pain as well as menstrual distress [288]. It was suggested that women with severe primary dysmenorrhea could manage severe dysmenorrhea with two vitamin K acupuncture point injections per year.

Finally, an interesting recent study examined the relationship of breakfast to the development of future reproductive diseases. Missing this first meal interferes with the start of the active phase during the circadian rhythm that is regulated by the central clock system. Since both food intake and the light/dark cycle are the main regulators of circadian rhythms, skipping breakfast can lead to changes in light stimulation within the central clock system [289]. The authors suggested that meal skipping affects the hypothalamic–pituitary–ovarian axis, impairs the reproductive rhythm, and leads to ovarian dysfunction. Young women who skip breakfast show significantly higher incidences of dysmenorrhea and irregular menstruation, suggesting that missing meals affects ovarian and uterine functions [289]. Since dysmenorrhea becomes more manifested in those with a history of dieting, the authors posited that inadequate dietary habits in adolescence become a trigger for the subsequent development of organic gynecological diseases. [289]. Thus, they suggested shifting the focus from therapeutic to prophylactic and from dietary content to dietary timing in the management of gynecological disorders in young women.

Further investigation, together with developing new methods, is recommended to test their hypothesis.

9. Conclusions

Gynecological diseases, like other diseases, have a causal relationship with some factors in the environment. These factors may be physical or/and social. Someone may suffer from gynecological diseases either due to her physical condition/exposure (e.g., nutritional status, environment, exposure to bacteria or viruses, etc.) or due to social conditions (education, income level, culture, etc.). So, while dealing with a gynecological disease clinically, it is recommended to look at these factors that might improve the outcome. In this article, we covered several dietary supplements and nutrients that may provide potential benefits upon implementation in preventive/therapeutic measures to control common gynecological diseases, including uterine fibroids, endometriosis, PCOS, infertility, menstrual disorders, and vaginal infections, as well as malignant cancers such as cervical cancer, endometrial cancer, and ovarian cancer. Nutrition has the most important lifelong environmental impact on human health. There are several studies indicating that fruits, tea, vegetables, as well as various dietary compounds can alter several signaling pathways involved in disease pathogenesis as well as impact cancer cells, such as the activation of tumor suppressor genes and an increase in apoptosis and the activity of cell survival proteins, thus playing a protective role against cancer. However, this research area needs more attention.

Author Contributions: Conceptualization, A.A.-H. and M.A. Authors of sections: Sources and writing original draft—M.C. and C.W.; gynecological cancers—S.E.; endometriosis and PCOS—H.S.; uterine fibroids and infertility—L.P.; menstrual disorders—H.E.; microbiome and infections—review and editing, M.A.; supervision, A.A.-H. and M.A.; funding acquisition, A.A.-H. All authors have read and agreed to the published version of the manuscript.

Funding: This study was supported in part by the National Institutes of Health grants R01 HD094378-04, R01 ES 028615-02, R01 HD100367-01, U54 MD007602, and R01 HD094380-02.

Institutional Review Board Statement: Not applicable.

Informed Consent Statement: Not applicable.

Data Availability Statement: Not applicable.

Conflicts of Interest: Ayman Al-Hendy has been a consultant and participated in advisory boards for Allergan plc, Bayer, Repros, Myovant, MD Stem Cells, AstraZeneca, Wyeth, and AbbVie. The rest of the authors declare no conflict of interest.

References

1. Izetbegovic, S.; Alajbegovic, J.; Mutevelic, A.; Pasagic, A.; Masic, I. Prevention of diseases in gynecology. *Int. J. Prev. Med.* **2013**, *4*, 1347–1358.
2. Kussmann, M.; Fay, L.B. Nutrigenomics and personalized nutrition: Science and concept. *Per. Med.* **2008**, *5*, 447–455. [CrossRef]
3. Herceg, Z. Epigenetics and cancer: Towards an evaluation of the impact of environmental and dietary factors. *Mutagenesis* **2007**, *22*, 91–103. [CrossRef]
4. Junien, C. Impact of diets and nutrients/drugs on early epigenetic programming. *J. Inherit. Metab. Dis.* **2006**, *29*, 359–365. [CrossRef]
5. Dolinoy, C.D.; Weidman, J.R.; Jirtle, R.L. Epigenetic gene regulation: Linking early developmental environment to adult disease. *Reprod. Toxicol.* **2007**, *23*, 297–307. [CrossRef]
6. Paluszczak, J.; Krajka-Kuzniak, V.; Baer-Dubowska, W. The effect of dietary polyphenols on the epigenetic regulation of gene expression in MCF7 breast cancer cells. *Toxicol. Lett.* **2010**, *192*, 119–125. [CrossRef] [PubMed]
7. Andreescu, N.; Puiu, M.; Niculescu, M. Effects of Dietary Nutrients on Epigenetic Changes in Cancer. *Methods Mol. Biol.* **2018**, *1856*, 121–139.
8. Stephen, H.E.; Chandra, A. Declining estimates of infertility in the United States: 1982–2002. *Fertil. Steril.* **2006**, *86*, 516–523. [CrossRef] [PubMed]
9. Braga, D.P.; Halpern, G.; Setti, A.S.; Figueira, R.C.; Iaconelli, A., Jr.; Borges, E., Jr. The impact of food intake and social habits on embryo quality and the likelihood of blastocyst formation. *Reprod. Biomed. Online* **2015**, *31*, 30–38. [CrossRef] [PubMed]

10. Chavarro, J.E.; Rich-Edwards, J.W.; Rosner, B.A.; Willett, W.C. Protein intake and ovulatory infertility. *Am. J. Obstet. Gynecol.* **2008**, *198*, 210–e1. [CrossRef] [PubMed]
11. Gaskins, J.A.; Chavarro, J.E. Diet and fertility: A review. *Am. J. Obstet. Gynecol.* **2018**, *218*, 379–389. [CrossRef] [PubMed]
12. Czeizel, E.A.; Bartfai, Z.; Banhidy, F. Primary prevention of neural-tube defects and some other congenital abnormalities by folic acid and multivitamins: History, missed opportunity and tasks. *Ther. Adv. Drug Saf.* **2011**, *2*, 173–188. [CrossRef] [PubMed]
13. García-Fernández, E.; Rico-Cabanas, L.; Rosgaard, N.; Estruch, R.; Bach-Faig, A. Mediterranean diet and cardiodiabesity: A review. *Nutrients* **2014**, *6*, 3474–3500. [CrossRef] [PubMed]
14. Karayiannis, D.; Kontogianni, M.D.; Mendorou, C.; Mastrominas, M.; Yiannakouris, N. Adherence to the Mediterranean diet and IVF success rate among non-obese women attempting fertility. *Hum. Reprod.* **2018**, *33*, 494–502. [CrossRef] [PubMed]
15. Vujkovic, M.; de Vries, J.H.; Lindemans, J.; Macklon, N.S.; van der Spek, P.J.; Steegers, E.A.; Steegers-Theunissen, R.P. The preconception Mediterranean dietary pattern in couples undergoing in vitro fertilization/intracytoplasmic sperm injection treatment increases the chance of pregnancy. *Fertil. Steril.* **2010**, *94*, 2096–2101. [CrossRef]
16. Twigt, J.M.; Bolhuis, M.E.; Steegers, E.A.; Hammiche, F.; Van Inzen, W.G.; Laven, J.S.; Steegers-Theunissen, R.P. The preconception diet is associated with the chance of ongoing pregnancy in women undergoing IVF/ICSI treatment. *Hum. Reprod.* **2012**, *27*, 2526–2531. [CrossRef]
17. Gaskins, A.J.; Chiu, Y.H.; Williams, P.L.; Keller, M.G.; Toth, T.L.; Hauser, R.; Chavarro, J.E.; EARTH Study Team. Maternal whole grain intake and outcomes of in vitro fertilization. *Fertil. Steril.* **2016**, *105*, 1503–1510e4. [CrossRef]
18. Mumford, S.L.; Browne, R.W.; Kim, K.; Nichols, C.; Wilcox, B.; Silver, R.M.; Connell, M.T.; Holland, T.L.; Kuhr, D.L.; Omosigho, U.R.; et al. Preconception plasma phospholipid fatty acids and fecundability. *J. Clin. Endocrinol. Metab.* **2018**, *103*, 4501–4510. [CrossRef]
19. Saldeen, P.; Saldeen, T. Women and omega-3 Fatty acids. *Obstet. Gynecol. Surv.* **2004**, *59*, 722–730. [CrossRef]
20. Abadia, L.; Gaskins, A.J.; Chiu, Y.H.; Williams, P.L.; Keller, M.; Wright, D.L.; Souter, I.; Hauser, R.; Chavarro, J.E.; Enviroment and Reproductive Health Study Team. Serum 25-hydroxyvitamin D concentrations and treatment outcomes of women undergoing assisted reproduction. *Am. J. Clin. Nutr.* **2016**, *104*, 729–735.
21. Polyzos, N.P.; Anckaert, E.; Guzman, L.; Schiettecatte, J.; Van Landuyt, L.; Camus, M.; Smitz, J.; Tournaye, H. Vitamin D deficiency and pregnancy rates in women undergoing single embryo, blastocyst stage, transfer (SET) for IVF/ICSI. *Hum. Reprod.* **2014**, *29*, 2032–2040. [CrossRef] [PubMed]
22. Chavarro, J.E.; Rich-Edwards, J.W.; Rosner, B.; Willett, W.C. A prospective study of dairy foods intake and anovulatory infertility. *Hum. Reprod.* **2007**, *22*, 1340–1347. [CrossRef]
23. Arefi, S.; Khalili, G.; Iranmanesh, H.; Farifteh, F.; Hosseini, A.; Fatemi, H.M.; Lawrenz, B. Is the ovarian reserve influenced by vitamin D deficiency and the dress code in an infertile Iranian population? *J. Ovarian Res.* **2018**, *11*, 1–6. [CrossRef]
24. Mg, S.; Brown, J.; Clarke, J.; Rj, H. Antioxidants for female subfertility. *Cochrane Database Syst. Rev.* **2013**, *8*, CD007807.
25. Ruder, E.H.; Hartman, T.J.; Reindollar, R.H.; Goldman, M.B. Female dietary antioxidant intake and time to pregnancy among couples treated for unexplained infertility. *Fertil. Steril.* **2014**, *101*, 759–766. [CrossRef] [PubMed]
26. Marco, M.L.; Heeney, D.; Binda, S.; Cifelli, C.J.; Cotter, P.D.; Foligné, B.; Gänzle, M.; Kort, R.; Pasin, G.; Pihlanto, A.; et al. Health benefits of fermented foods: Microbiota and beyond. *Curr. Opin. Biotechnol.* **2017**, *44*, 94–102. [CrossRef]
27. Atassi, F.; Brassart, D.; Grob, P.; Graf, F.; Servin, A.L. Lactobacillus strains isolated from the vaginal microbiota of healthy women inhibit Prevotella bivia and Gardnerella vaginalis in coculture and cell culture. *FEMS Immunol. Med. Microbiol.* **2006**, *48*, 424–432. [CrossRef]
28. Rose, W.A., II; McGowin, C.L.; Spagnuolo, R.A.; Eaves-Pyles, T.D.; Popov, V.L.; Pyles, R.B. Commensal bacteria modulate innate immune responses of vaginal epithelial cell multilayer cultures. *PLoS ONE* **2012**, *7*, e32728. [CrossRef] [PubMed]
29. Younis, N.S.; Mahasneh, A. Probiotics and the envisaged role in treating human infertility. *Middle E. Fertil. Soc. J.* **2020**, *25*, 1–9. [CrossRef]
30. Bhandari, P.; Prabha, V. Evaluation of profertility effect of probiotic Lactobacillus plantarum 2621 in a murine model. *Indian J. Med. Res.* **2015**, *142*, 79–84.
31. Rocha, A.L.; Oliveira, F.R.; Azevedo, R.C.; Silva, V.A.; Peres, T.M.; Candido, A.L.; Gomes, K.B.; Reis, F.M. Recent advances in the understanding and management of polycystic ovary syndrome. *F1000Research* **2019**, *8*, 565. [CrossRef]
32. Esfandyari, S.; Chugh, R.M.; Park, H.S.; Hobeika, E.; Ulin, M.; Al-Hendy, A. Mesenchymal Stem Cells as a Bio Organ. for Treatment of Female Infertility. *Cells* **2020**, *9*, 2253. [CrossRef] [PubMed]
33. Esfandyari, S. miRNA-92a suppresses androgen-producing steroidogenic genes expression in h295r, a human pcos in-vitro theca-like cell model. *Fertil. Steril.* **2020**, *114*, e349–e350. [CrossRef]
34. Azziz, R.; Woods, K.S.; Reyna, R.; Key, T.J.; Knochenhauer, E.S.; Yildiz, B.O. The prevalence and features of the polycystic ovary syndrome in an unselected population. *J. Clin. Endocrinol. Metab.* **2004**, *89*, 2745–2749. [CrossRef]
35. Faghfoori, Z.; Fazelian, S.; Shadnoush, M.; Goodarzi, R. Nutritional management in women with polycystic ovary syndrome: A review study. *Diabetes Metab. Syndr. Clin. Res. Rev.* **2017**, *11*, S429–S432. [CrossRef]
36. Douglas, C.C.; Gower, B.A.; Darnell, B.E.; Ovalle, F.; Oster, R.A.; Azziz, R. Role of diet in the treatment of polycystic ovary syndrome. *Fertil. Steril.* **2006**, *85*, 679–688. [CrossRef]
37. Goss, A.M.; Gower, B.; Soleymani, T.; Stewart, M.; Pendergrass, M.; Lockhart, M.; Krantz, O.; Dowla, S.; Bush, N.; Barry, V.G.; et al. Effects of weight loss during a very low carbohydrate diet on specific adipose tissue depots and insulin sensitivity in older adults with obesity: A randomized clinical trial. *Nutr. Metab.* **2020**, *17*, 1–12. [CrossRef]

38. Kasim-Karakas, S.E.; Almario, R.U.; Gregory, L.; Wong, R.; Todd, H.; Lasley, B.L. Metabolic and endocrine effects of a polyunsaturated fatty acid-rich diet in polycystic ovary syndrome. *J. Clin. Endocrinol. Metab.* **2004**, *89*, 615–620. [CrossRef] [PubMed]
39. Teegarden, D.; Donkin, S.S. Vitamin D: Emerging new roles in insulin sensitivity. *Nutr. Res. Rev.* **2009**, *22*, 82–92. [CrossRef]
40. He, C.; Lin, Z.; Robb, S.W.; Ezeamama, A.E. Serum vitamin D levels and polycystic ovary syndrome: A systematic review and meta-analysis. *Nutrients* **2015**, *7*, 4555–4577. [CrossRef]
41. Ott, J.; Wattar, L.; Kurz, C.; Seemann, R.; Huber, J.C.; Mayerhofer, K.; Vytiska-Binstorfer, E. Parameters for calcium metabolism in women with polycystic ovary syndrome who undergo clomiphene citrate stimulation: A prospective cohort study. *Eur. J. Endocrinol.* **2012**, *166*, 897. [CrossRef]
42. Wojtusik, J.; Johnson, P.A. Vitamin D regulates anti-Mullerian hormone expression in granulosa cells of the hen. *Biol. Reprod.* **2012**, *86*, 1–7. [CrossRef] [PubMed]
43. Iliodromiti, S.; Kelsey, T.W.; Anderson, R.A.; Nelson, S.M. Can anti-Müllerian hormone predict the diagnosis of polycystic ovary syndrome? A systematic review and meta-analysis of extracted data. *J. Clin. Endocrinol. Metab.* **2013**, *98*, 3332–3340. [CrossRef]
44. Elhusseini, H.; Lizneva, D.; Gavrilova-Jordan, L.; Eziba, N.; Abdelaziz, M.; Brakta, S.; Halder, S.; Al-Hebdy, A. Vitamin d and female reproduction. In *A Critical Evaluation of Vitamin D: Basic Overview*; Gower, S., Ed.; IntechOpen: London, UK, 2017; p. 297.
45. Irani, M.; Minkoff, H.; Seifer, D.B.; Merhi, Z. Vitamin D increases serum levels of the soluble receptor for advanced glycation end products in women with PCOS. *J. Clin. Endocrinol. Metab.* **2014**, *99*, E886–E890. [CrossRef]
46. Legro, R.S.; Arslanian, S.A.; Ehrmann, D.A.; Hoeger, K.M.; Murad, M.H.; Pasquali, R.; Welt, C.K. Diagnosis and treatment of polycystic ovary syndrome: An Endocrine Society clinical practice guideline. *J. Clin. Endocrinol. Metab.* **2013**, *98*, 4565–4592. [CrossRef]
47. Rodriguez Paris, V.; Bertoldo, M.J. The mechanism of androgen actions in PCOS etiology. *Med. Sci.* **2019**, *7*, 89. [CrossRef]
48. Zhang, X.; Zheng, Y.; Guo, Y.; Lai, Z. The effect of low carbohydrate diet on polycystic ovary syndrome: A meta-analysis of randomized controlled trials. *Int. J. Endocrinol* **2019**. [CrossRef]
49. Ebrahimi, R.; Bahiraee, A.; Niazpour, F.; Emamgholipour, S.; Meshkani, R. The role of microRNAs in the regulation of insulin signaling pathway with respect to metabolic and mitogenic cascades: A review. *J. Cell. Biochem.* **2019**, *120*, 19290–19309. [CrossRef] [PubMed]
50. Emamgholipour, S.; Ebrahimi, R.; Bahiraee, A.; Niazpour, F.; Meshkani, R. Acetylation and insulin resistance: A focus on metabolic and mitogenic cascades of insulin signaling. *Crit. Rev. Clin. Lab. Sci.* **2020**, *57*, 196–214. [CrossRef]
51. Moran, L.J.; Noakes, M.; Clifton, P.M.; Tomlinson, L.; Norman, R.J. Dietary composition in restoring reproductive and metabolic physiology in overweight women with polycystic ovary syndrome. *J. Clin. Endocrinol. Metab.* **2003**, *88*, 812–819. [CrossRef] [PubMed]
52. Jamilian, M.; Asemi, Z. The effects of soy isoflavones on metabolic status of patients with polycystic ovary syndrome. *TJ Clin. Endocrinol. Metab.* **2016**, *101*, 3386–3394. [CrossRef]
53. Khani, B.; Mehrabian, F.; Khalesi, E.; Eshraghi, A. Effect of soy phytoestrogen on metabolic and hormonal disturbance of women with polycystic ovary syndrome. *J. Res. Med. Sci. Off. J. Isfahan Univ. Med. Sci.* **2011**, *16*, 297.
54. Tehrani, H.G.; Allahdadian, M.; Zarre, F.; Ranjbar, H.; Allahdadian, F. Effect of green tea on metabolic and hormonal aspect of polycystic ovarian syndrome in overweight and obese women suffering from polycystic ovarian syndrome: A clinical trial. *J. Educ. Health Promot.* **2017**, *6*, 36. [CrossRef] [PubMed]
55. Armanini, D.; Mattarello, M.J.; Fiore, C.; Bonanni, G.; Scaroni, C.; Sartorato, P.; Palermo, M. Licorice reduces serum testosterone in healthy women. *Steroids* **2004**, *69*, 763–766. [CrossRef]
56. MCalderon-Montano, J.; Burgos-Morón, E.; Pérez-Guerrero, C.; López-Lázaro, M. A review on the dietary flavonoid kaempferol. *Mini Rev. Med. Chem.* **2011**, *11*, 298–344. [CrossRef]
57. Tabrizi, F.P.; Hajizadeh-Sharafabad, F.; Vaezi, M.; Jafari-Vayghan, H.; Alizadeh, M.; Maleki, V. Quercetin and polycystic ovary syndrome, current evidence and future directions: A systematic review. *J. Ovarian Res.* **2020**, *13*, 11. [CrossRef]
58. Shah, K.N.; Patel, S.S. Phosphatidylinositide 3-kinase inhibition: A new potential target for the treatment of polycystic ovarian syndrome. *Pharm. Biol.* **2016**, *54*, 975–983. [CrossRef]
59. Wang, Z.; Zhai, D.; Zhang, D.; Bai, L.; Yao, R.; Yu, J.; Cheng, W.; Yu, C. Quercetin decreases insulin resistance in a polycystic ovary syndrome rat model by improving inflammatory microenvironment. *Reprod. Sci.* **2017**, *24*, 682–690. [CrossRef]
60. Rezvan, N.; Moini, A.; Gorgani-Firuzjaee, S.; Hosseinzadeh-Attar, M.J. Oral quercetin supplementation enhances adiponectin receptor transcript expression in polycystic ovary syndrome patients: A randomized placebo-controlled double-blind clinical trial. *Cell J.* **2018**, *19*, 627.
61. Khorshidi, M.; Moini, A.; Alipoor, E.; Rezvan, N.; Gorgani-Firuzjaee, S.; Yaseri, M.; Hosseinzadeh-Attar, M.J. The effects of quercetin supplementation on metabolic and hormonal parameters as well as plasma concentration and gene expression of resistin in overweight or obese women with polycystic ovary syndrome. *Phytother. Res.* **2018**, *32*, 2282–2289. [CrossRef]
62. Oh, J.S.; Kim, H.; Vijayakumar, A.; Kwon, O.; Choi, Y.J.; Huh, K.B.; Chang, N. Association between dietary flavanones intake and lipid profiles according to the presence of metabolic syndrome in Korean women with type 2 diabetes mellitus. *Nutr. Res. Pract.* **2016**, *10*, 67–73. [CrossRef]
63. Romualdi, D.; Costantini, B.; Campagna, G.; Lanzone, A.; Guido, M. Is there a role for soy isoflavones in the therapeutic approach to polycystic ovary syndrome? Results from a pilot study. *Fertil. Steril.* **2008**, *90*, 1826–1833. [CrossRef]

64. Banaszewska, B.; Wrotyńska-Barczyńska, J.; Spaczynski, R.Z.; Pawelczyk, L.; Duleba, A.J. Effects of resveratrol on polycystic ovary syndrome: A double-blind, randomized, placebo-controlled trial. *J. Clin. Endocrinol. Metab.* **2016**, *101*, 4322–4328. [CrossRef]
65. Günalan, E.; Yaba, A.; Yılmaz, B. The effect of nutrient supplementation in the management of polycystic ovary syndrome-associated metabolic dysfunctions: A critical review. *J. Turk. Ger. Gynecol. Assoc.* **2018**, *19*, 220. [CrossRef]
66. Anderson, R.A. Chromium in the prevention and control of diabetes. *Diab. Metab.* **2000**, *26*, 22–28.
67. Chakraborty, P.; Ghosh, S.; Goswami, S.K.; Kabir, S.N.; Chakravarty, B.; Jana, K. Altered trace mineral milieu might play an aetiological role in the pathogenesis of polycystic ovary syndrome. *Biol. Trace Elem. Res.* **2013**, *152*, 9–15. [CrossRef]
68. Lucidi, R.S.; Thyer, A.C.; Easton, C.A.; Holden, A.E.; Schenken, R.S.; Brzyski, R.G. Effect of chromium supplementation on insulin resistance and ovarian and menstrual cyclicity in women with polycystic ovary syndrome. *Fertil. Steril.* **2005**, *84*, 1755–1757. [CrossRef] [PubMed]
69. Jamilian, M.; Asemi, Z. Chromium supplementation and the effects on metabolic status in women with polycystic ovary syndrome: A randomized, double-blind, placebo-controlled trial. *Ann. Nutr. Metab.* **2015**, *67*, 42–48. [CrossRef]
70. Jamilian, M.; Bahmani, F.; Siavashani, M.A.; Mazloomi, M.; Asemi, Z.; Esmaillzadeh, A. The effects of chromium supplementation on endocrine profiles, biomarkers of inflammation, and oxidative stress in women with polycystic ovary syndrome: A randomized, double-blind, placebo-controlled trial. *Biol. Trace Elem. Res.* **2016**, *172*, 72–78. [CrossRef] [PubMed]
71. Ullah, G.; Jung, P.; Machaca, K. Modeling Ca2+ signaling differentiation during oocyte maturation. *Cell Calcium* **2007**, *42*, 556–564. [CrossRef] [PubMed]
72. Mazloomi, S.; Sharifi, F.; Hajihosseini, R.; Kalantari, S.; Mazloomzadeh, S. Association between hypoadiponectinemia and low serum concentrations of calcium and vitamin D in women with polycystic ovary syndrome. *ISRN Endocrinol.* **2012**. [CrossRef] [PubMed]
73. Dehghani Firouzabadi, R.; Aflatoonian, A.; Modarresi, S.; Sekhavat, L.; MohammadTaheri, S. Therapeutic effects of calcium & vitamin D supplementation in women with PCOS. *Complement. Ther. Clin. Pract.* **2012**, *18*, 85–88.
74. Mirone, M.; Giannetta, E.; Isidori, A. Selenium and reproductive function. A systematic review. *J. Endocrinol. Invest.* **2013**, *36*, 28–36.
75. Coskun, A.; Arikan, T.; Kilinc, M.; Arikan, D.C.; Ekerbiçer, H.Ç. Plasma selenium levels in Turkish women with polycystic ovary syndrome. *Eur. J. Obstet. Gynecol. Reprod. Biol.* **2013**, *168*, 183–186. [CrossRef]
76. Modarres, S.Z.; Heidar, Z.; Foroozanfard, F.; Rahmati, Z.; Aghadavod, E.; Asemi, Z. The effects of selenium supplementation on gene expression related to insulin and lipid in infertile polycystic ovary syndrome women candidate for in vitro fertilization: A randomized, double-blind, placebo-controlled trial. *Biol. Trace Elem. Res.* **2018**, *183*, 218–225. [CrossRef]
77. Jamilian, M.; Razavi, M.; Fakhrie Kashan, Z.; Ghandi, Y.; Bagherian, T.; Asemi, Z. Metabolic response to selenium supplementation in women with polycystic ovary syndrome: A randomized, double-blind, placebo-controlled trial. *Clin. Endocrinol.* **2015**, *82*, 885–891. [CrossRef]
78. Tubek, S. Zinc supplementation or regulation of its homeostasis: Advantages and threats. *Biol. Trace Elem. Res.* **2007**, *119*, 1–9. [CrossRef]
79. Beletate, V.; el Dib, R.; Atallah, Á.N. Zinc supplementation for the prevention of type 2 diabetes mellitus. *Cochrane Datab. Syst. Rev.* **2007**, *1*, CD005525. [CrossRef]
80. Guler, I.; Himmetoglu, O.; Turp, A.; Erdem, A.; Erdem, M.; Onan, M.A.; Taskiran, C.; Taslipinar, M.Y.; Guner, H. Zinc and homocysteine levels in polycystic ovarian syndrome patients with insulin resistance. *Biol. Trace Elem. Res.* **2014**, *158*, 297–304. [CrossRef]
81. Saris, N.E.; Mervaala, E.; Karppanen, H.; Khawaja, J.A.; Lewenstam, A. Magnesium: An update on physiological, clinical and analytical aspects. *Clin. Chim. Acta* **2000**, *294*, 1–26. [CrossRef]
82. Rumawas, M.E.; McKeown, N.M.; Rogers, G.; Meigs, J.B.; Wilson, P.W.; Jacques, P.F. Magnesium intake is related to improved insulin homeostasis in the framingham offspring cohort. *J. Am. Coll. Nutr.* **2006**, *25*, 486–492. [CrossRef]
83. Ryan, L.G.; Syrop, C.H.; van Voorhis, B.J. Role, epidemiology, and natural history of benign uterine mass lesions. *Clin. Obstet. Gynecol.* **2005**, *48*, 312–324. [CrossRef]
84. Ulin, M.; Ali, M.; Chaudhry, Z.T.; Al-Hendy, A.; Yang, Q. Uterine fibroids in menopause and perimenopause. *Menopause* **2020**, *27*, 238–242. [CrossRef]
85. Wu, J.M.; Wechter, M.E.; Geller, E.J.; Nguyen, T.V.; Visco, A.G. Hysterectomy rates in the United States, 2003. *Obstet. Gynecol.* **2007**, *110*, 1091–1095. [CrossRef]
86. Cardozo, E.R.; Clark, A.D.; Banks, N.K.; Henne, M.B.; Stegmann, B.J.; Segars, J.H. The estimated annual cost of uterine leiomyomata in the United States. *Am. J. Obstet. Gynecol.* **2012**, *206*, 211e1. [CrossRef] [PubMed]
87. Ciebiera, M.; Ali, M.; Prince, L.; Jackson-Bey, T.; Atabiekov, I.; Zgliczyński, S.; Al-Hendy, A. The Evolving Role of Natural Compounds in the Medical Treatment of Uterine Fibroids. *J. Clin. Med.* **2020**, *9*, 1479. [CrossRef]
88. Ali, M.; Esfandyari, S.; Al-Hendy, A. Evolving role of microRNAs in uterine fibroid pathogenesis: Filling the gap! *Fertil. Steril.* **2020**, *113*, 1167–1168. [CrossRef]
89. Laughlin, K.S.; Schroeder, J.C.; Baird, D.D. New directions in the epidemiology of uterine fibroids. *Semin. Reprod. Med.* **2010**, *28*, 204–217. [CrossRef]
90. Tinelli, A.; Vinciguerra, M.; Malvasi, A.; Andjić, M.; Babović, I.; Sparić, R. Uterine Fibroids and Diet. *Int. J. Environ. Res. Publ. Health* **2021**, *18*, 1066. [CrossRef]

91. Mozaffarian, D.; Pischon, T.; Hankinson, S.E.; Rifai, N.; Joshipura, K.; Willett, W.C.; Rimm, E.B. Dietary intake of trans fatty acids and systemic inflammation in women. *Am. J. Clin. Nutr.* **2004**, *79*, 606–612. [CrossRef]
92. Wu, H.A.; Pike, M.C.; Stram, D.O. Meta-analysis: Dietary fat intake, serum estrogen levels, and the risk of breast cancer. *J. Natl. Cancer Inst.* **1999**, *91*, 529–534. [CrossRef] [PubMed]
93. Baird, D.D.; Patchel, S.A.; Saldana, T.M.; Umbach, D.M.; Cooper, T.; Wegienka, G.; Harmon, Q.E. Uterine fibroid incidence and growth in an ultrasound-based, prospective study of young African Americans. *Am. J. Obstet. Gynecol.* **2020**, *223*, 402e1. [CrossRef] [PubMed]
94. Kristal, R.A.; Shattuck, A.L.; Patterson, R.E. Differences in fat-related dietary patterns between black, Hispanic and White women: Results from the women's health trial feasibility study in minority populations. *Pub. Health Nutr.* **1999**, *2*, 253–262. [CrossRef]
95. Rosenberg, L.; Adams-Campbell, L.; Palmer, J.R. The black women's health study: A follow-up study for causes and preventions of illness. *J. Am. Med. Wom. Assoc.* **1995**, *50*, 56–58.
96. Wise, L.A.; Radin, R.G.; Kumanyika, S.K.; Ruiz-Narvaez, E.A.; Palmer, J.R.; Rosenberg, L. Prospective study of dietary fat and risk of uterine leiomyomata. *Am. J. Clin. Nutr.* **2014**, *99*, 1105–1116. [CrossRef]
97. Brasky, T.M.; Bethea, T.N.; Wesselink, A.K.; Wegienka, G.R.; Baird, D.D.; Wise, L.A. Dietary fat intake and risk of uterine leiomyomata: A prospective ultrasound study. *Am. J. Epidemiol.* **2020**, *189*, 1538–1546. [CrossRef]
98. Harris, H.R.; Eliassen, A.H.; Doody, D.R.; Terry, K.L.; Missmer, S.A. Dietary fat intake, erythrocyte fatty acids, and risk of uterine fibroids. *Fertil. Steril.* **2020**, *114*, 837–847. [CrossRef] [PubMed]
99. Wegienka, G. Are uterine leiomyoma a consequence of a chronically inflammatory immune system? *Med. Hypotheses* **2012**, *79*, 226–231. [CrossRef] [PubMed]
100. Chiaffarino, F.; Parazzini, F.; La Vecchia, C.; Chatenoud, L.; Di Cintio, E.; Marsico, S. Diet. and uterine myomas. *Obstet. Gynecol.* **1999**, *94*, 395–398. [PubMed]
101. Nagata, C.; Nakamura, K.; Oba, S.; Hayashi, M.; Takeda, N.; Yasuda, K. Association of intakes of fat, dietary fibre, soya isoflavones and alcohol with uterine fibroids in Japanese women. *Br. J. Nutr.* **2009**, *101*, 1427–1431. [CrossRef] [PubMed]
102. Islam, M.S.; Castellucci, C.; Fiorini, R.; Greco, S.; Gagliardi, R.; Zannotti, A.; Giannubilo, S.R.; Ciavattini, A.; Frega, N.G.; Pacetti, D.; et al. Omega-3 fatty acids modulate the lipid profile, membrane architecture, and gene expression of leiomyoma cells. *J. Cell. Physiol.* **2018**, *233*, 7143–7156. [CrossRef] [PubMed]
103. Kant, K.A.; Graubard, B.I. Ethnicity is an independent correlate of biomarkers of micronutrient intake and status in American adults. *J. Nutr.* **2007**, *137*, 2456–2463. [CrossRef] [PubMed]
104. Timbo, B.B.; Ross, M.P.; McCarthy, P.V.; Lin, C.T. Dietary supplements in a national survey: Prevalence of use and reports of adverse events. *J. Am. Diet. Assoc.* **2006**, *106*, 1966–1974. [CrossRef] [PubMed]
105. Wise, L.A.; Radin, R.G.; Palmer, J.R.; Kumanyika, S.K.; Boggs, D.A.; Rosenberg, L. Intake of fruit, vegetables, and carotenoids in relation to risk of uterine leiomyomata. *Am. J. Clin. Nutr.* **2011**, *94*, 1620–1631. [CrossRef] [PubMed]
106. He, Y.; Zeng, Q.; Dong, S.; Qin, L.; Li, G.; Wang, P. Associations between uterine fibroids and lifestyles including diet, physical activity and stress: A case-control study in China. *Asia Pac. J. Clin. Nutr.* **2013**, *22*, 109–117. [PubMed]
107. Sahin, K.; Ozercan, R.; Onderci, M.; Sahin, N.; Gursu, M.F.; Khachik, F.; Sarkar, F.H.; Munkarah, A.; Ali-Fehmi, R.; Kmak, D.; et al. Lycopene supplementation prevents the development of spontaneous smooth muscle tumors of the oviduct in Japanese quail. *Nutr. Cancer* **2004**, *50*, 181–189. [CrossRef] [PubMed]
108. Setchell, K.D.; Cassidy, A. Dietary isoflavones: Biological effects and relevance to human health. *J. Nutr.* **1999**, *129*, 758S–767S. [CrossRef] [PubMed]
109. Greco, S.; Islam, M.S.; Zannotti, A.; Carpini, G.D.; Giannubilo, S.R.; Ciavattini, A.; Petraglia, F.; Ciarmela, P. Quercetin and indole-3-carbinol inhibit extracellular matrix expression in human primary uterine leiomyoma cells. *Reprod. Biomed. Online* **2020**, *40*, 593–602. [CrossRef]
110. Lila, M.A.; Burton-Freeman, B.; Grace, M.; Kalt, W. Unraveling Anthocyanin Bioavailability for Human Health. *Annu. Rev. Food Sci. Technol.* **2016**, *7*, 375–393. [CrossRef] [PubMed]
111. Wang, S.Y.; Feng, R.; Lu, Y.; Bowman, L.; Ding, M. Inhibitory effect on activator protein-1, nuclear factor-kappaB, and cell transformation by extracts of strawberries (Fragaria x ananassa Duch.). *J. Agric. Food Chem.* **2005**, *53*, 4187–4193. [CrossRef]
112. Giampieri, F.; Islam, M.S.; Greco, S.; Gasparrini, M.; Forbes Hernandez, T.Y.; Delli Carpini, G.; Giannubilo, S.R.; Ciavattini, A.; Mezzetti, B.; Capocasa, F.; et al. Romina: A powerful strawberry with in vitro efficacy against uterine leiomyoma cells. *J. Cell. Physiol.* **2019**, *234*, 7622–7633. [CrossRef] [PubMed]
113. Islam, M.S.; Giampieri, F.; Janjusevic, M.; Gasparrini, M.; Forbes-Hernandez, T.Y.; Mazzoni, L.; Greco, S.; Giannubilo, S.R.; Ciavattini, A.; Mezzetti, B.; et al. Anthocyanin rich strawberry extract induces apoptosis and ROS while decreases glycolysis and fibrosis in human uterine leiomyoma cells. *Oncotarget* **2017**, *8*, 23575–23587. [CrossRef] [PubMed]
114. Kim, D.C.; Ramachandran, S.; Baek, S.H.; Kwon, S.H.; Kwon, K.Y.; Cha, S.D.; Bae, I.; Cho, C.H. Induction of growth inhibition and apoptosis in human uterine leiomyoma cells by isoliquiritigenin. *Reprod. Sci.* **2008**, *15*, 552–558. [CrossRef]
115. Moore, A.B.; Castro, L.; Yu, L.; Zheng, X.; Di, X.; Sifre, M.I.; Kissling, G.E.; Newbold, R.R.; Bortner, C.D.; Dixon, D. Stimulatory and inhibitory effects of genistein on human uterine leiomyoma cell proliferation are influenced by the concentration. *Hum. Reprod.* **2007**, *22*, 2623–2631. [CrossRef] [PubMed]

116. Di, X.; Yu, L.; Moore, A.B.; Castro, L.; Zheng, X.; Hermon, T.; Dixon, D. A low concentration of genistein induces estrogen receptor-alpha and insulin-like growth factor-I receptor interactions and proliferation in uterine leiomyoma cells. *Hum. Reprod.* **2008**, *23*, 1873–1883. [CrossRef]
117. Beydoun, M.A.; Gary, T.L.; Caballero, B.H.; Lawrence, R.S.; Cheskin, L.J.; Wang, Y. Ethnic differences in dairy and related nutrient consumption among US adults and their association with obesity, central obesity, and the metabolic syndrome. *Am. J. Clin. Nutr.* **2008**, *87*, 1914–1925. [CrossRef]
118. Lu, W.; Chen, H.; Niu, Y.; Wu, H.; Xia, D.; Wu, Y. Dairy products intake and cancer mortality risk: A meta-analysis of 11 population-based cohort studies. *Nutr. J.* **2016**, *15*, 91. [CrossRef]
119. Shen, Y.; Xu, Q.; Xu, J.; Ren, M.L.; Cai, Y.L. Environmental exposure and risk of uterine leiomyoma: An epidemiologic survey. *Eur. Rev. Med. Pharmacol. Sci.* **2013**, *17*, 3249–3256.
120. Wise, L.A.; Radin, R.G.; Palmer, J.R.; Kumanyika, S.K.; Rosenberg, L. A prospective study of dairy intake and risk of uterine leiomyomata. *Am. J. Epidemiol.* **2010**, *171*, 221–232. [CrossRef]
121. Wise, L.A.; Ruiz-Narváez, E.A.; Haddad, S.A.; Rosenberg, L.; Palmer, J.R. Polymorphisms in vitamin D-related genes and risk of uterine leiomyomata. *Fertil. Steril.* **2014**, *102*, 503–510.e1. [CrossRef]
122. Ciebiera, M.; Ali, M.; Prince, L.; Zgliczyński, S.; Jakiel, G.; Al-Hendy, A. The Significance of Measuring Vitamin D Serum Levels in Women with Uterine Fibroids. *Reprod. Sci.* **2020**. [CrossRef]
123. Al-Hendy, A.; Diamond, M.P.; El-Sohemy, A.; Halder, S.K. 1,25-dihydroxyvitamin D3 regulates expression of sex steroid receptors in human uterine fibroid cells. *J. Clin. Endocrinol. Metab.* **2015**, *100*, E572–E582. [CrossRef]
124. Ciebiera, M.; Ali, M.; Zgliczyńska, M.; Skrzypczak, M.; Al-Hendy, A. Vitamins and uterine fibroids: Current data on pathophysiology and possible clinical relevance. *Int. J. Mol. Sci.* **2020**, *21*, 5528. [CrossRef]
125. Ali, M.; Al-Hendy, A.; Yang, Q. Vitamin D, a promising natural compound with anti-uterine fibroid characteristics. *Fertil. Steril.* **2019**, *111*, 268–269. [CrossRef]
126. Elkafas, H.; Ali, M.; Elmorsy, E.; Kamel, R.; Thompson, W.E.; Badary, O.; Al-Hendy, A.; Yang, Q. Vitamin d3 ameliorates dna damage caused by developmental exposure to endocrine disruptors in the uterine myometrial stem cells of Eker rats. *Cells* **2020**, *9*, 1459. [CrossRef]
127. Ali, M.; Shahin, S.M.; Sabri, N.A.; Al-Hendy, A.; Yang, Q. Hypovitaminosis D exacerbates the DNA damage load in human uterine fibroids, which is ameliorated by vitamin D3 treatment. *Acta Pharmacol. Sin.* **2019**, *40*, 957–970. [CrossRef]
128. ElHusseini, H.; Elkafas, H.; Abdelaziz, M.; Halder, S.; Atabiekov, I.; Eziba, N.; Ismail, N.; El Andaloussi, A.; Al-Hendy, A. Diet.-induced vitamin D deficiency triggers inflammation and DNA damage profile in murine myometrium. *Int. J. Women's Health* **2018**, *10*, 503–514. [CrossRef] [PubMed]
129. Sheng, B.; Song, Y.; Liu, Y.; Jiang, C.; Zhu, X. Association between vitamin D and uterine fibroids: A study protocol of an open-label, randomised controlled trial. *BMJ Open* **2020**, *10*, e038709. [CrossRef] [PubMed]
130. Prins, G.S.; Hu, W.Y.; Shi, G.B.; Hu, D.P.; Majumdar, S.; Li, G.; Huang, K.; Nelles, J.L.; Ho, S.M.; Walker, C.L.; et al. Bisphenol A promotes human prostate stem-progenitor cell self-renewal and increases in vivo carcinogenesis in human prostate epithelium. *Endocrinology* **2014**, *155*, 805–817. [CrossRef] [PubMed]
131. Bariani, M.V.; Rangaswamy, R.; Siblini, H.; Yang, Q.; Al-Hendy, A.; Zota, A.R. The role of endocrine-disrupting chemicals in uterine fibroid pathogenesis. *Curr. Opin. Endocrinol. Diabetes Obes.* **2020**, *27*, 380–387. [CrossRef] [PubMed]
132. Johnstone, E.B.; Louis, G.M.; Parsons, P.J.; Steuerwald, A.J.; Palmer, C.D.; Chen, Z.; Sun, L.; Hammoud, A.O.; Dorais, J.; Peterson, C.M. Increased urinary cobalt and whole blood concentrations of cadmium and lead in women with uterine leiomyomata: Findings from the ENDO Study. *Reprod. Toxicol.* **2014**, *49*, 27–32. [CrossRef] [PubMed]
133. Jackson, L.W.; Zullo, M.D.; Goldberg, J.M. The association between heavy metals, endometriosis and uterine myomas among premenopausal women: National Health and Nutrition Examination Survey 1999–2002. *Hum. Reprod.* **2008**, *23*, 679–687. [CrossRef] [PubMed]
134. Maybin, J.A.; Critchley, H.O. Menstrual physiology: Implications for endometrial pathology and beyond. *Hum. Reprod. Update* **2015**, *21*, 748–761. [CrossRef]
135. Karamian, A.; Paktinat, S.; Esfandyari, S.; Nazarian, H.; Ali Ziai, S.; Zarnani, A.H.; Salehpour, S.; Hosseinirad, H.; Karamian, A.; Novin, M.G. Pyrvinium pamoate induces in-vitro suppression of IL-6 and IL-8 produced by human endometriotic stromal cells. *Hum. Exp. Toxicol.* **2020**, *4*, 649–660.
136. Nnoaham, K.E.; Hummelshoj, L.; Webster, P.; d'Hooghe, T.; de Cicco Nardone, F.; de Cicco Nardone, C.; Jenkinson, C.; Kennedy, S.H.; Zondervan, K.T.; Study, W.E. Impact of endometriosis on quality of life and work productivity: A multicenter study across ten countries. *Fertil. Steril.* **2011**, *96*, 366–373e8. [CrossRef]
137. Taylor, R.N.; Lebovic, D.I.; Mueller, M.D. Angiogenic factors in endometriosis. *Ann. N. Y. Acad. Sci. USA* **2002**, *955*, 89–100. [CrossRef]
138. Husby, G.K.; Haugen, R.S.; Moen, M.H. Diagnostic delay in women with pain and endometriosis. *Acta Obstet. Gynecol. Scand.* **2003**, *82*, 649–653. [CrossRef] [PubMed]
139. Sourial, S.; Tempest, N.; Hapangama, D.K. Theories on the pathogenesis of endometriosis. *Int. J. Reprod. Med.* **2014**, *2014*, 179515. [CrossRef]
140. Youoeflu, S.; Jahanian Sadatmahallch, S.; Mottaghi, A.; Kazemnejad, A. The association of food consumption and nutrient intake with endometriosis risk in Iranian women: A case-control study. *Int. J. Reprod. BioMed.* **2019**, *17*, 661.

141. Aris, A.; Paris, K. Hypothetical link between endometriosis and xenobiotics-associated genetically modified food. *Gynecol. Obstet. Fertil.* **2010**, *38*, 747–753.
142. Khanaki, K.; Nouri, M.; Ardekani, A.M.; Ghassemzadeh, A.; Shahnazi, V.; Sadeghi, M.R.; Darabi, M.; Mehdizadeh, A.; Dolatkhah, H.; Saremi, A.; et al. Evaluation of the relationship between endometriosis and omega-3 and omega-6 polyunsaturated fatty acids. *Iran. J. Biomed. J.* **2012**, *16*, 38.
143. Halpern, G.; Schor, E.; Kopelman, A. Nutritional aspects related to endometriosis. *Rev. Assoc. Méd. Brasil.* **2015**, *61*, 519–523. [CrossRef]
144. Lasco, A.; Catalano, A.; Benvenga, S. Improvement of primary dysmenorrhea caused by a single oral dose of vitamin D: Results of a randomized, double-blind, placebo-controlled study. *Arch. Intern. Med.* **2012**, *172*, 366–367. [CrossRef] [PubMed]
145. Almassinokiani, F.; Khodaverdi, S.; Solaymani-Dodaran, M.; Akbari, P.; Pazouki, A. Effects of vitamin D on endometriosis-related pain: A double-blind clinical trial. *Med. Sci. Monit. Int. Med. J. Exper. Clin. Res.* **2016**, *22*, 4960. [CrossRef] [PubMed]
146. Ngô, C.; Chéreau, C.; Nicco, C.; Weill, B.; Chapron, C.; Batteux, F. Reactive oxygen species controls endometriosis progression. *Am. J. Pathol.* **2009**, *175*, 225–234. [CrossRef] [PubMed]
147. Porpora, M.G.; Brunelli, R.; Costa, G.; Imperiale, L.; Krasnowska, E.K.; Lundeberg, T.; Nofroni, I.; Piccioni, M.G.; Pittaluga, E.; Ticino, A.; et al. A promise in the treatment of endometriosis: An observational cohort study on ovarian endometrioma reduction by N-acetylcysteine. *Evid. Based Complement. Altern. Med.* **2013**, *2013*, 240702. [CrossRef] [PubMed]
148. Park, S.; Lim, W.; Bazer, F.W.; Whang, K.Y.; Song, G. Quercetin inhibits proliferation of endometriosis regulating cyclin D1 and its target microRNAs in vitro and in vivo. *J. Nutr. Biochem.* **2019**, *63*, 87–100. [CrossRef] [PubMed]
149. Cao, Y.; Zhuang, M.F.; Yang, Y.; Xie, S.W.; Cui, J.G.; Cao, L.; Zhang, T.T.; Zhu, Y. Preliminary study of quercetin affecting the hypothalamic-pituitary-gonadal axis on rat endometriosis model. *Evid. Based Complement. Altern. Med.* **2014**, *2014*, 781684. [CrossRef] [PubMed]
150. Ergenoğlu, A.M.; Yeniel, A.Ö.; Erbaş, O.; Aktuğ, H.; Yildirim, N.; Ulukuş, M.; Taskiran, D. Regression of endometrial implants by resveratrol in an experimentally induced endometriosis model in rats. *Reprod. Sci.* **2013**, *20*, 1230–1236. [CrossRef]
151. Khodarahmian, M.; Amidi, F.; Moini, A.; Kashani, L.; Salahi, E.; Danaii-Mehrabad, S.; Nashtaei, M.S.; Mojtahedi, M.F.; Esfandyari, S.; Sobhani, A. A randomized exploratory trial to assess the effects of resveratrol on VEGF and TNF-α 2 expression in endometriosis women. *J. Reprod. Immunol.* **2020**, *143*, 103248. [CrossRef]
152. Zhou, A.; Hong, Y.; Lv, Y. Sulforaphane attenuates endometriosis in rat models through inhibiting pi3k/akt signaling pathway. *Dose Res.* **2019**, *17*, 1559325819855538. [CrossRef]
153. Valipour, J.; Nashtaei, M.S.; Khosravizadeh, Z.; Mahdavinezhad, F.; Nekoonam, S.; Esfandyari, S.; Amidi, F. Effect of sulforaphane on apoptosis, reactive oxygen species and lipids peroxidation of human sperm during cryopreservation. *Cryobiology* **2021**, *99*, 122–130. [CrossRef]
154. Stephens, F.B.; Constantin-Teodosiu, D.; Greenhaff, P.L. New insights concerning the role of carnitine in the regulation of fuel metabolism in skeletal muscle. *J. Pshycol.* **2007**, *581*, 431–444. [CrossRef]
155. Tselekidou, E.D.; Vassiliadis, S.; Athanassakis, I. Establishment or Aggravation of Endometriosis by L-Carnitine: The Role of Pge1 and Pge2 in the Endometriosis-Induction Process. New Developments in Endometriosis. Available online: https://www.createspace.com (accessed on 15 January 2021).
156. Gerbase, A.C.; Rowley, J.T.; Heymann, D.H.; Berkley, S.F.; Piot, P. Global prevalence and incidence estimates of selected curable STDs. *Sex Transm. Infect.* **1998**, *74*, S12–S16.
157. Onisto, M.; Fasolato, S.; Veggian, R.; Caenazzo, C.; Garbisa, S. Hormonal and basement membrane markers for immunoidentification of cultured human trophoblast cells. *Int. J. Gynaecol. Obstet.* **1989**, *30*, 145–153. [CrossRef]
158. Rabiu, K.A.; Adewunmi, A.A.; Akinlusi, F.M.; Akinola, O.I. Female reproductive tract infections: Understandings and care seeking behaviour among women of reproductive age in Lagos, Nigeria. *BMC Women's Health.* **2010**, *10*, 8. [CrossRef]
159. Moreno, I.; Simon, C. Relevance of assessing the uterine microbiota in infertility. *Fertil. Steril.* **2018**, *110*, 337–343. [CrossRef]
160. Heil, B.A.; Paccamonti, D.L.; Sones, J.L. Role for the mammalian female reproductive tract microbiome in pregnancy outcomes. *Physiol. Genomics* **2019**, *51*, 390–399. [CrossRef]
161. Krawinkel, M.B. Interaction of nutrition and infections globally: An overview. *Ann. Nutr. Metab.* **2012**, *61*, 39–45. [CrossRef]
162. Cassotta, M.; Forbes-Hernández, T.Y.; Calderón Iglesias, R.; Ruiz, R.; Elexpuru Zabaleta, M.; Giampieri, F.; Battino, M. Links between nutrition, infectious diseases, and microbiota: Emerging technologies and opportunities for human-focused research. *Nutrients* **2020**, *12*, 1827. [CrossRef]
163. Molenaar, M.C.; Singer, M.; Ouburg, S. The two-sided role of the vaginal microbiome in Chlamydia trachomatis and Mycoplasma genitalium pathogenesis. *J. Reprod. Immunol.* **2018**, *130*, 11–17. [CrossRef]
164. Tuddenham, S.; Ghanem, K.G. A microbiome variable in the HIV-prevention equation. *Science* **2017**, *356*, 907–908. [CrossRef]
165. Martin, D.H.; Marrazzo, J.M. The vaginal microbiome: Current understanding and future directions. *J. Infect. Dis.* **2016**, *214*, S36–S41. [CrossRef]
166. Borgogna, J.L.; Shardell, M.D.; Yeoman, C.J.; Ghanem, K.G.; Kadriu, H.; Ulanov, A.V.; Gaydos, C.A.; Hardick, J.; Robinson, C.K.; Bavoil, P.M.; et al. The association of Chlamydia trachomatis and Mycoplasma genitalium infection with the vaginal metabolome. *Sci. Rep.* **2020**, *10*, 3420. [CrossRef]

167. Ng, K.Y.; Mingels, R.; Morgan, H.; Macklon, N.; Cheong, Y. In vivo oxygen, temperature and pH dynamics in the female reproductive tract and their importance in human conception: A systematic review. *Hum. Reprod. Update* **2018**, *24*, 15–34. [CrossRef]
168. Van Oostrum, N.; De Sutter, P.; Meys, J.; Verstraelen, H. Risks associated with bacterial vaginosis in infertility patients: A systematic review and meta-analysis. *Hum. Reprod.* **2013**, *28*, 1809–1815. [CrossRef]
169. Koumans, E.H.; Sternberg, M.; Bruce, C.; McQuillan, G.; Kendrick, J.; Sutton, M.; Markowitz, L.E. The prevalence of bacterial vaginosis in the United States, 2001-2004; associations with symptoms, sexual behaviors, and reproductive health. *Sex. Transm. Dis.* **2007**, *34*, 864–869. [CrossRef] [PubMed]
170. Thoma, M.E.; Klebanoff, M.A.; Rovner, A.J.; Nansel, T.R.; Neggers, Y.; Andrews, W.W.; Schwebke, J.R. Bacterial vaginosis is associated with variation in dietary indices. *J. Nutr.* **2011**, *141*, 1698–1704. [CrossRef] [PubMed]
171. Smart, S.; Singal, A.; Mindel, A. Social and sexual risk factors for bacterial vaginosis. *Sex. Transm. Infect.* **2004**, *80*, 58–62. [CrossRef] [PubMed]
172. Neggers, Y.H.; Nansel, T.R.; Andrews, W.W.; Schwebke, J.R.; Yu, K.F.; Goldenberg, R.L.; Klebanoff, M.A. Dietary intake of selected nutrients affects bacterial vaginosis in women. *J. Nutr.* **2007**, *137*, 2128–2133. [CrossRef]
173. Bodnar, L.M.; Krohn, M.A.; Simhan, H.N. Maternal vitamin D deficiency is associated with bacterial vaginosis in the first trimester of pregnancy. *J. Nutr.* **2009**, *139*, 1157–1161. [CrossRef]
174. Mitchell, C.; Marrazzo, J. Bacterial vaginosis and the cervicovaginal immune response. *Am. J. Reprod. Immunol.* **2014**, *71*, 555–563. [CrossRef] [PubMed]
175. Dunlop, A.L.; Taylor, R.N.; Tangpricha, V.; Fortunato, S.; Menon, R. Maternal vitamin D, folate, and polyunsaturated fatty acid status and bacterial vaginosis during pregnancy. *Infect. Dis. Obstet. Gynecol.* **2011**, *2011*, 216217. [CrossRef]
176. Hensel, K.J.; Randis, T.M.; Gelber, S.E.; Ratner, A.J. Pregnancy-specific association of vitamin D deficiency and bacterial vaginosis. *Am. J. Obstet. Gynecol.* **2011**, *204*, 41-e1. [CrossRef]
177. Taheri, M.; Baheiraei, A.; Foroushani, A.R.; Nikmanesh, B.; Modarres, M. Treatment of vitamin D deficiency is an effective method in the elimination of asymptomatic bacterial vaginosis: A placebo-controlled randomized clinical trial. *Indian J. Med. Res.* **2015**, *141*, 799–806.
178. Al-Ghazzewi, F.H.; Tester, R.F. Biotherapeutic agents and vaginal health. *J. Appl. Microbiol.* **2016**, *121*, 18–27. [CrossRef]
179. Tuominen, H.; Rautava, S.; Syrjänen, S.; Collado, M.C.; Rautava, J. HPV infection and bacterial microbiota in the placenta, uterine cervix and oral mucosa. *Sci. Rep.* **2018**, *8*, 9787. [CrossRef]
180. Atashili, J.; Poole, C.; Ndumbe, P.M.; Adimora, A.A.; Smith, J.S. Bacterial vaginosis and HIV acquisition: A meta-analysis of published studies. *AIDS* **2008**, *22*, 1493–1501. [CrossRef]
181. Allsworth, J.E.; Lewis, V.A.; Peipert, J.F. Viral sexually transmitted infections and bacterial vaginosis: 2001–2004 national health and nutrition examination survey data. *Sex. Transm. Dis.* **2008**, *35*, 791–796. [CrossRef]
182. White, M.C.; Hayes, N.S.; Richardson, L.C. Public health's future role in cancer survivorship. *Am. J. Prev. Med.* **2015**, *49*, S550–S553. [CrossRef]
183. Dunn, B.K.; Kramer, B.S. Cancer prevention: Lessons learned and future directions. *Trends Cancer* **2016**, *2*, 713–722. [CrossRef] [PubMed]
184. Sundstrom, K.; Elfstrom, K.M. Advances in cervical cancer prevention: Efficacy, effectiveness, elimination? *PLoS MED* **2020**, *17*, e1003035. [CrossRef]
185. MacKintosh, M.L.; Crosbie, E.J. Prevention strategies in endometrial carcinoma. *Curr. Oncol. Rep.* **2018**, *20*, 101. [CrossRef]
186. Temkin, S.M.; Bergstrom, J.; Samimi, G.; Minasian, L. Ovarian cancer prevention in high.-risk women. *Clin. Obstet. Gynecol.* **2017**, *60*, 738–757. [CrossRef]
187. Szewczuk, M.; Gasiorowska, E.; Matysiak, K.; Nowak-Markwitz, E. The role of artificial nutrition in gynecological cancer therapy. *Ginekol. Pol.* **2019**, *90*, 167–172. [CrossRef]
188. Koshiyama, M. The effects of the dietary and nutrient intake on gynecologic cancers. *Healthcare* **2019**, *7*, 88. [CrossRef]
189. Key, T.J.; Bradbury, K.E.; Perez-Cornago, A.; Sinha, R.; Tsilidis, K.K.; Tsugane, S. Diet, nutrition, and cancer risk: What do we know and what is the way forward? *BMJ* **2020**, *368*, 368. [CrossRef]
190. Ferenczy, A.; Franco, E. Persistent human papillomavirus infection and cervical neoplasia. *Lancet Oncol.* **2002**, *3*, 11–16. [CrossRef]
191. Stebbing, J.; Hart, C.A. Antioxidants and cancer. *Lancet Oncol.* **2011**, *12*, 996. [CrossRef]
192. Tomita, L.Y.; Roteli-Martins, C.M.; Villa, L.L.; Franco, E.L.; Cardoso, M.A. Associations of dietary dark-green and deep-yellow vegetables and fruits with cervical intraepithelial neoplasia: Modification by smoking. *Br. J. Nutr.* **2011**, *105*, 928–937. [CrossRef] [PubMed]
193. Siegel, E.M.; Salemi, J.L.; Villa, L.L.; Ferenczy, A.; Franco, E.L.; Giuliano, A.R. Dietary consumption of antioxidant nutrients and risk of incident cervical intraepithelial neoplasia. *Gynecol. Oncol.* **2010**, *118*, 289–294. [CrossRef]
194. Jia, Y.; Hu, T.; Hang, C.Y.; Yang, R.; Li, X.; Chen, Z.L.; Mei, Y.D.; Zhang, Q.H.; Huang, K.C.; Xiang, Q.Y.; et al. Case-control study of diet in patients with cervical cancer or precancerosis in Wufeng, a high incidence region in China. *Asian Pac. J. Cancer Prev.* **2012**, *13*, 5299–5302. [CrossRef] [PubMed]
195. Guo, L.; Zhu, H.; Lin, C.; Che, J.; Tian, X.; Han, S.; Zhao, H.; Zhu, Y.; Mao, D. Associations between antioxidant vitamins and the risk of invasive cervical cancer in Chinese women: A case-control study. *Sci. Rep.* **2015**, *5*, 13607. [CrossRef]

196. Giuliano, A.R.; Siegel, E.M.; Roe, D.J.; Ferreira, S.; Luiza Baggio, M.; Galan, L.; Duarte-Franco, E.; Villa, L.L.; Rohan, T.E.; Marshall, J.R.; et al. Dietary intake and risk of persistent human papillomavirus (HPV) infection: The Ludwig-McGill HPV natural history study. *J. Infect. Dis.* **2003**, *188*, 1508–1516. [CrossRef]
197. Ono, A.; Koshiyama, M.; Nakagawa, M.; Watanabe, Y.; Ikuta, E.; Seki, K.; Oowaki, M. The preventive effect of dietary antioxidants on cervical cancer development. *Medicina* **2020**, *56*, 604. [CrossRef]
198. Yeo, A.S.; Schiff, M.A.; Montoya, G.; Masuk, M.; van Asselt-King, L.; Becker, T.M. Serum micronutrients and cervical dysplasia in Southwestern American Indian women. *Nutr. Cancer* **2000**, *38*, 141–150. [CrossRef]
199. Huang, X.; Chen, C.; Zhu, F.; Zhang, Y.; Feng, Q.; Li, J.; Yu, Q.; Zhong, Y.; Luo, S.; Gao, J. Association between dietary vitamin A and HPV infection in American women: Data from NHANES 2003–2016. *Biomed Res. Int.* **2020**, *2020*, 4317610. [CrossRef] [PubMed]
200. Rizvi, S.; Raza, S.T.; Faizal Ahmed, A.A.; Abbas, S.; Mahdi, F. The role of vitamin e in human health and some diseases. *Sultan Qaboos Univ. Med. J.* **2014**, *14*, e157–e165. [PubMed]
201. Hu, X.; Li, S.; Zhou, L.; Zhao, M.; Zhu, X. Effect of vitamin E supplementation on uterine cervical neoplasm: A meta-analysis of case-control studies. *PLoS ONE* **2017**, *12*, e0183395. [CrossRef]
202. Vahedpoor, Z.; Jamilian, M.; Bahmani, F.; Aghadavod, E.; Karamali, M.; Kashanian, M.; Asemi, Z. Effects of long-term vitamin d supplementation on regression and metabolic status of cervical intraepithelial neoplasia: A randomized, double-blind, placebo-controlled trial. *Horm. Cancer* **2017**, *8*, 58–67. [CrossRef]
203. Hernandez, B.Y.; McDuffie, K.; Wilkens, L.R.; Kamemoto, L.; Goodman, M.T. Diet and premalignant lesions of the cervix: Evidence of a protective role for folate, riboflavin, thiamin, and vitamin B12. *Cancer Causes Control* **2003**, *14*, 859–870. [CrossRef] [PubMed]
204. Zoberi, I.; Bradbury, C.M.; Curry, H.A.; Bisht, K.S.; Goswami, P.C.; Roti, J.L.; Gius, D. Radiosensitizing and anti-proliferative effects of resveratrol in two human cervical tumor cell lines. *Cancer Lett.* **2002**, *175*, 165–173. [CrossRef]
205. Silva, G.Á.; Nunes, R.A.; Morale, M.G.; Boccardo, E.; Aguayo, F.; Termini, L. Oxidative stress: Therapeutic approaches for cervical cancer treatment. *Clinics* **2018**, *73*, e548s. [CrossRef] [PubMed]
206. Venkatraman, M.; Anto, R.J.; Nair, A.; Varghese, M.; Karunagaran, D. Biological and chemical inhibitors of NF-kappaB sensitize SiHa cells to cisplatin-induced apoptosis. *Mol. Carcinog.* **2005**, *44*, 51–59. [CrossRef]
207. Ciebiera, M.; Łukaszuk, K.; Męczekalski, B.; Ciebiera, M.; Wojtyła, C.; Słabuszewska-Jóźwiak, A.; Jakiel, G. Alternative oral agents in prophylaxis and therapy of uterine fibroids-an up-to-date review. *Int. J. Mol. Sci.* **2017**, *18*, 2586. [CrossRef] [PubMed]
208. Min, K.J.; Kwon, T.K. Anticancer effects and molecular mechanisms of epigallocatechin-3-gallate. *Integr. Med. Res.* **2014**, *3*, 16–24. [CrossRef] [PubMed]
209. Pennant, M.E.; Mehta, R.; Moody, P.; Hackett, G.; Prentice, A.; Sharp, S.J.; Lakshman, R. Premenopausal abnormal uterine bleeding and risk of endometrial cancer. *BJOG* **2017**, *124*, 404–411. [CrossRef]
210. Setiawan, V.W.; Yang, H.P.; Pike, M.C.; McCann, S.E.; Yu, H.; Xiang, Y.B.; Wolk, A.; Wentzensen, N.; Weiss, N.S.; Webb, P.M.; et al. Type I and II endometrial cancers: Have they different risk factors? *J. Clin. Oncol.* **2013**, *31*, 2607–2618. [CrossRef]
211. Morice, P.; Leary, A.; Creutzberg, C.; Abu-Rustum, N.; Darai, E. Endometrial cancer. *Lancet* **2016**, *387*, 1094–1108. [CrossRef]
212. Leslie, K.K.; Thiel, K.W.; Goodheart, M.J.; De Geest, K.; Jia, Y.; Yang, S. Endometrial cancer. *Obstet. Gynecol. Clin. N. Am.* **2012**, *39*, 255–268. [CrossRef]
213. Bandera, E.V.; Gifkins, D.M.; Moore, D.F.; McCullough, M.L.; Kushi, L.H. Antioxidant vitamins and the risk of endometrial cancer: A dose-response meta-analysis. *Cancer Causes Control* **2009**, *20*, 699–711. [CrossRef]
214. Cui, X.; Rosner, B.; Willett, W.C.; Hankinson, S.E. Antioxidant intake and risk of endometrial cancer: Results from the Nurses' Health Study. *Int. J. Cancer* **2011**, *128*, 1169–1178. [CrossRef]
215. Acmaz, G.; Aksoy, H.; Albayrak, E.; Baser, M.; Ozyurt, S.; Aksoy, U.; Unal, D. Evaluation of endometrial precancerous lesions in postmenopausal obese women—A high risk group? *Asian Pac. J. Cancer Prev.* **2014**, *15*, 195–198. [CrossRef] [PubMed]
216. Brasky, T.M.; Neuhouser, M.L.; Cohn, D.E.; White, E. Associations of long-chain omega-3 fatty acids and fish intake with endometrial cancer risk in the VITamins and Lifestyle cohort. *Am. J. Clin. Nutr.* **2014**, *99*, 599–608. [CrossRef] [PubMed]
217. Rinaldi, S.; Peeters, P.H.; Bezemer, I.D.; Dossus, L.; Biessy, C.; Sacerdote, C.; Berrino, F.; Panico, S.; Palli, D.; Tumino, R.; et al. Relationship of alcohol intake and sex steroid concentrations in blood in pre- and post-menopausal women: The European prospective investigation into cancer and nutrition. *Cancer Causes Control* **2006**, *17*, 1033–1043. [CrossRef] [PubMed]
218. Fedirko, V.; Jenab, M.; Rinaldi, S.; Biessy, C.; Allen, N.E.; Dossus, L.; Onland-Moret, N.C.; Schütze, M.; Tjønneland, A.; Hansen, L.; et al. Alcohol drinking and endometrial cancer risk in the European Prospective Investigation into cancer and nutrition (EPIC) study. *Ann. Epidemiol.* **2013**, *23*, 93–98. [CrossRef] [PubMed]
219. Rossi, M.; Edefonti, V.; Parpinel, M.; Lagiou, P.; Franchi, M.; Ferraroni, M.; Decarli, A.; Zucchetto, A.; Serraino, D.; Dal Maso, L.; et al. Proanthocyanidins and other flavonoids in relation to endometrial cancer risk: A case-control study in Italy. *Br. J. Cancer* **2013**, *109*, 1914–1920. [CrossRef] [PubMed]
220. Messina, M.J.; Persky, V.; Setchell, K.D.; Barnes, S. Soy intake and cancer risk: A review of the in vitro and in vivo data. *Nutr. Cancer* **1994**, *21*, 113–131. [CrossRef]
221. Wang, L.; Lee, I.M.; Zhang, S.M.; Blumberg, J.B.; Buring, J.E.; Sesso, H.D. Dietary intake of selected flavonols, flavones, and flavonoid-rich foods and risk of cancer in middle-aged and older women. *Am. J. Clin. Nutr.* **2009**, *89*, 905–912. [CrossRef]

222. Bandera, E.V.; Williams, M.G.; Sima, C.; Bayuga, S.; Pulick, K.; Wilcox, H.; Soslow, R.; Zauber, A.G.; Olson, S.H. Phytoestrogen consumption and endometrial cancer risk: A population-based case-control study in New Jersey. *Cancer Causes Control* **2009**, *20*, 1117–1127. [CrossRef]
223. Ollberding, N.J.; Lim, U.; Wilkens, L.R.; Setiawan, V.W.; Shvetsov, Y.B.; Henderson, B.E.; Kolonel, L.N.; Goodman, M.T. Legume, soy, tofu, and isoflavone intake and endometrial cancer risk in postmenopausal women in the multiethnic cohort study. *J. Natl. Cancer Inst.* **2012**, *104*, 67–76. [CrossRef]
224. Zhang, G.Q.; Chen, J.L.; Liu, Q.; Zhang, Y.; Zeng, H.; Zhao, Y. Soy intake is associated with lower endometrial cancer risk: A systematic review and meta-analysis of observational studies. *Medicine* **2015**, *94*, e2281. [CrossRef]
225. Zhong, X.S.; Ge, J.; Chen, S.W.; Xiong, Y.Q.; Ma, S.J.; Chen, Q. Association between dietary isoflavones in soy and legumes and endometrial cancer: A systematic review and meta-analysis. *J. Acad. Nutr. Diet.* **2018**, *118*, 637–651. [CrossRef] [PubMed]
226. Unfer, V.; Casini, M.L.; Costabile, L.; Mignosa, M.; Gerli, S.; Di Renzo, G.C. Endometrial effects of long-term treatment with phytoestrogens: A randomized, double-blind, placebo-controlled study. *Fertil. Steril.* **2004**, *82*, 145–148. [CrossRef] [PubMed]
227. Mohr, S.B.; Garland, C.F.; Gorham, E.D.; Grant, W.B.; Garland, F.C. Is ultraviolet B irradiance inversely associated with incidence rates of endometrial cancer: An ecological study of 107 countries. *Prev. Med.* **2007**, *45*, 327–331. [CrossRef]
228. McCullough, M.L.; Bandera, E.V.; Moore, D.F.; Kushi, L.H. Vitamin D and calcium intake in relation to risk of endometrial cancer: A systematic review of the literature. *Prev. Med.* **2008**, *46*, 298–302. [CrossRef] [PubMed]
229. Luo, H.; Rankin, G.O.; Li, Z.; DePriest, L.; Chen, Y.C. Kaempferol induces apoptosis in ovarian cancer cells through activating p53 in the intrinsic pathway. *Food Chem.* **2011**, *128*, 513–519. [CrossRef] [PubMed]
230. Chuwa, A.H.; Sone, K.; Oda, K.; Tanikawa, M.; Kukita, A.; Kojima, M.; Oki, S.; Fukuda, T.; Takeuchi, M.; Miyasaka, A.; et al. Kaempferol, a natural dietary flavonoid, suppresses 17beta-estradiol-induced survivin expression and causes apoptotic cell death in endometrial cancer. *Oncol. Lett.* **2018**, *16*, 6195–6201.
231. Yang, T.O.; Crowe, F.; Cairns, B.J.; Reeves, G.K.; Beral, V. Tea and coffee and risk of endometrial cancer: Cohort study and meta-analysis. *Am. J. Clin. Nutr.* **2015**, *101*, 570–578. [CrossRef]
232. Zhou, Q.; Li, H.; Zhou, J.G.; Ma, Y.; Wu, T.; Ma, H. Green tea, black tea consumption and risk of endometrial cancer: A systematic review and meta-analysis. *Arch. Gynecol. Obstet.* **2016**, *293*, 143–155. [CrossRef] [PubMed]
233. Coburn, S.B.; Bray, F.; Sherman, M.E.; Trabert, B. International patterns and trends in ovarian cancer incidence, overall and by histologic subtype. *Int. J. Cancer* **2017**, *140*, 2451–2460. [CrossRef]
234. Jayson, G.C.; Kohn, E.C.; Kitchener, H.C.; Ledermann, J.A. Ovarian cancer. *Lancet* **2014**, *384*, 1376–1388. [CrossRef]
235. Goff, B.A.; Mandel, L.; Muntz, H.G.; Melancon, C.H. Ovarian carcinoma diagnosis. *Cancer* **2000**, *89*, 2068–2075. [CrossRef]
236. Kisielewski, R.; Mazurek, A.; Laudański, P.; Tołwińska, A. Inflammation and ovarian cancer—Current views. *Ginekol. Pol.* **2013**, *84*, 293–297. [CrossRef] [PubMed]
237. Shivappa, N.; Hébert, J.R.; Rosato, V.; Rossi, M.; Montella, M.; Serraino, D.; La Vecchia, C. Dietary inflammatory index and ovarian cancer risk in a large Italian case-control study. *Cancer Causes Control* **2016**, *27*, 897–906. [CrossRef]
238. Dolecek, T.A.; McCarthy, B.J.; Joslin, C.E.; Peterson, C.E.; Kim, S.; Freels, S.A.; Davis, F.G. Prediagnosis food patterns are associated with length of survival from epithelial ovarian cancer. *J. Am. Diet. Assoc.* **2010**, *110*, 369–382. [CrossRef]
239. Playdon, M.C.; Nagle, C.M.; Ibiebele, T.I.; Ferrucci, L.M.; Protani, M.M.; Carter, J.; Hyde, S.E.; Neesham, D.; Nicklin, J.L.; Mayne, S.T.; et al. Pre-diagnosis diet and survival after a diagnosis of ovarian cancer. *Br. J. Cancer* **2017**, *116*, 1627–1637. [CrossRef]
240. Qiu, W.; Lu, H.; Qi, Y.; Wang, X. Dietary fat intake and ovarian cancer risk: A meta-analysis of epidemiological studies. *Oncotarget* **2016**, *7*, 37390–37406. [CrossRef]
241. Bandera, E.V.; King, M.; Chandran, U.; Paddock, L.E.; Rodriguez-Rodriguez, L.; Olson, S.H. Phytoestrogen consumption from foods and supplements and epithelial ovarian cancer risk: A population-based case control study. *BMC Wom. Health* **2011**, *11*, 40. [CrossRef] [PubMed]
242. Neill, A.S.; Ibiebele, T.I.; Lahmann, P.H.; Hughes, M.C.; Nagle, C.M.; Webb, P.M. Dietary phyto-oestrogens and the risk of ovarian and endometrial cancers: Findings from two Australian case-control studies. *Br. J. Nutr.* **2014**, *111*, 1430–1440. [CrossRef] [PubMed]
243. Hedelin, M.; Löf, M.; Andersson, T.M.; Adlercreutz, H.; Weiderpass, E. Dietary phytoestrogens and the risk of ovarian cancer in the women's lifestyle and health cohort study. *Cancer Epidemiol. Biomarkers Prev.* **2011**, *20*, 308–317. [CrossRef] [PubMed]
244. Hua, X.; Yu, L.; You, R.; Yang, Y.; Liao, J.; Chen, D.; Yu, L. Association among Dietary flavonoids, flavonoid subclasses and ovarian cancer risk: A meta-analysis. *PLoS ONE* **2016**, *11*, e0151134. [CrossRef] [PubMed]
245. Shafabakhsh, R.; Asemi, Z. Quercetin: A natural compound for ovarian cancer treatment. *J. Ovarian Res.* **2019**, *12*, 55. [CrossRef]
246. Luo, H.; Rankin, G.O.; Liu, L.; Daddysman, M.K.; Jiang, B.H.; Chen, Y.C. Kaempferol inhibits angiogenesis and VEGF expression through both HIF dependent and independent pathways in human ovarian cancer cells. *Nutr. Cancer* **2009**, *61*, 554–563. [CrossRef]
247. Huang, H.; Chen, A.Y.; Ye, X.; Guan, R.; Rankin, G.O.; Chen, Y.C. Galangin, a flavonoid from lesser galangal, induced apoptosis via p53-dependent pathway in ovarian cancer cells. *Molecules* **2020**, *25*, 1579. [CrossRef]
248. Lin, Y.G.; Kunnumakkara, A.B.; Nair, A.; Merritt, W.M.; Han, L.Y.; Armaiz-Pena, G.N.; Kamat, A.A.; Spannuth, W.A.; Gershenson, D.M.; Lutgendorf, S.K.; et al. Curcumin inhibits tumor growth and angiogenesis in ovarian carcinoma by targeting the nuclear factor-kappaB pathway. *Clin. Cancer Res.* **2007**, *13*, 3423–3430. [CrossRef] [PubMed]
249. Pourhanifeh, M.H.; Darvish, M.; Tabatabaeian, J.; Fard, M.R.; Mottaghi, R.; Azadchehr, M.J.; Jahanshahi, M.; Sahebkar, A.; Mirzaei, H. Therapeutic role of curcumin and its novel formulations in gynecological cancers. *J. Ovarian Res.* **2020**, *13*, 30. [CrossRef]

250. Wahl, H.; Tan, L.; Griffith, K.; Choi, M.; Liu, J.R. Curcumin enhances Apo2L/TRAIL-induced apoptosis in chemoresistant ovarian cancer cells. *Gynecol. Oncol.* **2007**, *105*, 104–112. [CrossRef] [PubMed]
251. He, M.; Wang, D.; Zou, D.; Wang, C.; Lopes-Bastos, B.; Jiang, W.G.; Chester, J.; Zhou, Q.; Cai, J. Re-purposing of curcumin as an anti-metastatic agent for the treatment of epithelial ovarian cancer: In vitro model using cancer stem cell enriched ovarian cancer spheroids. *Oncotarget* **2016**, *7*, 86374–86387. [CrossRef] [PubMed]
252. Yallapu, M.M.; Maher, D.M.; Sundram, V.; Bell, M.C.; Jaggi, M.; Chauhan, S.C. Curcumin induces chemo/radio-sensitization in ovarian cancer cells and curcumin nanoparticles inhibit ovarian cancer cell growth. *J. Ovarian Res.* **2010**, *3*, 11. [CrossRef]
253. Sun, Y.; Xun, K.; Wang, Y.; Chen, X. A systematic review of the anticancer properties of berberine, a natural product from Chinese herbs. *Anticancer Drugs* **2009**, *20*, 757–769. [CrossRef]
254. Liu, L.; Fan, J.; Ai, G.; Liu, J.; Luo, N.; Li, C.; Cheng, Z. Berberine in combination with cisplatin induces necroptosis and apoptosis in ovarian cancer cells. *Biol. Res.* **2019**, *52*, 37. [CrossRef] [PubMed]
255. Tse, A.K.; Wan, C.K.; Shen, X.L.; Yang, M.; Fong, W.F. Honokiol inhibits TNF-alpha-stimulated NF-kappaB activation and NF-kappaB-regulated gene expression through suppression of IKK activation. *Biochem. Pharmacol.* **2005**, *70*, 1443–1457. [CrossRef]
256. Lee, J.S.; Sul, J.Y.; Park, J.B.; Lee, M.S.; Cha, E.Y.; Ko, Y.B. Honokiol induces apoptosis and suppresses migration and invasion of ovarian carcinoma cells via AMPK/mTOR signaling pathway. *Int. J. Mol. Med.* **2019**, *43*, 1969–1978. [CrossRef] [PubMed]
257. Wu, S.H.; Wu, T.Y.; Hsiao, Y.T.; Lin, J.H.; Hsu, S.C.; Hsia, T.C.; Yang, S.T.; Hsu, W.H.; Chung, J.G. Bufalin induces cell death in human lung cancer cells through disruption of DNA damage response pathways. *Am. J. Chin. Med.* **2014**, *42*, 729–742. [CrossRef] [PubMed]
258. Su, S.; Dou, H.; Wang, Z.; Zhang, Q. Bufalin inhibits ovarian carcinoma via targeting mTOR/HIF-alpha pathway. *Basic Clin. Pharmacol. Toxicol.* **2020**. [CrossRef]
259. Kosuge, T.; Adachi, T.; Kamiya, H. Isolation of tetramethylpyrazine from culture of Bacillus natto, and biosynthetic pathways of tetramethylpyrazine. *Nature* **1962**, *195*, 1103. [CrossRef] [PubMed]
260. Zhang, H.; Ding, S.; Xia, L. Ligustrazine inhibits the proliferation and migration of ovarian cancer cells via regulating miR-211. *Biosci. Rep.* **2020**, *41*, BSR20200199. [CrossRef] [PubMed]
261. Ciebiera, M.; Włodarczyk, M.; Ciebiera, M.; Zaręba, K.; Łukaszuk, K.; Jakiel, G. Vitamin D and Uterine Fibroids-Review of the Literature and Novel Concepts. *Int. J. Mol. Sci.* **2018**, *19*, 2051. [CrossRef]
262. Dovnik, A.; Dovnik, N.F. Vitamin D and ovarian cancer: Systematic review of the literature with a focus on molecular mechanisms. *Cells* **2020**, *9*, 335. [CrossRef]
263. Song, X.; Li, Z.; Ji, X.; Zhang, D. Calcium intake and the risk of ovarian cancer: A meta-analysis. *Nutrients* **2017**, *9*, 679. [CrossRef] [PubMed]
264. Livdans-Forret, A.B.; Harvey, P.J.; Larkin-Thier, S.M. Menorrhagia: A synopsis of management focusing on herbal and nutritional supplements, and chiropractic. *J. Can. Chiropr. Assoc.* **2007**, *51*, 235–246.
265. Geller, S.E.; Studee, L. Botanical and dietary supplements for menopausal symptoms: What works, what does not. *J Wom. Health* **2005**, *14*, 634–649. [CrossRef] [PubMed]
266. Low, M.S.; Speedy, J.; Styles, C.E.; De-Regil, L.M.; Pasricha, S.R. Daily iron supplementation for improving anaemia, iron status and health in menstruating women. *Cochrane Datab. Syst. Rev.* **2016**, *4*, CD009747. [CrossRef] [PubMed]
267. Lithgow, D.M.; Politzer, W.M. Vitamin A in the treatment of menorrhagia. *S. Afr. Med. J.* **1977**, *51*, 91–93.
268. Ayre, J.E.; Bauld, W.A. Thiamine deficiency and high. estrogen findings in uterine cancer and in menorrhagia. *Science* **1946**, *103*, 441–445. [CrossRef]
269. Cohen, J.D.; Rubin, H.W. Functional menorrhagia: Treatment with bioflavonoids and vitamin C. *Curr. Ther. Res. Clin. Exp.* **1960**, *2*, 539–542. [PubMed]
270. Morrow, C.; Naumburg, E.H. Dysmenorrhea. *Prim. Care* **2009**, *36*, 19–32. [CrossRef]
271. Dennehy, C.E. The use of herbs and dietary supplements in gynecology: An evidence-based review. *J. Midwifery Women's Health* **2006**, *51*, 402–409. [CrossRef]
272. Bajalan, Z.; Alimoradi, Z.; Moafi, F. Nutrition as a potential factor of primary dysmenorrhea: A systematic review of observational studies. *Gynecol. Obstet. Invest.* **2019**, *84*, 209–224. [CrossRef]
273. Pattanittum, P.; Kunyanone, N.; Brown, J.; Sangkomkamhang, U.S.; Barnes, J.; Seyfoddin, V.; Marjoribanks, J. Dietary supplements for dysmenorrhoea. *Cochrane Database Syst. Rev.* **2016**, *3*, CD002124. [CrossRef]
274. Naz, M.S.; Kiani, Z.; Fakari, F.R.; Ghasemi, V.; Abed, M.; Ozgoli, G. The effect of micronutrients on pain management of primary dysmenorrhea: A systematic review and meta-analysis. *J. Caring Sci.* **2020**, *9*, 47–56.
275. Shin, H.J.; Na, H.S.; Do, S.H. Magnesium and Pain. *Nutrients* **2020**, *9*, 2184. [CrossRef] [PubMed]
276. Chiang, Y.F.; Hung, H.C.; Chen, H.Y.; Huang, K.C.; Lin, P.H.; Chang, J.Y.; Huang, T.C.; Hsia, S.M. The inhibitory effect of extra virgin olive oil and its active compound oleocanthal on prostaglandin-induced uterine hypercontraction and pain-ex vivo and in vivo study. *Nutrients* **2020**, *12*, 3012. [CrossRef]
277. Lee, H.W.; Ang, L.; Lee, M.S.; Alimoradi, Z.; Kim, E. Fennel for reducing pain in primary dysmenorrhea: A systematic review and meta-analysis of randomized controlled trials. *Nutrients* **2020**, *12*, 3438. [CrossRef] [PubMed]
278. Nagata, C.; Hirokawa, K.; Shimizu, N.; Shimizu, H. Associations of menstrual pain with intakes of soy, fat and dietary fiber in Japanese women. *Eur. J. Clin. Nutr.* **2005**, *59*, 88–92. [CrossRef]

279. Mehrpooya, M.; Eshraghi, A.; Rabiee, S.; Larki-Harchegani, A.; Ataei, S. Comparison the effect of fish-oil and calcium supplementation on treatment of primary dysmenorrhea. *Rev. Recent Clin. Trials* **2017**, *12*, 148–153. [CrossRef]
280. Sadeghi, N.; Paknezhad, F.; Rashidi Nooshabadi, M.; Kavianpour, M.; Jafari Rad, S.; Khadem Haghighian, H. Vitamin E and fish oil, separately or in combination, on treatment of primary dysmenorrhea: A double-blind, randomized clinical trial. *Gynecol. Endocrinol.* **2018**, *34*, 804–808. [CrossRef]
281. Lerchbaum, E.; Rabe, T. Vitamin D and female fertility. *Curr. Opin. Obstet. Gynecol.* **2014**, *26*, 145–150. [CrossRef] [PubMed]
282. Bahrami, A.; Avan, A.; Sadeghnia, H.R.; Esmaeili, H.; Tayefi, M.; Ghasemi, F.; Nejati Salehkhani, F.; Arabpour-Dahoue, M.; Rastgar-Moghadam, A.; Ferns, G.A.; et al. High. dose vitamin D supplementation can improve menstrual problems, dysmenorrhea, and premenstrual syndrome in adolescents. *Gynecol. Endocrinol.* **2018**, *34*, 659–663. [CrossRef]
283. Abdi, F.; Amjadi, M.A.; Zaheri, F.; Rahnemaei, F.A. Role of vitamin D and calcium in the relief of primary dysmenorrhea: A systematic review. *Obstet. Gynecol. Sci.* **2021**, *64*, 13–26. [CrossRef] [PubMed]
284. Zhang, Y.; Mao, X.; Su, J.; Geng, Y.; Guo, R.; Tang, S.; Li, J.; Xiao, X.; Xu, H.; Yang, H. A network pharmacology-based strategy deciphers the underlying molecular mechanisms of Qixuehe Capsule in the treatment of menstrual disorders. *Chin. Med.* **2017**, *12*, 23. [CrossRef] [PubMed]
285. Zekavat, O.R.; Karimi, M.Y.; Amanat, A.; Alipour, F. A randomised controlled trial of oral zinc sulphate for primary dysmenorrhoea in adolescent females. *Aust. N. Z. J. Obstet. Gynaecol.* **2015**, *55*, 369–373. [CrossRef]
286. Nasiadek, M.; Stragierowicz, J.; Klimczak, M.; Kilanowicz, A. The role of zinc in selected female reproductive system disorders. *Nutrients* **2020**, *12*, 2464. [CrossRef] [PubMed]
287. Chao, M.T.; Wade, C.M.; Booth, S.L. Increase in plasma phylloquinone concentrations following acupoint injection for the treatment of primary dysmenorrhea. *J. Acupunct. Meridian. Stud.* **2014**, *7*, 151–154. [CrossRef]
288. Wade, C.; Wang, L.; Zhao, W.J.; Cardini, F.; Kronenberg, F.; Gui, S.Q.; Ying, Z.; Zhao, N.Q.; Chao, M.T.; Yu, J. Acupuncture point injection treatment of primary dysmenorrhoea: A randomised, double blind, controlled study. *BMJ Open* **2016**, *6*, e008166. [CrossRef]
289. Fujiwara, T.; Ono, M.; Mieda, M.; Yoshikawa, H.; Nakata, R.; Daikoku, T.; Sekizuka-Kagami, N.; Maida, Y.; Ando, H.; Fujiwara, H. Adolescent dietary habit-induced obstetric and gynecologic disease (ADHOGD) as a new hypothesis-possible involvement of clock system. *Nutrients* **2020**, *12*, 1294. [CrossRef]

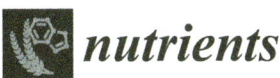

Review

Nutrition in Menopausal Women: A Narrative Review

Thais R. Silva [1,2], Karen Oppermann [3], Fernando M. Reis [4,*] and Poli Mara Spritzer [1,2,*]

1. Gynecological Endocrinology Unit, Division of Endocrinology, Hospital de Clínicas de Porto Alegre, Rua Ramiro Barcelos 2350, Porto Alegre 90035-003, Brazil; thaisrasia@gmail.com
2. Laboratory of Molecular Endocrinology, Department of Physiology, Federal University of Rio Grande do Sul, Porto Alegre 90035-003, Brazil
3. Medical School of Universidade de Passo Fundo, São Vicente de Paulo Hospital, Passo Fundo 99052-900, Brazil; karenoppermann@gmail.com
4. Division of Human Reproduction, Hospital das Clínicas, Department of Obstetrics and Gynecology, Universidade Federal de Minas Gerais, Belo Horizonte 30130-100, Brazil
* Correspondence: fmreis@ufmg.br (F.M.R.); spritzer@ufrgs.br (P.M.S.); Tel.: +55-51-3359-8027 (P.M.S.)

Abstract: Among the various aspects of health promotion and lifestyle adaptation to the postmenopausal period, nutritional habits are essential because they concern all women, can be modified, and impact both longevity and quality of life. In this narrative review, we discuss the current evidence on the association between dietary patterns and clinical endpoints in postmenopausal women, such as body composition, bone mass, and risk markers for cardiovascular disease. Current evidence suggests that low-fat, plant-based diets are associated with beneficial effects on body composition, but further studies are needed to confirm these results in postmenopausal women. The Mediterranean diet pattern along with other healthy habits may help the primary prevention of bone, metabolic, and cardiovascular diseases in the postmenopausal period. It consists on the use of healthy foods that have anti-inflammatory and antioxidant properties, and is associated with a small but significant decrease in blood pressure, reduction of fat mass, and improvement in cholesterol levels. These effects remain to be evaluated over a longer period of time, with the assessment of hard outcomes such as bone fractures, diabetes, and coronary ischemia.

Keywords: menopause; nutrition; body composition; bone; cardiovascular risk

1. Introduction

Menopause is literally the ceasing of menstruation, but a broader definition includes "the permanent cessation of menstrual cycles following the loss of ovarian follicular activity" [1]. Climacteric is the transitional phase from the first signs of ovarian senescence until its complete installation. Among the various endocrine changes that characterize the progressive loss of ovarian function and ultimately lead to menopause, the most important is the decrease of circulating levels of ovarian steroids. The loss of luteal phase progesterone due to missed ovulation may cause menstrual irregularity and heavy menstrual bleeding in the late premenopausal years, while the subsequent decrease of estradiol levels due to follicular exhaustion is related to vasomotor symptoms, and the cause of urogenital atrophy, bone loss, and increased cardiovascular and metabolic risk [2,3]. Although menopause is a conspicuous event, the menopausal transition may span several years and the health impact of postmenopausal hypoestrogenism can extend for decades, even when symptoms are no longer present [4,5].

Menopause is associated with increased prevalence of obesity, metabolic syndrome, cardiovascular disease, and osteoporosis [3]. Weight gain is observed among midlife women and has been ascribed to both chronological aging and to the menopause transition [6]. Recent data from a large population-based cohort in the United States [7] reinforced the idea that weight gain is not only related to the menopause transition, even though the fat mass increases rapidly in this phase. In this sense, a population-based study that

Citation: Silva, T.R.; Oppermann, K.; Reis, F.M.; Spritzer, P.M. Nutrition in Menopausal Women: A Narrative Review. *Nutrients* **2021**, *13*, 2149. https://doi.org/10.3390/nu13072149

Academic Editor: Leanne M. Redman

Received: 21 May 2021
Accepted: 18 June 2021
Published: 23 June 2021

Publisher's Note: MDPI stays neutral with regard to jurisdictional claims in published maps and institutional affiliations.

Copyright: © 2021 by the authors. Licensee MDPI, Basel, Switzerland. This article is an open access article distributed under the terms and conditions of the Creative Commons Attribution (CC BY) license (https://creativecommons.org/licenses/by/4.0/).

we conducted in southern Brazil showed that sedentariness rather than menopause is associated with a two-fold increased risk of overweight/obesity [8]. Therefore, exercise along with calorie restriction should be recommended in all those postmenopausal women with excess weight, for reductions in metabolic and cardiovascular risk [9].

The ability to switch from fat utilization during fasting to carbohydrate utilization during hyperinsulinemia is defined as metabolic flexibility [10]. Gonadal hormones might regulate metabolic flexibility at the level of the mitochondria, determining how nutrients are converted into energy [11]. In postmenopausal women, metabolic flexibility diminishes due to estrogen reduction and more fat accumulates in central depots [12].

The integral health care of menopausal women should therefore emphasize lifestyle assessment and counseling to counterbalance the negative effects of estrogen deficiency on general well-being and minimize the risk of metabolic syndrome, osteoporosis, bone fractures, and vascular events [2,3]. Among the various aspects of health promotion and lifestyle adaptation to the postmenopausal period, nutritional habits are essential because they concern all women, can be modified, and impact both longevity and quality of life. In this narrative review, we shall discuss the current evidence on the association between dietary patterns and clinical endpoints in postmenopausal women, such as body composition, bone mass, and risk markers for cardiovascular disease (CVD), including studies of risk association and/or effects of dietary interventions and thereby providing novel insight into the establishment of optimal dietary guidelines for healthy postmenopausal period.

In order to find relevant publications, a search was conducted in Pubmed with combinations of keywords and Medical Subject Headings (MeSH) "Diet", "Recommended Dietary Allowances", "Diet, Mediterranean", "Diet, Fat-Restricted", "Diet, Carbohydrate-Restricted", "Glycemic Index", "Body Composition", "Menopause", "Postmenopause", and "Cardiovascular Diseases". All articles published up to February 2021 were considered for eligibility.

2. Dietary Intake and Clinical Endpoints in Menopausal Women

2.1. Body Composition

In the menopausal transition, lowering estrogen levels have been associated with loss of lean body mass (LBM) and increase in fat mass (FM) [13,14]. In the longitudinal Study of Women's Health Across the Nation, LBM loss during the menopausal transition averaged 0.5% (a mean annual absolute decrease of 0.2 kg), and FM increased by 1.7% per year (mean annual absolute increase of 0.45 kg) [7]. Body composition changes in this population were associated with increased risk of coronary heart disease, potentially compromising the woman's health as a whole. In the National Health and Nutrition Examination Survey (NHANES), participants with low LBM and high FM had the highest cardiovascular and total mortality risk [15].

2.1.1. Dietary Intake and Lean Body Mass in Postmenopausal Women
Dietary Protein

Ageing increases dietary protein requirements [16,17] because skeletal muscles reduce their capacity of activating protein synthesis in response to anabolic stimuli, possibly due to insulin resistance [18,19]. In fact, observational studies have indicated that higher protein intake is associated with higher LBM in postmenopausal women [20–22]. In the Women's Health Initiative study, higher protein intake (1.2 g/kg body weight) was associated with a 32% lower risk of frailty and better physical function [23]. The mean protein intake associated with higher skeletal muscle mass index in postmenopausal women was 1.6 g/kg body weight [22], although the Institute of Medicine recommends for all ages the protein allowance of 0.8 g/kg body weight [24]. Because observational results are unable to determine the direction of cause and effect, randomized controlled trials (RCT) have been developed to validate this hypothesis. A meta-analysis of 36 RCTs with 1682 participants concluded that protein supplementation, from 6 to 78 weeks, does not lead to increase in LBM in non-frail community-dwelling older adults [25]. The few available interventional studies focusing on postmenopausal women have shown that high protein intake did not promote LBM gain when compared to recommended dietary allowance (RDA) (Table 1) [26,27]. Indeed, beyond the metabolic and physiological changes of aging that may alter protein metabolism [28], the current evidence suggests that RDA may be sufficient to maintain LBM in older women.

While LBM maintenance cannot be attributed to high dietary protein intake in healthy postmenopausal women, it could be associated, at least in part, with healthy dietary patterns, such as the Mediterranean diet (MD).

Mediterranean Dietary Pattern

Through acting directly in oxidative stress [29], inflammation [30,31], and insulin resistance [18,19], regarded as risk factors for muscle catabolism, the MD components have been associated with better muscle measurements in postmenopausal women [32–34].

In a recent review, Granic et al. [35] hypothesized that the 'myoprotective' effect of the MD could be linked to higher intake of plant-based foods because they combine nutrients that act together to preserve the muscles. In a previous work, we have also proposed a model for the potential benefits of MD on body composition in postmenopausal women. The presence of antioxidants like beta-carotene, as well as vitamins C and E protects from deleterious effects of oxidative stress, while magnesium improves energy metabolism, transmembrane transport, and skeletal muscle function [34] (Figure 1).

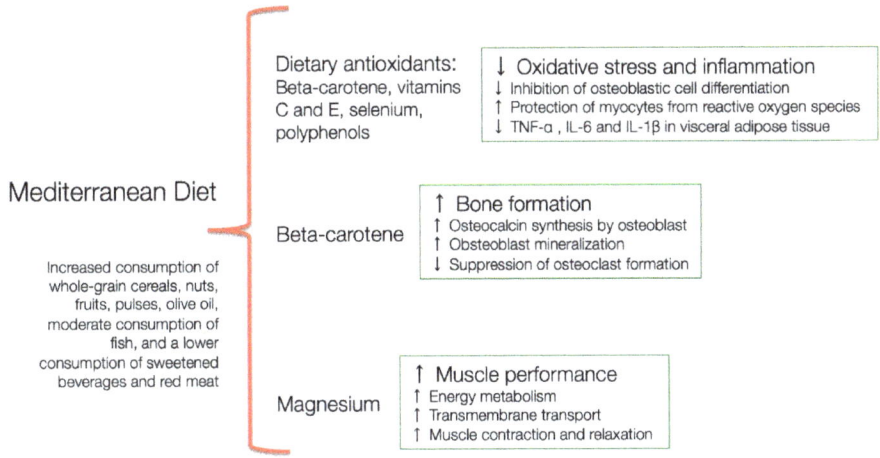

Figure 1. Potential benefits of Mediterranean diet on body composition in postmenopausal women. Redrawn and modified from [34].

However, studies about MD intervention focusing on LBM gain or maintenance in postmenopausal women were not available until now, expressing an important gap regarding this issue. Therefore, further research is needed on the potential effects of non-protein nutrients on muscle health in older women.

2.1.2. Dietary Intake and Fat Mass in Postmenopausal Women

Dietary Carbohydrate, Whole Grains, and Glycemic Index

The role of dietary carbohydrate for promoting FM loss remains to be elucidated. In obese individuals, a previous systematic review has shown that mild low carbohydrate diet (40% of total energy) was not associated with decrease in fat mass [36]. Recently, a randomized control trial with 57 women (age 40 ± 3.5 years, BMI 31.1 ± 2.6 kg·m^{-2}) yielded similar results, with low-carbohydrate-high-fat diet having no superior effect on FM in comparison to a normal diet [37]. However, some carbohydrate sources can be beneficial, while others are not, depending at least in part on their fiber content [38]. In an RCT with 81 men and 32 postmenopausal women, the consumption of whole grains during six weeks had positive effects on the resting metabolic rate and stool energy excretion, which influenced favorably the energy balance [39]. Indeed, this study adds support for dietary guidance recommending the consumption of whole grains instead of refined grains in order to reduce adiposity [40], although there are very few interventional studies focusing on postmenopausal women.

Complementing additional ways of characterizing carbohydrate foods, such as fiber and whole grain content, glycemic index (GI) should also be considered particularly important in reducing total body FM and managing weight [38]. Eating a meal with high GI elicits a quick pancreatic response to the rising blood glucose levels, with intense insulin secretion that rapidly lowers blood glucose and causes hunger and overeating [41]. In fact, a Cochrane systematic review including data from 202 overweight or obese men and women in six RCTs reported a significantly greater decrease in total FM in the low GI diet than in control diet groups [42]. Specifically in postmenopausal women, a clinical trial with low GI (<55) dietary intervention, aimed to balance energy needs, has shown that, despite similar energy intake and resting metabolic rates during the six months of follow-up, all participants lost total body and regional FM [43].

Mediterranean Dietary Pattern

An umbrella review of meta-analyses reported evidence suggesting greater effectiveness of MD in reducing body weight and waist circumference when compared to control diets [44]. However, the evidence regarding the MD effect on FM was scarce. In a cross-sectional study with 176 perimenopausal women from the FLAMENCO project, a higher MD adherence, an increased consumption of whole-grain cereals, nuts, fruits, pulses, whole dairy products, and olive oil, and a lower consumption of sweetened beverages were associated with lower FM [45] (Figure 1). In a non-controlled clinical trial, 89 women (46 in reproductive age and 43 postmenopausal) were prescribed hypocaloric traditional MD for eight weeks and obtained an average reduction of 2.3 kg in FM, suggesting that postmenopausal women can lose FM with this diet in the same way as younger women [46]. However, the potential role of MD in reducing FM in comparison to other dietary patterns needs to be further evaluated.

In contrast, The Women's Health Initiative Dietary Modification trial have found that a low-fat ($\leq$20% of total energy) diet was related with greater reductions in percentage body fat and FM after one and three years of follow-up [47]. Indeed, trials where participants, men and women, were randomized to a lower fat intake ($\leq$30% of total energy) showed a consistent, stable but small effect on percentage body fat compared with higher fat arms, as published in a Cochrane systematic review [48]. Despite MD being associated with higher dietary fat intake, both MD and low-fat diet are often associated with increased intake of vegetables, fruits and grains. Recently, a crossover RCT showed that a plant-based, low-fat diet promoted greater decrease in FM than an animal-based, ketogenic diet [49]. However, the study enrolled only 20 adults and the primary outcome was daily ad libitum energy intake between each two-week diet period. In summary, low-fat, plant-based diets are associated with beneficial effects on FM, and future studies are needed to confirm these results in postmenopausal women.

2.2. Bone Health

The decrease in bone mineral density (BMD) that accompanies aging is related to declining reproductive hormone concentrations [50,51]. BMD loss accelerates markedly along the late perimenopause, when menses become more irregular [52].

Several studies have shown the importance of adequate calcium and vitamin D intake for better BMD and prevention of osteoporosis and fractures in older adults [53]. However, the recommended daily intake of calcium for older adults ranges from 700 mg in the UK [54] to 1200 mg in the US [55], and the North American Menopause Society actually recommends 1000 to 1500 mg of dietary calcium per day to postmenopausal women [56]. Available evidence from completed RCTs provided no support for the use of vitamin D or calcium supplementations alone to prevent fractures. On the other hand, daily supplementation with both vitamin D (400–800 IU/day) and calcium (1000–1200 mg/day) was a more promising strategy [57].

Besides, analysis of isolated nutrients is not sufficient to reveal the complex interactions between nutrients and non-nutrients contained in food. Therefore, the study of dietary patterns, particularly the MD pattern, has been proposed to investigate the relationship between diet and BMD.

Previous studies showed that better adherence to the MD is positively associated with BMD in middle-aged and elderly people [58] and in postmenopausal women [34,59]. Recent findings from an RCT undertaken across five European centers support these results from observational studies. In this trial, a MD-like diet prescribed for one year and accompanied by individual advice and supplies of the required foods produced a significant decrease in the rate of BMD loss among people with osteoporosis, compared to a group that received only informative leaflets [60].

The potential benefits of the MD for BMD may result from the combined presence of nutrients and non-nutrients components. Dietary intake of carotenoids has been associated with BMD [61]. Indeed, beta-carotene seems to suppress osteoclast formation and bone resorption [62]. Vitamin K also plays a role in bone formation through osteocalcin synthesis by osteoblasts, which is a vitamin K dependent protein [63]. However, concerns have been raised about the integrity of some vitamin K supplementation studies [64]. In addition, a recent RCT of vitamin K (MK-7) or placebo supplementation in postmenopausal women observed no difference in bone turnover markers and microstructure between the groups during three years of follow-up [65]. Regarding vitamin C, a recent meta-analysis of observational studies reported that greater dietary vitamin C intake was associated with a lower risk of hip fracture and osteoporosis, as well as higher BMD at femoral neck and lumbar spine [66]. Moreover, a review of Mendelian randomization-based studies examined potential associations between serum nutritional factors and BMD. Higher selenium levels positively influence BMD at specific skeletal sites, suggesting that selenium plays a crucial role in bone metabolism [67]. Therefore, an adequate consumption of beta-carotene, vitamin C, and selenium trough MD could lead to better BMD (Figure 1). In contrast, processed food pattern (high intakes of meat pies, hamburgers, beer, sweets, fruit juice, processed meats, snacks, spirits, pizza and low intake of cruciferous vegetables) was inversely associated with bone mineral content in a cohort study with 347 women (aged 36–57 years) [68].

In a nutshell, the data above suggest that a MD pattern, combined with other healthy lifestyle habits, may be a useful non-pharmacological strategy for the primary prevention of osteoporosis and fractures in the postmenopausal period.

2.3. Cardiovascular Risk

The estrogens secreted by the ovaries during the reproductive period exert protective effects on vascular endothelial function as well as on lipid metabolism. After menopause, the relative estrogen deprivation contributes to increase vascular tone through both endocrine and autonomic mechanisms that converge impaired nitric oxide dependent vasodilation [1,69].

While CVD risk increases with menopause, this is difficult to distinguish from the effect of ageing [70]. Nonetheless, the use of menopausal hormone therapy (MHT) has been associated with protective effect against coronary artery calcification [71] and slower progression of carotid artery intima-media thickness, both of which are markers of subclinical CVD [72].

Postmenopausal women have two to three times higher prevalence of metabolic syndrome, compared to similar aged premenopausal women [73]. The changes on cardiovascular risk begin during the perimenopause period. Menopause transition results in lipid profile changes, with a 10–15% higher LDL-cholesterol and triglyceride levels and slightly lower HDL cholesterol levels [74]. This period also accounts for an increase in BMI and abdominal adiposity, with postmenopausal women presenting approximately five times the risk of central obesity compared to premenopausal women [13] (Figure 2). The presence of central obesity has been associated with decreased heart rate variability, another marker of subclinical CVD [75].

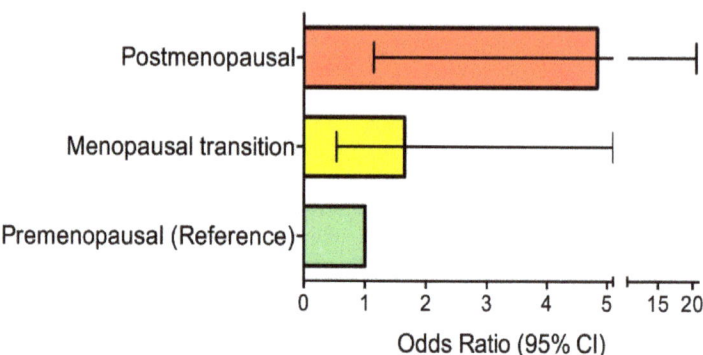

Figure 2. Adjusted odds ratios (with 95% confidence intervals) for central adiposity, defined as waist circumference ≥ 88 cm, in women in the menopausal transition and postmenopausal women. Adapted from [13].

Furthermore, there is an increase in blood pressure after menopause that may be a direct effect of hormonal changes on the vasculature and metabolic changes with ageing [69]. Sodium sensitivity increases during menopausal transition, frequently leading to intermittent fluid retention (edema of the legs, hands, and lower eyelids), contributing to higher cardiovascular risks [76].

Diet is a major modifiable risk factor for CVD. The traditional approach of nutritional epidemiology focuses on the potential impacts of individual foods or nutrients. Scientific societies recommend the following healthy dietary pattern to decrease the risk of major chronic diseases and increase overall wellbeing (Table 2): protein sources primarily from plants, nuts, fish, or alternative sources of omega-3 fatty acids; fat mostly from unsaturated plant sources; carbohydrates primarily from whole grains; at least five servings of fruits and vegetables per day; and moderate dairy consumption as an option [77].

The American Heart Association (AHA) suggests the following dietary targets to improve cardiovascular health: fruits ≥ 4.5 cups/day, fish and shellfish ≥ 200 g/week, sodium ≤ 1500 mg/day, sugar-sweetened beverages ≤ 36 fl oz/week, whole grains 3 or more 1-oz-equivalent servings/day, nuts, seeds, and legumes ≥ 4 servings/week (Table 2) [78–80]. In a recent meta-analysis of cohort studies, higher intakes of fruit and vegetables were associated with lower mortality rates, supporting current dietary recommendations to increase intake of fruits and vegetables, but not fruit juices and potatoes [81].

Table 1. Randomized controlled trials about the effect of high protein diets on LBM in postmenopausal women.

Author/Year	Country	Arms/Comparators	Duration	Participants	Interventions	LBM Analyses
Igley, 2009	USA	HP: 1.2 g/kg body weight NP: 0.9 g/kg body weight	12 weeks	36 postmenopausal women and men age = 61 ± 1 years	HP diet + resistance training vs. NP diet + resistance training	LBM increased: 1.1 ± 0.2 kg no difference between the groups
Rossato, 2017	Brazil	HP: 1.2 g/kg body weight NP: 0.8 g/kg body weight	10 weeks	23 postmenopausal women age = 63.2 ± 7.8 years	HP diet + resistance training vs. NP diet + resistance training	HP LBM: 37.1 ± 6.2 to 38.4 ± 6.5 kg NP LBM: 37.6 ± 6.2 to 38.8 ± 6.4 kg no difference between the groups ($p = 0.572$)
Silva, 2020	Brazil	HP: 1.6 g/kg body weight NP: 0.8 g/kg body weight	6 months	26 postmenopausal women age = 70.8 ± 3.6 years	HP diet vs. NP diet	HP LBM: 35.6 ± 0.7 to 35.7 ± 0.7 kg NP LBM: 35.3 ± 0.7 to 35.4 ± 0.7 kg no difference between the groups ($p = 0.683$)

LBM: lean body mass; HP: high protein diet; NP: normal protein diet.

Table 2. Healthy diet recommendations.

Guideline	Proteins		Fats		Carbohydrates	
	Yes	No or Moderate	Yes	No	Yes	No
EAT Lancet Commission [7]	• Protein from plants • Legumes Nuts • Fish • Fruits	• Red meat • Processed meat • Poultry and eggs • Dairy products	• Fat mostly from unsaturated plant sources	• Saturated fats • Partly hydrogenated oils	• Carbohydrates primarily from whole grains	• Refined grains • Sugar
American Heart Association [8]	• Fish ≥ 200 g/week	• Processed meats ≤ 100 g/week	• Nuts, seeds, and legumes ≥ 4 servings/week	• Saturated fat ≤ 7% energy	• Whole grains ≥ 3 servings/day • Fruits ≥ 4.5 cups/day	• Sodium ≤ 1500 mg/d • Sugar-sweetened beverages ≤ 36 fl oz/week

Although diet could be a powerful intervention to reduce cardiovascular risks in postmenopausal women, the studies could not clearly demonstrate this action on the arteries. The Study of Women's Health Across the Nation [82] evaluated the prospective associations between empirically derived dietary patterns during midlife and subclinical carotid atherosclerosis later in life among women. After extensively adjusting for covariates, higher adherences to Western dietary patterns (e.g., rich in dairy products, pizza, read meat, and salad dressing and poor in fruits, skimmed milk, legumes, cruciferous vegetables, and tomatoes) were associated with increased common carotid artery intima-media thickness (CCA-IMT). Prudent diet (e.g., including dark yellow vegetables, green leafy vegetables, cruciferous vegetables, legumes, and fruits and avoiding whole milk, margarine, organ meats, sweets, and beer) was not associated with CCA-IMT. The adoption of a diet low in red meat, processed meat, deep-fried products, and sugar-sweetened beverages among midlife women is associated with a lower future risk of atherosclerosis.

Low-energy diet is also recommended for postmenopausal women to prevent metabolic alterations [83]. In a cross-sectional study of 4984 women aged 30–79 years, three dietary patterns (Western, healthy, and traditional) were identified. In a stratified analysis by menopausal status, the inverse association of the healthy dietary pattern (characterized by high factor loadings with green-yellow vegetables, healthy-protein foods, seaweeds, and bonefish) and metabolic syndrome was statistically significant only among postmenopausal women. In assessing each component of metabolic syndrome, the healthy dietary pattern was found to be protective for blood pressure and triglyceride levels among premenopausal women and for obesity and HDL-cholesterol levels among postmenopausal women [84].

A reduction in energy expenditure during midlife can also cause obesity during menopause [83]. According to a four-year follow-up study, the decrease in physical activity began two years before menopause. Aging resulted in gained subcutaneous abdominal fat over time to all women, however, only those who became postmenopausal had a significant increase in visceral abdominal fat [13,85].

In a population-based cross-sectional study involving 292 Brazilian women, we have shown a higher risk of overweight/obesity for inactive women. Sedentariness increased the risk of diabetes mellitus and metabolic syndrome after adjustment for menopausal status and other potential confounders [8]. In addition, active postmenopausal women seem to have healthier dietary choices than their sedentary counterparts, such as foods with higher intake of protein and lower intake of chips and refined grains [86].

During the menopause transition there is a tendency to weight gain accompanied by an increase in central fat distribution that continues into the post-menopause [13,87]. For postmenopausal women, sedentary lifestyle and a diet with carbohydrate intake accounting for more than 55% of total energy contribute to higher cardiovascular risk, according to high sensitivity C-reactive protein levels [88].

The best diet for weight loss is still debatable, whether low-fat, low-carbohydrate, or high-protein diet, with no evident superiority of one over the others for the specific purpose of losing weight [87]. The obesity-management guidelines from the American College of Cardiology/American Heart Association Task Force on Practice Guidelines and the Obesity Society recommend a daily caloric deficit of 500 to 750 kcal, which for most women means eating 1200 to 1500 kcal/d, and is expected to result in an average weight loss 0.5 to 0.75 kg/wk [89].

Although the differences on cardiometabolic risk are small, the macronutrient composition of the weight loss diet may affect some intermediate outcomes. Low-fat diets tend to reduce low-density lipoprotein (LDL) cholesterol levels, while low-carbohydrate diets may be more effective to low triglycerides and increase high-density lipoprotein cholesterol levels [87].

Nevertheless, MD has the advantage of combining weight loss with CVD risk reduction [90]. This diet reduces the consumption of saturated animal fats in favor of unsaturated vegetable fats and a high intake of polyphenols and n-3 fatty acids with anti-inflammatory and antioxidant properties [91]. The phenolic compounds (polyphenols) are presented in extra virgin olive oil, whole grain cereals, nuts, legumes, vegetables, red wine, and fruits. Due to their antioxidant and anti-inflammatory properties, the synergistic consumption of these Mediterranean foods could represent an ideal nutritional pattern in menopause [92]. Evidence from observational studies and randomized trials consistently shows a small but significant decrease in LDL cholesterol as well as systolic and diastolic blood pressure in association with the MD. This diet has also been linked to reduced risk of CVD (including coronary disease) and CVD death among different female cohorts, although more evidence is required for these outcomes in postmenopausal women [93].

Concerning weight loss, the effect of hypocaloric MD is compared with a low-fat diet, a low-carbohydrate diet and the American Diabetes Association diet [90]. On top of that, peri- and postmenopausal women showed a high adherence to MD [92], which could increase the results on weight and cardio-metabolic profile.

In addition, we recently reported higher isoflavone dietary intake may be associated with lower risk of subclinical CVD, as assessed by CCA-IMT status, independently of endogenous estradiol levels and BMI [94]. Isoflavones might have beneficial effects by its anti-inflammatory and antioxidant properties, through the production of equol, an active metabolite formed from daidzin/daidzein by gut microbiota [95].

In general, the changes in weight and fat distribution in women are associated with aging and mainly with the decrease in estradiol levels during peri- and post-menopause. There are also changes in physical activity contributing to the accumulation of weight and body fat. At the same time, changes in cholesterol and triglyceride levels also favor increased cardiovascular risk.

In summary, physical activity and diet are modifiable factors in the quest for cardiovascular protection. Weight loss diets in overweight or obese women improve the metabolic syndrome in its various parameters. MD is composed of healthy foods that have anti-inflammatory and antioxidant properties. In addition to these benefits, it seems to incorporate greater adherence of women over time. These effects remain to be evaluated over a longer period of time, with the study of hard outcomes such as coronary ischemia.

3. Summary and Research Perspectives

- Menopausal transition has been associated with loss of BMD, LBM and increase of FM;
- RDA for protein intake may be sufficient to maintain LBM; Mediterranean diet components could be linked with better LBM;
- Low-carbohydrate-high-fat diet should not be recommended in order to reduce FM;
- In overweight or obese women, low GI diet could lead to greater decrease in FM than control diets;
- Future studies evaluating the effects of low-fat, plant-based diets on FM in postmenopausal women are needed;
- Mediterranean diet might significantly reduce the rate of BMD loss in women with osteoporosis;
- Calcium, vitamin D, vitamin K, selenium, magnesium, and beta-carotene adequate intake could be linked with better BMD in postmenopausal women;
- Diet is a major modifiable risk factor for CVD and could be a powerful intervention to reduce cardiovascular risks in postmenopausal women;
- Low-energy diet is recommended for postmenopausal women to prevent metabolic disturbance;
- Low-fat diets may lead to greater improvement in LDL cholesterol levels, whereas low-carbohydrate diets may result in greater improvement in triglyceride and HDL cholesterol levels;
- Mediterranean diet is associated with a small but significant decrease in blood pressure and reduced CVD risk of among different female cohorts, although more evidence is required for these outcomes in postmenopausal women.

Author Contributions: Conceptualization, P.M.S.; manuscript drafting, T.R.S., K.O., and F.M.R.; writing—review and editing, K.O., F.M.R., and P.M.S.; funding acquisition, P.M.S. All authors have read and agreed to the published version of the manuscript.

Funding: This work is supported by the Brazilian National Institute of Hormones and Women's Health/Conselho Nacional de Desenvolvimento Científico e Tecnológico (CNPq INCT 465482/2014-7) and Fundação de Amparo à Pesquisa do Rio Grande do Sul (FAPERGS INCT 17/2551-0000519-8).

Institutional Review Board Statement: Not applicable.

Informed Consent Statement: Not applicable.

Data Availability Statement: Not applicable.

Conflicts of Interest: The authors have no conflict of interest related to the present review.

References

1. Davis, S.R.; Lambrinoudaki, I.; Lumsden, M.; Mishra, G.D.; Pal, L.; Rees, M.; Santoro, N.; Simoncini, T. Menopause. *Nat. Rev. Dis. Primers* **2015**, *1*, 15004. [CrossRef] [PubMed]
2. El Khoudary, S.R.; Aggarwal, B.; Beckie, T.M.; Hodis, H.N.; Johnson, A.E.; Langer, R.D.; Limacher, M.C.; Manson, J.E.; Stefanick, M.L.; Allison, M.A. Menopause Transition and Cardiovascular Disease Risk: Implications for Timing of Early Prevention: A Scientific Statement From the American Heart Association. *Circulation* **2020**, *142*, e506–e532. [CrossRef] [PubMed]
3. Nappi, R.E.; Simoncini, T. Menopause transition: A golden age to prevent cardiovascular disease. *Lancet Diabetes Endocrinol.* **2021**, *9*, 135–137. [CrossRef]
4. Biglia, N.; Cagnacci, A.; Gambacciani, M.; Lello, S.; Maffei, S.; Nappi, R.E. Vasomotor symptoms in menopause: A biomarker of cardiovascular disease risk and other chronic diseases? *Climacteric J. Int. Menopause Soc.* **2017**, *20*, 306–312. [CrossRef]
5. Harlow, S.D.; Gass, M.; Hall, J.E.; Lobo, R.; Maki, P.; Rebar, R.W.; Sherman, S.; Sluss, P.M.; de Villiers, T.J. Executive summary of the Stages of Reproductive Aging Workshop + 10: Addressing the unfinished agenda of staging reproductive aging. *Menopause* **2012**, *19*, 387–395. [CrossRef]
6. Davis, S.R.; Castelo-Branco, C.; Chedraui, P.; Lumsden, M.A.; Nappi, R.E.; Shah, D.; Villaseca, P. Understanding weight gain at menopause. *Climacteric J. Int. Menopause Soc.* **2012**, *15*, 419–429. [CrossRef]
7. Greendale, G.A.; Sternfeld, B.; Huang, M.; Han, W.; Karvonen-Gutierrez, C.; Ruppert, K.; Cauley, J.A.; Finkelstein, J.S.; Jiang, S.F.; Karlamangla, A.S. Changes in body composition and weight during the menopause transition. *JCI Insight* **2019**, *4*. [CrossRef]
8. Colpani, V.; Oppermann, K.; Spritzer, P.M. Association between habitual physical activity and lower cardiovascular risk in premenopausal, perimenopausal, and postmenopausal women: A population-based study. *Menopause* **2013**, *20*, 525–531. [CrossRef]
9. Cheng, C.C.; Hsu, C.Y.; Liu, J.F. Effects of dietary and exercise intervention on weight loss and body composition in obese postmenopausal women: A systematic review and meta-analysis. *Menopause* **2018**, *25*, 772–782. [CrossRef]
10. Kelley, D.E.; Mandarino, L.J. Fuel selection in human skeletal muscle in insulin resistance: A reexamination. *Diabetes* **2000**, *49*, 677–683. [CrossRef]
11. Irwin, R.W.; Yao, J.; Hamilton, R.T.; Cadenas, E.; Brinton, R.D.; Nilsen, J. Progesterone and estrogen regulate oxidative metabolism in brain mitochondria. *Endocrinology* **2008**, *149*, 3167–3175. [CrossRef]
12. Eaton, S.A.; Sethi, J.K. Immunometabolic Links between Estrogen, Adipose Tissue and Female Reproductive Metabolism. *Biology* **2019**, *8*, 8. [CrossRef]
13. Donato, G.B.; Fuchs, S.C.; Oppermann, K.; Bastos, C.; Spritzer, P.M. Association between menopause status and central adiposity measured at different cutoffs of waist circumference and waist-to-hip ratio. *Menopause* **2006**, *13*, 280–285. [CrossRef]
14. Rolland, Y.M.; Perry, H.M., 3rd; Patrick, P.; Banks, W.A.; Morley, J.E. Loss of appendicular muscle mass and loss of muscle strength in young postmenopausal women. *J. Gerontol. Ser. A Biol. Sci. Med. Sci.* **2007**, *62*, 330–335. [CrossRef]
15. Srikanthan, P.; Horwich, T.B.; Tseng, C.H. Relation of Muscle Mass and Fat Mass to Cardiovascular Disease Mortality. *Am. J. Cardiol.* **2016**, *117*, 1355–1360. [CrossRef]
16. Bauer, J.; Biolo, G.; Cederholm, T.; Cesari, M.; Cruz-Jentoft, A.J.; Morley, J.E.; Phillips, S.; Sieber, C.; Stehle, P.; Teta, D.; et al. Evidence-based recommendations for optimal dietary protein intake in older people: A position paper from the PROT-AGE Study Group. *J. Am. Med. Dir. Assoc.* **2013**, *14*, 542–559. [CrossRef] [PubMed]
17. Richter, M.; Baerlocher, K.; Bauer, J.M.; Elmadfa, I.; Heseker, H.; Leschik-Bonnet, E.; Stangl, G.; Volkert, D.; Stehle, P. Revised Reference Values for the Intake of Protein. *Ann. Nutr. Metab.* **2019**, *74*, 242–250. [CrossRef]
18. Francaux, M.; Demeulder, B.; Naslain, D.; Fortin, R.; Lutz, O.; Caty, G.; Deldicque, L. Aging Reduces the Activation of the mTORC1 Pathway after Resistance Exercise and Protein Intake in Human Skeletal Muscle: Potential Role of REDD1 and Impaired Anabolic Sensitivity. *Nutrients* **2016**, *8*, 47. [CrossRef]
19. Markofski, M.M.; Dickinson, J.M.; Drummond, M.J.; Fry, C.S.; Fujita, S.; Gundermann, D.M.; Glynn, E.L.; Jennings, K.; Paddon-Jones, D.; Reidy, P.T.; et al. Effect of age on basal muscle protein synthesis and mTORC1 signaling in a large cohort of young and older men and women. *Exp. Gerontol.* **2015**, *65*, 1–7. [CrossRef]

20. Isanejad, M.; Mursu, J.; Sirola, J.; Kröger, H.; Rikkonen, T.; Tuppurainen, M.; Erkkilä, A.T. Dietary protein intake is associated with better physical function and muscle strength among elderly women. *Br. J. Nutr.* **2016**, *115*, 1281–1291. [CrossRef] [PubMed]
21. Meng, X.; Zhu, K.; Devine, A.; Kerr, D.A.; Binns, C.W.; Prince, R.L. A 5-year cohort study of the effects of high protein intake on lean mass and BMC in elderly postmenopausal women. *J. Bone Miner. Res.* **2009**, *24*, 1827–1834. [CrossRef]
22. Silva, T.R.; Spritzer, P.M. Skeletal muscle mass is associated with higher dietary protein intake and lower body fat in postmenopausal women: A cross-sectional study. *Menopause* **2017**, *24*, 502–509. [CrossRef]
23. Beasley, J.M.; LaCroix, A.Z.; Neuhouser, M.L.; Huang, Y.; Tinker, L.; Woods, N.; Michael, Y.; Curb, J.D.; Prentice, R.L. Protein intake and incident frailty in the Women's Health Initiative observational study. *J. Am. Geriatr. Soc.* **2010**, *58*, 1063–1071. [CrossRef] [PubMed]
24. Trumbo, P.; Schlicker, S.; Yates, A.A.; Poos, M. Dietary reference intakes for energy, carbohydrate, fiber, fat, fatty acids, cholesterol, protein and amino acids. *J. Am. Diet. Assoc.* **2002**, *102*, 1621–1630. [CrossRef]
25. Ten Haaf, D.S.M.; Nuijten, M.A.H.; Maessen, M.F.H.; Horstman, A.M.H.; Eijsvogels, T.M.H.; Hopman, M.T.E. Effects of protein supplementation on lean body mass, muscle strength, and physical performance in nonfrail community-dwelling older adults: A systematic review and meta-analysis. *Am. J. Clin. Nutr.* **2018**, *108*, 1043–1059. [CrossRef]
26. Iglay, H.B.; Apolzan, J.W.; Gerrard, D.E.; Eash, J.K.; Anderson, J.C.; Campbell, W.W. Moderately increased protein intake predominately from egg sources does not influence whole body, regional, or muscle composition responses to resistance training in older people. *J. Nutr. Health Aging* **2009**, *13*, 108–114. [CrossRef]
27. Rossato, L.T.; Nahas, P.C.; de Branco, F.M.S.; Martins, F.M.; Souza, A.P.; Carneiro, M.A.S.; Orsatti, F.L.; de Oliveira, E.P. Higher Protein Intake Does Not Improve Lean Mass Gain When Compared with RDA Recommendation in Postmenopausal Women Following Resistance Exercise Protocol: A Randomized Clinical Trial. *Nutrients* **2017**, *9*, 1007. [CrossRef] [PubMed]
28. Balagopal, P.; Rooyackers, O.E.; Adey, D.B.; Ades, P.A.; Nair, K.S. Effects of aging on in vivo synthesis of skeletal muscle myosin heavy-chain and sarcoplasmic protein in humans. *Am. J. Physiol.* **1997**, *273*, E790–E800. [CrossRef] [PubMed]
29. Baumann, C.W.; Kwak, D.; Liu, H.M.; Thompson, L.V. Age-induced oxidative stress: How does it influence skeletal muscle quantity and quality? *J. Appl. Physiol.* **2016**, *121*, 1047–1052. [CrossRef] [PubMed]
30. Cruz-Jentoft, A.J.; Romero-Yuste, S.; Chamizo Carmona, E.; Nolla, J.M. Sarcopenia, immune-mediated rheumatic diseases, and nutritional interventions. *Aging Clin. Exp. Res.* **2021**. [CrossRef]
31. Daussin, F.N.; Boulanger, E.; Lancel, S. From mitochondria to sarcopenia: Role of inflammaging and RAGE-ligand axis implication. *Exp. Gerontol.* **2021**, *146*, 111247. [CrossRef]
32. Isanejad, M.; Sirola, J.; Mursu, J.; Rikkonen, T.; Kröger, H.; Tuppurainen, M.; Erkkilä, A.T. Association of the Baltic Sea and Mediterranean diets with indices of sarcopenia in elderly women, OSPTRE-FPS study. *Eur. J. Nutr.* **2018**, *57*, 1435–1448. [CrossRef] [PubMed]
33. Kelaiditi, E.; Jennings, A.; Steves, C.J.; Skinner, J.; Cassidy, A.; MacGregor, A.J.; Welch, A.A. Measurements of skeletal muscle mass and power are positively related to a Mediterranean dietary pattern in women. *Osteoporos. Int.* **2016**, *27*, 3251–3260. [CrossRef] [PubMed]
34. Silva, T.R.D.; Martins, C.C.; Ferreira, L.L.; Spritzer, P.M. Mediterranean diet is associated with bone mineral density and muscle mass in postmenopausal women. *Climacteric J. Int. Menopause Soc.* **2019**, *22*, 162–168. [CrossRef]
35. Granic, A.; Sayer, A.A.; Robinson, S.M. Dietary Patterns, Skeletal Muscle Health, and Sarcopenia in Older Adults. *Nutrients* **2019**, *11*, 745. [CrossRef] [PubMed]
36. Hashimoto, Y.; Fukuda, T.; Oyabu, C.; Tanaka, M.; Asano, M.; Yamazaki, M.; Fukui, M. Impact of low-carbohydrate diet on body composition: Meta-analysis of randomized controlled studies. *Obes. Rev.* **2016**, *17*, 499–509. [CrossRef] [PubMed]
37. Valsdottir, T.D.; Øvrebø, B.; Falck, T.M.; Litleskare, S.; Johansen, E.I.; Henriksen, C.; Jensen, J. Low-Carbohydrate High-Fat Diet and Exercise: Effect of a 10-Week Intervention on Body Composition and CVD Risk Factors in Overweight and Obese Women-A Randomized Controlled Trial. *Nutrients* **2020**, *13*, 110. [CrossRef] [PubMed]
38. Augustin, L.S.; Kendall, C.W.; Jenkins, D.J.; Willett, W.C.; Astrup, A.; Barclay, A.W.; Björck, I.; Brand-Miller, J.C.; Brighenti, F.; Buyken, A.E.; et al. Glycemic index, glycemic load and glycemic response: An International Scientific Consensus Summit from the International Carbohydrate Quality Consortium (ICQC). *Nutr. Metab. Cardiovasc. Dis. NMCD* **2015**, *25*, 795–815. [CrossRef]
39. Karl, J.P.; Meydani, M.; Barnett, J.B.; Vanegas, S.M.; Goldin, B.; Kane, A.; Rasmussen, H.; Saltzman, E.; Vangay, P.; Knights, D.; et al. Substituting whole grains for refined grains in a 6-wk randomized trial favorably affects energy-balance metrics in healthy men and postmenopausal women. *Am. J. Clin. Nutr.* **2017**, *105*, 589–599. [CrossRef] [PubMed]
40. Pol, K.; Christensen, R.; Bartels, E.M.; Raben, A.; Tetens, I.; Kristensen, M. Whole grain and body weight changes in apparently healthy adults: A systematic review and meta-analysis of randomized controlled studies. *Am. J. Clin. Nutr.* **2013**, *98*, 872–884. [CrossRef]
41. Ludwig, D.S. Dietary glycemic index and obesity. *J. Nutr.* **2000**, *130*, 280s–283s. [CrossRef] [PubMed]
42. Thomas, D.E.; Elliott, E.J.; Baur, L. Low glycaemic index or low glycaemic load diets for overweight and obesity. *Cochrane Database Syst. Rev.* **2007**, Cd005105. [CrossRef]
43. Silva, T.R.; Lago, S.C.; Yavorivski, A.; Ferreira, L.L.; Fighera, T.M.; Spritzer, P.M. Effects of high protein, low-glycemic index diet on lean body mass, strength, and physical performance in late postmenopausal women: A randomized controlled trial. *Menopause* **2020**, *28*, 307–317. [CrossRef]

44. Dinu, M.; Pagliai, G.; Casini, A.; Sofi, F. Mediterranean diet and multiple health outcomes: An umbrella review of meta-analyses of observational studies and randomised trials. *Eur. J. Clin. Nutr.* **2018**, *72*, 30–43. [CrossRef] [PubMed]
45. Flor-Alemany, M.; Marín-Jiménez, N.; Nestares, T.; Borges-Cosic, M.; Aranda, P.; Aparicio, V.A. Mediterranean diet, tobacco consumption and body composition during perimenopause. The FLAMENCO project. *Maturitas* **2020**, *137*, 30–36. [CrossRef]
46. Lombardo, M.; Perrone, M.A.; Guseva, E.; Aulisa, G.; Padua, E.; Bellia, C.; Della-Morte, D.; Iellamo, F.; Caprio, M.; Bellia, A. Losing Weight after Menopause with Minimal Aerobic Training and Mediterranean Diet. *Nutrients* **2020**, *12*, 2471. [CrossRef]
47. Carty, C.L.; Kooperberg, C.; Neuhouser, M.L.; Tinker, L.; Howard, B.; Wactawski-Wende, J.; Beresford, S.A.; Snetselaar, L.; Vitolins, M.; Allison, M.; et al. Low-fat dietary pattern and change in body-composition traits in the Women's Health Initiative Dietary Modification Trial. *Am. J. Clin. Nutr.* **2011**, *93*, 516–524. [CrossRef] [PubMed]
48. Hooper, L.; Abdelhamid, A.S.; Jimoh, O.F.; Bunn, D.; Skeaff, C.M. Effects of total fat intake on body fatness in adults. *Cochrane Database Syst. Rev.* **2020**, *6*, Cd013636. [CrossRef] [PubMed]
49. Hall, K.D.; Guo, J.; Courville, A.B.; Boring, J.; Brychta, R.; Chen, K.Y.; Darcey, V.; Forde, C.G.; Gharib, A.M.; Gallagher, I.; et al. Effect of a plant-based, low-fat diet versus an animal-based, ketogenic diet on ad libitum energy intake. *Nat. Med.* **2021**, *27*, 344–353. [CrossRef] [PubMed]
50. Silva, T.R.; Franz, R.; Maturana, M.A.; Spritzer, P.M. Associations between body composition and lifestyle factors with bone mineral density according to time since menopause in women from Southern Brazil: A cross-sectional study. *BMC Endocr. Disord.* **2015**, *15*, 71. [CrossRef]
51. Sowers, M.R.; Jannausch, M.; McConnell, D.; Little, R.; Greendale, G.A.; Finkelstein, J.S.; Neer, R.M.; Johnston, J.; Ettinger, B. Hormone predictors of bone mineral density changes during the menopausal transition. *J. Clin. Endocrinol. Metab.* **2006**, *91*, 1261–1267. [CrossRef]
52. Finkelstein, J.S.; Brockwell, S.E.; Mehta, V.; Greendale, G.A.; Sowers, M.R.; Ettinger, B.; Lo, J.C.; Johnston, J.M.; Cauley, J.A.; Danielson, M.E.; et al. Bone mineral density changes during the menopause transition in a multiethnic cohort of women. *J. Clin. Endocrinol. Metab.* **2008**, *93*, 861–868. [CrossRef]
53. Bischoff-Ferrari, H.A.; Dawson-Hughes, B.; Baron, J.A.; Burckhardt, P.; Li, R.; Spiegelman, D.; Specker, B.; Orav, J.E.; Wong, J.B.; Staehelin, H.B.; et al. Calcium intake and hip fracture risk in men and women: A meta-analysis of prospective cohort studies and randomized controlled trials. *Am. J. Clin. Nutr.* **2007**, *86*, 1780–1790. [CrossRef]
54. Salmon, J. Excerpts from Dietary Reference Values for Food Energy and Nutrients for the United Kingdom: Introduction to the Guide and Summary Tables. *Nutr. Rev.* **1992**, *50*, 90–93. [CrossRef]
55. Institute of Medicine (US) Committee to Review Dietary Reference Intakes for Vitamin D and Calcium. The National Academies Collection: Reports funded by National Institutes of Health. In *Dietary Reference Intakes for Calcium and Vitamin D*; National Academies Press (US) Copyright©, 2021; Ross, A.C., Taylor, C.L., Yaktine, A.L., Del Valle, H.B., Eds.; National Academy of Sciences: Washington, DC, USA, 2011.
56. Society, N.A.M. The role of calcium in peri- and postmenopausal women: 2006 position statement of the North American Menopause Society. *Menopause* **2006**, *13*, 862–877; quiz 878–880. [CrossRef]
57. Yao, P.; Bennett, D.; Mafham, M.; Lin, X.; Chen, Z.; Armitage, J.; Clarke, R. Vitamin D and Calcium for the Prevention of Fracture: A Systematic Review and Meta-analysis. *JAMA Netw. Open* **2019**, *2*, e1917789. [CrossRef]
58. Chen, G.D.; Dong, X.W.; Zhu, Y.Y.; Tian, H.Y.; He, J.; Chen, Y.M. Adherence to the Mediterranean diet is associated with a higher BMD in middle-aged and elderly Chinese. *Sci. Rep.* **2016**, *6*, 25662. [CrossRef]
59. Erkkilä, A.T.; Sadeghi, H.; Isanejad, M.; Mursu, J.; Tuppurainen, M.; Kröger, H. Associations of Baltic Sea and Mediterranean dietary patterns with bone mineral density in elderly women. *Public Health Nutr.* **2017**, *20*, 2735–2743. [CrossRef]
60. Jennings, A.; Cashman, K.D.; Gillings, R.; Cassidy, A.; Tang, J.; Fraser, W.; Dowling, K.G.; Hull, G.L.J.; Berendsen, A.A.M.; de Groot, L.; et al. A Mediterranean-like dietary pattern with vitamin D3 (10 µg/d) supplements reduced the rate of bone loss in older Europeans with osteoporosis at baseline: Results of a 1-y randomized controlled trial. *Am. J. Clin. Nutr.* **2018**, *108*, 633–640. [CrossRef]
61. Regu, G.M.; Kim, H.; Kim, Y.J.; Paek, J.E.; Lee, G.; Chang, N.; Kwon, O. Association between Dietary Carotenoid Intake and Bone Mineral Density in Korean Adults Aged 30–75 Years Using Data from the Fourth and Fifth Korean National Health and Nutrition Examination Surveys (2008–2011). *Nutrients* **2017**, *9*, 1025. [CrossRef] [PubMed]
62. Wang, F.; Wang, N.; Gao, Y.; Zhou, Z.; Liu, W.; Pan, C.; Yin, P.; Yu, X.; Tang, M. β-Carotene suppresses osteoclastogenesis and bone resorption by suppressing NF-κB signaling pathway. *Life Sci.* **2017**, *174*, 15–20. [CrossRef]
63. Atkins, G.J.; Welldon, K.J.; Wijenayaka, A.R.; Bonewald, L.F.; Findlay, D.M. Vitamin K promotes mineralization, osteoblast-to-osteocyte transition, and an anticatabolic phenotype by {gamma}-carboxylation-dependent and -independent mechanisms. *Am. J. Physiol. Cell Physiol.* **2009**, *297*, C1358–C1367. [CrossRef]
64. Avenell, A.; Grey, A.; Gamble, G.D.; Bolland, M.J. Concerns About the Integrity of the Yamaguchi Osteoporosis Prevention Study (YOPS) Report, Am J Med. 2004;117:549-555. *Am. J. Med.* **2020**, *133*, e311–e314. [CrossRef] [PubMed]
65. Rønn, S.H.; Harsløf, T.; Oei, L.; Pedersen, S.B.; Langdahl, B.L. The effect of vitamin MK-7 on bone mineral density and microarchitecture in postmenopausal women with osteopenia, a 3-year randomized, placebo-controlled clinical trial. *Osteoporos. Int.* **2021**, *32*, 185–191. [CrossRef]

66. Zeng, L.F.; Luo, M.H.; Liang, G.H.; Yang, W.Y.; Xiao, X.; Wei, X.; Yu, J.; Guo, D.; Chen, H.Y.; Pan, J.K.; et al. Can Dietary Intake of Vitamin C-Oriented Foods Reduce the Risk of Osteoporosis, Fracture, and BMD Loss? Systematic Review With Meta-Analyses of Recent Studies. *Front. Endocrinol.* **2019**, *10*, 844. [CrossRef]
67. Qu, Z.; Yang, F.; Yan, Y.; Hong, J.; Wang, W.; Li, S.; Jiang, G.; Yan, S. Relationship between Serum Nutritional Factors and Bone Mineral Density: A Mendelian Randomization Study. *J. Clin. Endocrinol. Metab.* **2021**, *106*, e2434–e2443. [CrossRef]
68. Wu, F.; Wills, K.; Laslett, L.L.; Oldenburg, B.; Jones, G.; Winzenberg, T. Associations of dietary patterns with bone mass, muscle strength and balance in a cohort of Australian middle-aged women. *Br. J. Nutr.* **2017**, *118*, 598–606. [CrossRef]
69. Maas, A.; Rosano, G.; Cifkova, R.; Chieffo, A.; van Dijken, D.; Hamoda, H.; Kunadian, V.; Laan, E.; Lambrinoudaki, I.; Maclaran, K.; et al. Cardiovascular health after menopause transition, pregnancy disorders, and other gynaecologic conditions: A consensus document from European cardiologists, gynaecologists, and endocrinologists. *Eur. Heart J.* **2021**, *42*, 967–984. [CrossRef]
70. O'Keeffe, L.M.; Kuh, D.; Fraser, A.; Howe, L.D.; Lawlor, D.; Hardy, R. Age at period cessation and trajectories of cardiovascular risk factors across mid and later life. *Heart* **2020**, *106*, 499–505. [CrossRef]
71. Oppermann, K.; Colpani, V.; Spritzer, P.M. Risk factors associated with coronary artery calcification in midlife women: A population-based study. *Gynecol. Endocrinol.* **2019**, *35*, 904–908. [CrossRef] [PubMed]
72. Manson, J.E.; Allison, M.A.; Rossouw, J.E.; Carr, J.J.; Langer, R.D.; Hsia, J.; Kuller, L.H.; Cochrane, B.B.; Hunt, J.R.; Ludlam, S.E.; et al. Estrogen therapy and coronary-artery calcification. *N. Engl. J. Med.* **2007**, *356*, 2591–2602. [CrossRef]
73. Hallajzadeh, J.; Khoramdad, M.; Izadi, N.; Karamzad, N.; Almasi-Hashiani, A.; Ayubi, E.; Qorbani, M.; Pakzad, R.; Hasanzadeh, A.; Sullman, M.J.M.; et al. Metabolic syndrome and its components in premenopausal and postmenopausal women: A comprehensive systematic review and meta-analysis on observational studies. *Menopause* **2018**, *25*, 1155–1164. [CrossRef]
74. Choi, Y.; Chang, Y.; Kim, B.K.; Kang, D.; Kwon, M.J.; Kim, C.W.; Jeong, C.; Ahn, Y.; Park, H.Y.; Ryu, S.; et al. Menopausal stages and serum lipid and lipoprotein abnormalities in middle-aged women. *Maturitas* **2015**, *80*, 399–405. [CrossRef] [PubMed]
75. Franz, R.; Maturana, M.A.; Magalhães, J.A.; Moraes, R.S.; Spritzer, P.M. Central adiposity and decreased heart rate variability in postmenopause: A cross-sectional study. *Climacteric J. Int. Menopause Soc.* **2013**, *16*, 576–583. [CrossRef]
76. Ji, H.; Kim, A.; Ebinger, J.E.; Niiranen, T.J.; Claggett, B.L.; Bairey Merz, C.N.; Cheng, S. Sex Differences in Blood Pressure Trajectories Over the Life Course. *JAMA Cardiol.* **2020**, *5*, 19–26. [CrossRef]
77. Willett, W.; Rockström, J.; Loken, B.; Springmann, M.; Lang, T.; Vermeulen, S.; Garnett, T.; Tilman, D.; DeClerck, F.; Wood, A.; et al. Food in the Anthropocene: The EAT-Lancet Commission on healthy diets from sustainable food systems. *Lancet* **2019**, *393*, 447–492. [CrossRef]
78. Arnett, D.K.; Blumenthal, R.S.; Albert, M.A.; Buroker, A.B.; Goldberger, Z.D.; Hahn, E.J.; Himmelfarb, C.D.; Khera, A.; Lloyd-Jones, D.; McEvoy, J.W.; et al. 2019 ACC/AHA Guideline on the Primary Prevention of Cardiovascular Disease: A Report of the American College of Cardiology/American Heart Association Task Force on Clinical Practice Guidelines. *Circulation* **2019**, *140*, e596–e646. [CrossRef]
79. Mozaffarian, D.; Benjamin, E.J.; Go, A.S.; Arnett, D.K.; Blaha, M.J.; Cushman, M.; Das, S.R.; de Ferranti, S.; Després, J.P.; Fullerton, H.J.; et al. Heart Disease and Stroke Statistics-2016 Update: A Report From the American Heart Association. *Circulation* **2016**, *133*, e38–e360. [CrossRef]
80. Mosca, L.; Benjamin, E.J.; Berra, K.; Bezanson, J.L.; Dolor, R.J.; Lloyd-Jones, D.M.; Newby, L.K.; Piña, I.L.; Roger, V.L.; Shaw, L.J.; et al. Effectiveness-based guidelines for the prevention of cardiovascular disease in women–2011 update: A guideline from the American Heart Association. *J. Am. Coll. Cardiol.* **2011**, *57*, 1404–1423. [CrossRef]
81. Wang, D.D.; Li, Y.; Bhupathiraju, S.N.; Rosner, B.A.; Sun, Q.; Giovannucci, E.L.; Rimm, E.B.; Manson, J.E.; Willett, W.C.; Stampfer, M.J.; et al. Fruit and Vegetable Intake and Mortality: Results From 2 Prospective Cohort Studies of US Men and Women and a Meta-Analysis of 26 Cohort Studies. *Circulation* **2021**, *143*, 1642–1654. [CrossRef]
82. Wang, D.; Karvonen-Gutierrez, C.A.; Jackson, E.A.; Elliott, M.R.; Appelhans, B.M.; Barinas-Mitchell, E.; Bielak, L.F.; Huang, M.H.; Baylin, A. Western Dietary Pattern Derived by Multiple Statistical Methods Is Prospectively Associated with Subclinical Carotid Atherosclerosis in Midlife Women. *J. Nutr.* **2020**, *150*, 579–591. [CrossRef]
83. Ko, S.H.; Kim, H.S. Menopause-Associated Lipid Metabolic Disorders and Foods Beneficial for Postmenopausal Women. *Nutrients* **2020**, *12*, 202. [CrossRef]
84. Cho, Y.A.; Kim, J.; Cho, E.R.; Shin, A. Dietary patterns and the prevalence of metabolic syndrome in Korean women. *Nutr. Metab. Cardiovasc. Dis. NMCD* **2011**, *21*, 893–900. [CrossRef]
85. Lovejoy, J.C.; Champagne, C.M.; de Jonge, L.; Xie, H.; Smith, S.R. Increased visceral fat and decreased energy expenditure during the menopausal transition. *Int. J. Obes.* **2008**, *32*, 949–958. [CrossRef]
86. Silva, T.R.; Alves, B.C.; Maturana, M.A.; Spritzer, P.M. Healthier dietary pattern and lower risk of metabolic syndrome in physically active postmenopausal women. *J. Am. Coll. Nutr.* **2013**, *32*, 287–295. [CrossRef]
87. Kapoor, E.; Collazo-Clavell, M.L.; Faubion, S.S. Weight Gain in Women at Midlife: A Concise Review of the Pathophysiology and Strategies for Management. *Mayo Clin. Proc.* **2017**, *92*, 1552–1558. [CrossRef] [PubMed]
88. Alves, B.C.; Silva, T.R.; Spritzer, P.M. Sedentary Lifestyle and High-Carbohydrate Intake are Associated with Low-Grade Chronic Inflammation in Post-Menopause: A Cross-sectional Study. *Rev. Bras. Ginecol. Obstet.* **2016**, *38*, 317–324. [CrossRef] [PubMed]

89. Jensen, M.D.; Ryan, D.H.; Apovian, C.M.; Ard, J.D.; Comuzzie, A.G.; Donato, K.A.; Hu, F.B.; Hubbard, V.S.; Jakicic, J.M.; Kushner, R.F.; et al. 2013 AHA/ACC/TOS guideline for the management of overweight and obesity in adults: A report of the American College of Cardiology/American Heart Association Task Force on Practice Guidelines and The Obesity Society. *J. Am. Coll. Cardiol.* **2014**, *63*, 2985–3023. [CrossRef] [PubMed]
90. Mancini, J.G.; Filion, K.B.; Atallah, R.; Eisenberg, M.J. Systematic Review of the Mediterranean Diet for Long-Term Weight Loss. *Am. J. Med.* **2016**, *129*, 407–415.e404. [CrossRef] [PubMed]
91. Thom, G.; Lean, M. Is There an Optimal Diet for Weight Management and Metabolic Health? *Gastroenterology* **2017**, *152*, 1739–1751. [CrossRef]
92. Pugliese, G.D.; Barrea, L.D.; Laudisio, D.D.; Aprano, S.D.; Castellucci, B.D.; Framondi, L.D.; Di Matteo, R.D.; Savastano, S.P.; Colao, A.P.; Muscogiuri, G.D. Mediterranean diet as tool to manage obesity in menopause: A narrative review. *Nutrients* **2020**, *79–80*, 110991. [CrossRef]
93. Cano, A.; Marshall, S.; Zolfaroli, I.; Bitzer, J.; Ceausu, I.; Chedraui, P.; Durmusoglu, F.; Erkkola, R.; Goulis, D.G.; Hirschberg, A.L.; et al. The Mediterranean diet and menopausal health: An EMAS position statement. *Maturitas* **2020**, *139*, 90–97. [CrossRef] [PubMed]
94. Ferreira, L.L.; Silva, T.R.; Maturana, M.A.; Spritzer, P.M. Dietary intake of isoflavones is associated with a lower prevalence of subclinical cardiovascular disease in postmenopausal women: Cross-sectional study. *J. Hum. Nutr. Diet.* **2019**, *32*, 810–818. [CrossRef] [PubMed]
95. Yoshikata, R.; Myint, K.Z.; Ohta, H.; Ishigaki, Y. Inter-relationship between diet, lifestyle habits, gut microflora, and the equol-producer phenotype: Baseline findings from a placebo-controlled intervention trial. *Menopause* **2019**, *26*, 273–285. [CrossRef] [PubMed]

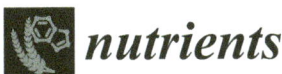

Review

Nutrition Strategy and Life Style in Polycystic Ovary Syndrome—Narrative Review

Małgorzata Szczuko [1,*], Justyna Kikut [1], Urszula Szczuko [1], Iwona Szydłowska [2], Jolanta Nawrocka-Rutkowska [3], Maciej Ziętek [3], Donatella Verbanac [4] and Luciano Saso [5]

1. Department of Human Nutrition and Metabolomics, Pomeranian Medical University in Szczecin, Broniewskiego 24 St, 71-460 Szczecin, Poland; justyna.kikut@pum.edu.pl (J.K.); urszula.szczuko@gmail.com (U.S.)
2. Department of Gynecology, Endocrinology and Gynecological Oncology, Pomeranian Medical University in Szczecin, Unii Lubelskiej 1 St, 71-256 Szczecin, Poland; iwona.szydlowska@pum.edu.pl
3. Department of Perinatology, Obstetrics and Gynecology Pomeranian Medical University in Szczecin, Siedlecka 2 St, 72-010 Police, Poland; jolanta.nawrocka@pum.edu.pl (J.N.-R.); maciej.zietek@pum.edu.pl (M.Z.)
4. Department of Medical Biochemistry and Hematology, Faculty of Pharmacy and Biochemistry, University of Zagreb, A. Kovačića 1, 10000 Zagreb, Croatia; donatella.verbanac@pharma.unizg.hr
5. Department of Physiology and Pharmacology "Vittorio Erspamer", Sapienza University, P. le Aldo Moro 5, 00185 Rome, Italy; luciano.saso@uniroma1.it
* Correspondence: malgorzata.szczuko@pum.edu.pl; Tel.: +48-91-441-4810; Fax: +48-91-441-4807

Abstract: Here we present an extensive narrative review of the broadly understood modifications to the lifestyles of women with polycystic ovary syndrome (PCOS). The PubMed database was analyzed, combining PCOS entries with causes, diseases, diet supplementation, lifestyle, physical activity, and use of herbs. The metabolic pathways leading to disturbances in lipid, carbohydrate, and hormonal metabolism in targeted patients are described. The article refers to sleep disorders, changes in mental health parameters, and causes of oxidative stress and inflammation. These conditions consistently lead to the occurrence of severe diseases in patients suffering from diabetes, the fatty degeneration of internal organs, infertility, atherosclerosis, cardiovascular diseases, dysbiosis, and cancer. The modification of lifestyles, diet patterns and proper selection of nutrients, pharmacological and natural supplementation in the form of herbs, and physical activity have been proposed. The progress and consequences of PCOS are largely modifiable and depend on the patient's approach, although we have to take into account also the genetic determinants.

Keywords: PCOS; reproduction; lifestyle; diet; sleep; supplementation; herbs supporting

1. Introduction

Polycystic ovary syndrome (PCOS) is the most common female endocrinopathy, affecting as many as 15% to 18% of women of reproductive age [1]. The definition of PCOS changed in 2003, when representatives of the European Society of Human Reproduction and American Society of Reproductive Medicine met in Rotterdam, The Netherlands. Currently, it is defined as a heterogeneous group with different phenotypes, which pose challenges in its treatment [2]. It seems, however, that some dependences and the tendency of the occurrence of the similar metabolic disorders are comparable [3].

Many studies have shown that higher hormone levels, gut microbiome composition, and plasma metabolomics are new parameters related to the PCOS phenotypes [4]. The clinical phenotypes can change over the life span with weight gain, and can coexist in the same patient. Individualized treatment remains the main approach, but grouping the phenotypes and following therapeutic recommendations may also prove to be clinically suitable. Precise recommendations should be implemented long before metabolic complications occur, which is particularly important for women with PCOS as they are predisposed

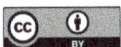

to developing endometrial and ovarian cancer [5,6]. Therefore, the therapeutic approaches aimed at using anti-inflammatory remedies in supplementing and supporting anticancer therapy are crucial. They can help in inactivating the cascade of the deteriorating signaling pathways. Through these, better survival, faster recovery, and the improvement of the patients' quality of life can be achieved.

1.1. Physiological Basis

The four main causes of the physiological basis of PCOS include:
- disorders of gonadotropin hormonal synthesis;
- the appearance of insulin resistance;
- the influence of the present excessive body fat; and finally,
- the metabolic pathways involved in PCOS (the secretion and activity of insulin, encoding for steroidogenesis, and other metabolic and hormonal pathways) (Figure 1) [7].

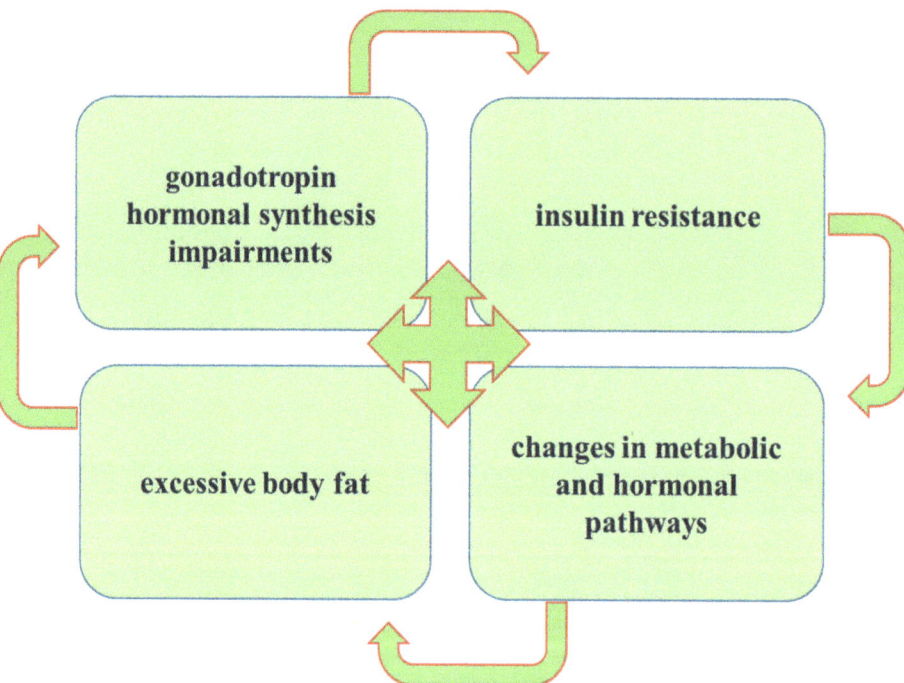

Figure 1. Main pathophysiological basis of polycystic ovary syndrome (PCOS)-disorders of gonadotropin hormonal synthesis, the appearance of insulin resistance, the influence of the present excessive body fat and oblique metabolic pathways involved in PCOS.

Appropriate functioning of the mechanisms responsible for the maturation of the ovarian follicle and its ovulation depends on the proper physiological activity of three organs: the hypothalamus, pituitary gland, and ovaries.

The mechanisms of hormonal regulation in the hypothalamic-pituitary-ovarian system take place through the axes of negative feedback: long, short and ultra short feedback. In the suprachiasmatic nucleus of the hypothalamus there are neurons synthesizing gonadotropin-releasing hormone (GnRH), which is released into the pituitary portal circulation in the median eminence. GnRH release is regulated by a network of interconnected neurons. Gonadoliberin is an example of a hormone secreted in a pulsatile rhythm, and the frequency of this rhythm determines the type of gonadotropin released. A low frequency of gonadoliberin pulses results in the secretion of follicle-stimulating hormone (FSH), while a high frequency results in the secretion of luteinizing hormone (LH) from the anterior lobe of the pituitary gland. LH is responsible for the luteinization of the corpus luteum, i.e., the transformation of granulosa cells into theca lutein cells which produce progesterone. In turn, FSH stimulates ovarian follicle maturation and estrogen secretion in the granulosa cells of ovarian follicles. It also increases the activity of aromatase, the enzyme responsible for converting androgens (testosteron and androstendion) to estrogens. When the concentration of luteinizing hormone increases relative to FSH, excessive androgen production occurs, which is more common in women with PCOS [8].

Insulin, both directly and indirectly, affects the pathogenesis of PCOS. It acts synergistically with luteinizing hormone, increasing the production of androgens (theca cells) and decreasing the liver synthesis of the main binding testosterone protein (SHBG), which results in testosterone circulating in the unbound, active form [8]. Excess body fat is involved in the development of PCOS in many ways. Adipose tissue cells (adipocytes) produce peptide hormones like resistin and leptin, as well as some inflammatory cytokines (IL-beta, TNF-alpha) [9].

The activity of leptin affects the function of the hypothalamus–pituitary gland–ovary axis by modifying the secretion of GnRH, LH, and FSH. Leptin is a signal for the hypothalamus to release LH, causing the secretion of pituitary GnRH, as well. This can result in excessive androgen synthesis. Adipose tissue, by secreting pro-inflammatory factors such as mentioned cytokines, contributes to the development of inflammation in PCOS and an increased amount of free radicals caused by hyperglycemia; excess adipose tissue and androgens contribute to the formation of chronic inflammation in PCOS [8].

The various clinical symptoms of the disease indicate that many metabolic pathways participate in PCOS development, including: secretion and activity of insulin, with genes encoding for insulin receptor (IR), insulin (INS), and insulin-like growth factor (IGF) and its receptor; genes encoding for steroidogenesis; genes responsible for the activity of cytochrome P450 (CYP 17, CYP 11 alpha); and other metabolic and hormonal pathways, with genes for androgenic receptor (AR), LH receptor, leptin, and follistatin [10]. Moderate adherence to an anti-inflammatory dietary pattern and the low glycemic index (GI) and low-fat dietary pattern, have protective effect on the odds of developing PCOS [11,12].

1.2. Improvement in Metabolic Pathways

1.2.1. Insulin Resistance

Weight gain mediates most of its direct medical sequelae through worsening insulin sensitivity.

Insulin resistance (IR) plays a key role in the development of metabolic dysfunction, including hypertension, dysglycemia, and dyslipidemia. A large amount of evidence supports a role of mitochondrial dysfunction in the development of IR, stimulated through ectopic fat deposition. Lipid-induced production of reactive oxygen species (ROS) within skeletal muscle promotes mitochondrial dysfunction and the development of IR [13]. Ultimately, IR underlies obesity-related conditions such as polycystic ovary syndrome (PCOS).

The cellular effects of insulin occur through two main post-receptor pathways: the phosphatidylinositol 3-kinase (PI3K) and the mitogen-activated protein kinase (MAPK) pathways [14]. The PI3K pathway regulates cellular intermediary metabolism, whereas the MAPK pathway controls growth processes and mitoses [14]. AKR1C3 expression in adipocytes leads to the occurrence of insulin resistance and hyperinsulinemia, then drives a vicious circle of intra-adipose androgen activation, lipid accumulation, and hyperinsulinemia [15]. Kauffman et al. suggested that ethnicity plays an additive effect on insulin resistance in PCOS. Mexican American women showed significantly higher insulin resistance compared with Caucasian American women [16].

1.2.2. Oxidative Stress and Chronic Inflammation

The association between body weight and IR is mediated through inflammatory pathways [17]. Obesity causes changes in the release of key cytokines and adipokines, which in turn manifest in paracrine and endocrine effects. The increased levels of leptin and plasminogen activator inhibitor-1 and the reduced release of adiponectin result in a generalized low-grade inflammatory response. This process is mediated by macrophages and other immune cells.

Increases in ROS generation, p47phox gene expression, and circulating thiobarbituric acid-reactive substances (TBARS) occur in PCOS in response to saturated fat ingestion independent of obesity. A diet rich in simple sugars, as well as saturated fatty acids additionally enhances the production of ROS by different mechanisms, including the influence on gut microbiota [18]. Circulating mononuclear cells and excess adipose tissue are separate and distinct contributors to oxidative stress in this disorder [19]. Lipid-stimulated oxidative stress may be a key driver of insulin resistance and hyperandrogenism in PCOS. Excess adipose tissue is a contributor to the pro-oxidant burden and an additional regulator of insulin action [19]. Moreover, the chronic exposure to androgens results in an increase in oxidative stress in islet cells, inducing mitochondrial dysfunction [20,21].

Superoxide is a ROS produced when NADPH is oxidized by membrane-bound NADPH oxidase [22]. Dysregulated ROS production from NADPH oxidase has been implicated in a variety of cardiovascular disorders, including endothelial dysfunction, atherosclerosis, and hypertension, which are observed in women with PCOS [23]. Peroxide-induced oxidative stress activates nuclear factor-κB (NF-κB), which is a cardinal inflammatory signal that increases tumor necrosis factor (TNF)-α gene transcription [24]. Oxidative stress in response to saturated fat ingestion is an intermediate step in stimulating TNF-α secretion from circulating leukocytes [19,25]. In our investigations, we also showed that women with PCOS exhibit increased TNF-α synthesis [4]. Women with PCOS with normal and low levels of androgens measured by the level of testosterone and free androgen index (FAI) were more susceptible to the development of oxidative stress and inflammation induced by TNF-α [26].

1.2.3. Anticancer Protection

Many studies have targeted the inactivation of the transcription factor (NRF2) as a therapeutic approach in various types of cancer [27]. NRF2 was first recognized in anticancer research as an inducer of several antioxidant enzymes. It can protect cells and tissues against many types of toxicant that interrupt essential biochemical processes and carcinogens by increasing the expression of cytoprotective genes [28]. NRF2 can act as a double-edged sword, being able to mediate both tumor-suppressive or pro-oncogenic functions depending on the specific biological context of its activation [29]. In line with this principle, the controlled activation of NRF2 might reduce the risk of cancer initiation and development in normal cells by scavenging ROS and by preventing genomic instability through decreased DNA damage. In contrast, already transformed cells with constitutive or prolonged activation of NRF2 signaling might represent a major clinical hurdle and exhibit an aggressive phenotype characterized by therapy resistance and unfavorable prognosis, requiring the use of NRF2 inhibitors [29].

It has been found that there are at least three pathways controlling the stability of NRF2. The first one depends on the cytosolic repressor KEAP1 [30]; the second is connected with the β-transducin repeat-containing protein (β-TrCP) [31]; while the third is related to the protein HRD1, which is an E3 ubiquitin ligase associated with the endoplasmic reticulum [32].

The abnormal activation of the NRF2/KEAP1 pathway promotes cancer development [33], metastasis formation [34], and even resistance to ovarian cancer therapy [35]. Mutations in the KEAP1 gene induce the hyper activation of the NRF2/KEAP1 pathway. Notably, KEAP1 missense or nonsense mutations were reported in endometrial carcinomas [36], as well as gall bladder [37], breast [38,39], cervical [40], and ovarian [41,42] cancers. MicroRNA miR-141 was the first-identified miRNA to directly repress KEAP1 levels in ovarian carcinoma cell lines [43].

1.3. Gut Microbiota Dysbiosis

The structural and functional dysbiosis of the gut microbiota in high-fat diet (HFD)-induced obesity was demonstrated in a mouse model [44]. The microbiota, through its metabolites, has multiple and complex effects on appetite, lipids, and carbohydrate metabolism and may influence body weight [44,45]. The gut microbiota can regulate about 10% of the host's transcriptome and genes involved in the immune response, proliferation, and metabolism [46]. Interest in dietary fiber, gut fermentation, and probiotics has led to extensive research in this field [47]. The role of dietary fiber was demonstrated to modulate gut microbiota dysbiosis in patients with type 2 diabetes [48]. The growth of *Bifidobacteria* correlates with insulin secretion and increased glucose tolerance, regulates IR, and helps reduce inflammation. Short-chain fatty acids (SCFAs) such as acetate and butirate produced by the beneficial gut flora influence glycemia through glucagon-like peptide 1 (GLP-1) and pancreatic polypeptide (PPY), which are intestinal hormones [45]. The hormone PYY is a peptide that acts as a paracrine substance to stimulate the feelings of satiety or hunger in the control center [49]. Due to the absolute role of metabolites such as SCFAs in the metabolism of lipids and carbohydrates, ensuring the good condition of the microbiota is one of the therapeutic goals [50] in combating inflammation at local and systemic levels [51], as well as infections of the urogenital tract [52].

2. Lifestyle Changes

Lifestyle change is the first line of treatment for the management of women with PCOS but is not an alternative to its pharmacological treatment [7]. Regular physical activity, maintaining appropriate body weight, following healthy dietary patterns and avoiding tobacco use is vital in prevention and treatment of metabolic disorders, and is included in clinical guidelines for various conditions. Focusing on overall wellbeing and mental health is a personal choice, and while it is not an immediate fix, it is an important step towards a more fulfilling life.

Nutritional counseling for PCOS patients has been one of the treatment methods for many years. However, strict caloric restrictions do not produce the expected long-term effects [53,54], and the isocaloric diet did not significantly improve the biochemical and anthropometric parameters even in combination with physical activity [55].

2.1. Diet

Analysis of the impact of lifestyle modification related to the share of energy from macronutrients (protein, fat, and carbohydrates) showed no significant differences in the levels of the analyzed parameters. However, a significant factor in these changes was the reduction in the caloric content of the diet [56] and the introduction of a reduced-calorie diet with a low GI [57]. Low GI (LGI) diets decreased homeostatic model assessment for insulin resistance (HOMA-IR), fasting insulin, total and low-density lipoprotein (LDL) cholesterol, triglycerides, waist circumference, and total testosterone compared with high GI (HGI) diets without affecting fasting glucose, HDL cholesterol, weight, or the free androgen index [58]. In addition, the inclusion of the LGI diet, punitive restrictions, and/or physical activity, and the supplementation of omega-3 increased HDL, sex hormone binding globulin (SHBG) synthesis, and reduction in body fat [8]. Gonzales et al. found that saturated fat acid (SFA) ingestion stimulates increases in circulating TNF-α and peripheral leukocytic suppressor of cytokine-3 (SOCS-3) expression [25]. Therefore, eliminating SFA from the diets of these patients is imperative. Dietary α-linolenic acid-rich flaxseed oil exerted beneficial effects on polycystic ovary syndrome through the sex steroid hormones–microbiota–inflammation axis in rats, but other sources of α-linolenic acid will probably produce an equally good effect [59].

The effects of soluble dietary fiber on SCFAs were demonstrated. Fermentable fiber has positive metabolic benefits on the gut microbiome with subsequent release of SCFAs [60]. Diets with a low GI may influence appetite-regulating hormones including ghrelin and glucagon [12,61]. Low-GI meals reduced ghrelin and increased glucagon in women with PCOS [61]. High fructose consumption (HFC) synergistically aggravated endocrine but not metabolic changes in PCOS, suggesting that (HFC) might deteriorate endocrine-related phenotypes in PCOS [62]. A meta-analysis and systematic review showed that the LGI diet is an effective, acceptable, and safe intervention for relieving IR, and professional dietary advice should be offered to all PCOS patients [63,64].

It seems that another reduced-GI diet modification is the ketogenic diet, which limits the consumption of total carbohydrates in favor of plant-based fat. The ketogenic diet (KD) improves the menstrual cycle, reducing blood glucose and body weight, improving liver function, and treating fatty liver in women with PCOS and liver dysfunction who were obese [65]. Even more interesting results were reported by Paoli et al. after using the KD for 12 weeks in women with PCOS [66]. The anthropometric and body composition measurements revealed a significant reduction in body weight (-9.43 kg), body mass index (BMI; -3.35), and fat-free body mass (8.29 kg). A significant decrease in glucose and insulin blood levels was observed, together with a significant improvement in HOMA-IR scores. A significant decrease of triglycerides, total cholesterol and LDL were observed along with a rise in HDL levels. The LH/FSH ratio, LH total and free testosterone, and DHEAS blood levels were also significantly reduced. Estradiol, progesterone and SHBG increased. The Ferriman Gallwey Score was slightly, although not significantly, reduced [66]. There was no significant association between parameters of hirsutism and the visceral adiposity index (VAI). Hirsutism is unlikely to be due to visceral adipocyte dysfunction [67]. Therefore, in PCOS patients with advanced obesity and/or obesity accompanied by full-blown metabolic syndrome, the introduction of a ketogenic diet may provide even better results than a diet with a LGI. Nonetheless, a general conclusion is that by following the main principles of a healthy diet, the physiological homeostasis can be managed, as well as faster recovery from disease achieved.

2.2. Physical Activity

Exercise training in the management of PCOS is becoming more recognized and accepted among professionals in the health sector and the patients. Physical training potentiates the effects caused by insulin sensitivity through the optimization of glucose transport and metabolism [68].

A recent meta-analysis found that improvements in health outcomes are more dependent on exercise intensity than dose. The results from this analysis support the use of exercise and that vigorous intensity exercise may have the greatest impact on cardiorespiratory fitness, insulin resistance, and body composition [69]. Insulin resistance, measured using the HOMA-IR and BMI showed a significant decrease with moderate and high certainty (MD-0.57; 95% confidence interval (CI), -0.98 to -0.16, and $p = 0.01$; MD-1.90, 95% CI -3.37, -0.42, and $p = 0.01$), respectively [70]. Other authors in a systematic review found that vigorous aerobic exercise and resistance training to improve insulin sensitivity and androgen measurements are warranted for women with PCOS. [71]. The minimum aerobic activity per week should be 120 min [69].

2.3. Sleep

Mental health disorders are highly prevalent in PCOS cases, which are associated with significantly more frequently experienced states of anxiety and depression, as well as sleep disorders [72]. Sleep disorders impact the etiology and development of the anxiety and depression seen in PCOS, so treating sleep-related conditions should be an integral part of treating women with PCOS [72]. Sleep deprivation has been connected with increased risk of IR, obesity, and type 2 diabetes (T2D) [73–75]. Although incompletely understood, the factors that mediate IR in response to sleep deprivation, likely implicated centrally regulated autonomic pathways, endocrine responses (e.g., changes in the key appetite hormones ghrelin and leptin), and inflammatory status. Mice experiencing sleep fragmentation (SF) showed white adipose tissue (WAT) inflammation and worsened IR, which resulted from enhanced disruption to the colonic epithelial barrier [76] and "gut leakage" syndrome which leads to LPS mediated inflammation [51]. Thus, SF-induced metabolic alterations may be mediated in part by concurrent changes in the gut microbiota, thereby providing an opportunity for gut-microbiome-targeted therapeutics [76]. The main pineal gland hormone melatonin is involved in the regulation of the circadian rhythm. In recent years, it was observed that a reduction in the melatonin levels of follicular fluid occurs in PCOS patients [77]. Melatonin receptors in the ovary and intrafollicular fluid adjust sex steroid secretion at different phases of ovarian follicular maturation. Melatonin is a strong antioxidant and an effective free-radical scavenger, which protects ovarian follicles during follicular maturation [77].

Based on current knowledge, it is plausible to conclude that sleep disorders can be considered as one of the first symptoms leading to the weakening of the body's protective properties and intensification of the pathways associated with insulin resistance in the course of PCOS.

2.4. Supplementation

The research showed that the vast majority of women with PCOS consume an improperly balanced diet, involving deficiencies in fiber, omega 3, calcium, magnesium, zinc, and vitamins (folic acid, vitamin C, vitamin B12, and vitamin D) [8]. An excess of nutrients was also noted in sucrase, sodium, total fats, saturated fatty acids, and cholesterol [8]. It was examined whether the deficiencies can be balanced with a correct calories-reduction diet with a lowered GI and it resulted positive regarding influence on the water-soluble vitamins [78,79]. In the case of most vitamin B, the increase in its supply with the diet led to the expected result in the form of its increased level in the plasma of women with PCOS. This effect was not observed for vitamin B3, and the levels of B2 and thiamine were not as satisfactory as in the case of the other, related vitamins [79]. It was documented that the insufficient supply of vitamin B3 is associated with the development of inflammatory conditions, leading to the associated diseases [80] as well as the increased risk of cardiovascular syndromes [81]. Women with PCOS may be treated with metformin, which normalizes glycemia, but its chronic intake is additionally associated with deficiencies in thiamine and cobalamin [82]. Therefore, it is a good idea to supplement with thiamine, which, by activating transketolase, contributing to the inhibition of mechanisms damaging blood vessels, reducing the risk of cardiovascular diseases [83,84].

While drawing attention to the potential properties of blood vessel protection in PCOS, supplementation with coenzyme Q10 also requires consideration. CoQ10 supplementation for 8 weeks had a beneficial effect on inflammatory and endothelial dysfunction markers in overweight and obese patients with PCOS [85].

When analyzing the available literature on supplementation in PCOS, attention should be paid to vitamin D, which increases insulin synthesis and release, increases insulin receptor expression, and increases insulin response to glucose transport [86]. Vitamin D indirectly influences carbohydrate metabolism by normalizing extracellular calcium and parathyroid hormone concentration. It also affects the expression of the genes of the metabolic pathways affecting systemic inflammation by inhibiting the synthesis of pro-inflammatory cytokines, which may contribute to the occurrence of IR [87]. Women with PCOS receiving 20,000 IU of cholecalciferol weekly benefited from improved carbohydrate metabolism. Decreases in fasting glucose, triglycerides, and estradiol were observed. Although no changes in androgen levels were observed, improvements in menstrual frequency were noted [88]. Combined magnesium, zinc, calcium, and vitamin D supplementation in another study led to a significant reduction in hirsutism and total testosterone compared with the placebo, but supplementation did not affect SHBG levels or the free androgen index (FAI) [89]. Conversely, the combination of vitamin D and fish oil reduced the parameters of inflammation in the body (serum C-reactive protein (CRP), downregulation of interleukin (IL)-1 genes) and total testosterone levels and has beneficial effect on mental health parameters measured by Beck's Depression Questionnaire [90].

Current results showed that myo-inositol is as effective as metformin in improving the clinical and metabolic profile of women with PCOS and the metabolic disorders associated with diabetes [91]. However, the administration of metformin is associated with side effects that are not experienced with inositol [92]. Inositol increases insulin sensitivity, normalizes androgens in the blood, improves glycemia, and affects numerous features of metabolic syndrome [93,94]. PCOS appears to involve increased epimerization of myo-inositol (MI) to d-chiro-inositol (DCI) in the ovary by insulin, the consequence of which is overproduction of DCI and deficiency of MI, which in turn affects the disturbance of FSH signaling and deterioration of the quality of oocytes [95]. Inositols (both isomers, both given separately and in combination) also have the potential to restore spontaneous ovulation and improve fertility in women with PCOS. An analysis of the literature showed supplementation with inositol as being a safe and, importantly, effective form of PCOS therapy, improving the development of ovarian follicles, oocyte maturation, and stimulation of pregnancy [96].

As in traditional medicine, natural substances such as isoquinoline alkaloids have been used to regulate the synthesis of androgens and the metabolism of lipids and carbohydrates, the introduction of berberine in patients with PCOS has been considered [97–99]. As with metformin, the beneficial metabolic effects of berberine in type II diabetes are related to the activation of adenosine monophosphate-activated protein kinase (AMPK). Berberine has good hypoglycemic and hypolipidemic effects, reduces body weight, and is an effective insulin sensitizer [100]. It also reduces the synthesis of steroid hormones and the expression of ovarian aromatase by acting on the hypothalamic–pituitary–ovarian axis, and improves the ovulation rate and the regulation of menstruation, thus increasing the pregnancy and live birth rates. In addition, studies showed that even with long-term use of berberine, its side effects are transient and mild (constipation, nausea) [101], which suggests that berberine may be a safe and promising compound for the treatment of PCOS patients [98,102].

Chromium is the basic element involved in the metabolism of carbohydrates and lipids; therefore, it has become one of the most commonly consumed dietary supplements in the USA [103]. The indications for its supplementation were once very broad; however, chrome is currently one of the most controversial components by which its influence is strongly undermined [104,105]. It was argued that it is not an essential micronutrient, but has potential benefits and/or side effects. By enhancing the insulin signaling pathway, increasing the activity of AMPK, and increasing cellular glucose uptake, it has a beneficial effect in PCOS patients in improving diabetes [106]. Decreases in the expressions of 3β-hydroxysteroid dehydrogenase and 17β-hydroxysteroid dehydrogenase were identified in adipose tissue, which were related to dehydroepiandrosterone [107].

The research, and the available literature, show that supplementation with zinc and selenium to counter deficiencies may be indicated in the case of at least some patients with PCOS. Due to intracellular signaling and structural functions, zinc plays a role in lipid and glucose metabolism and fertility [108]. Low zinc intake in obese people is associated with hyperinsulinemia, increased low-grade inflammation, and a worsened lipid profile. In addition, zinc ions can act in an insulin-mimetic manner in adipocytes, stimulating lipogenesis and glucose transport through the translocation of glucose transporter 4 (GLUT4) to the plasma membrane [109]. Zinc deficiency may play a significant role in the pathogenesis of PCOS and may be a prognostic marker of PCOS. Studies showed that the average serum zinc levels of PCOS patients are significantly lower compared with healthy controls [110]. In addition, serum zinc levels were shown to be lower in PCOS patients with impaired glucose tolerance than in PCOS patients with normal glucose tolerance. [110]. Selenium is associated with a lower level of CRP. It has anti-inflammatory and antioxidant properties [111]. Finally, it is necessary to supplement the omega-3 fatty acids, which tend to lack in the diet of PCOS women. However, with the balanced diet, supplementation can be regarded as a seasonal intervention [112]. Polyunsaturated fatty acids (PUFAs) enhance the reproductive performance in PCOS by increasing the expression of steroidogenesis enzymes, which are related to hormone secretion and ovarian functions, and the protein levels of CYP51, CYP19, StAR, and 3β-HSD [113]. In summary, supplementing the diet is an individual subject that requires dietary consultation with the patient, and its active participation and compliance is desirable for the overall improvement of the metabolic equilibrium. A properly balanced diet and a healthy lifestyle should be the first element of PCOS therapy.

2.5. Herbs Supporting Treatment

A balanced diet to support insulin management is the most important treatment for PCOS; drinking infusions of some herbs would therefore be a very good complement to the therapy, such as *Aloe vera*, cinnamon (*Cinnamomum verum*), green tea (*Camellia sinensi*), and chamomile (*Matricaria chamomilla*), and white mulberry (*Morus alba*) [114]. There are medical herbs can affect the lipid profile, blood glucose, and IR [115]. Because these herbs have properties of regulating lipid and carbohydrate metabolism they can be used by all phenotypes of PCOS women. Several of the herbs also have endocrine properties, these were the ones mentioned earlier: green tea [116] and marjoram (*Maiorana hortensis*) are some of the herbs whose effects include improvements in hormonal levels, ovaries weight, insulin sensitivity, antioxidants, and anti-inflammatory parameters [117,118].

Another group of herbs is indicated especially for women with PCOS with biochemical evidence of increased levels of androgens: green mint (*Mentha spicata* L.), which has an antiandrogenic effect and restores follicular development in ovarian tissue [119,120]; licorice smooth (*Glycyrrhiza glabra*) has been used in the treatment of PCOS because of its antiandrogen and estrogen-like activity. Licorice root appears to be effective in reducing excess testosterone as it blocks the conversion of androstenedione. Glycyrrhetinic acid and metabolites block 11 beta-hydroxysteroid dehydrogenase type 2 and bind mineralocorticoid receptors directly, acting as agonists [121,122]. However, licorice is not a flawless solution, having the potential to induce hypertension, hypokalemia, and metabolic alkalosis [123]. People with high cortisol levels should, therefore, avoid this preparation. The available literature suggests a role of herbal drugs in the action against 5-alpha-reductase enzyme, inhibiting it and reducing hair loss [124]. *Serenoa repens*, *Camellia sinensis*, *Rosmarinus officinalis*, and *Glycyrrhiza glabra* can also lower androgen levels and inhibit androgenetic alopecia [124]. *Vitex agnus-castus* is a good regulator of the menstrual cycle and has been used in traditional medicine for centuries [125]. The best-studied dietary phytoestrogens are the flaxseed lignans [126]. The lignan content of flax-seed (*Linum usitatissimum*) may alter the activity of key enzymes involved in estrogen synthesis (e.g., aromatase) to modulate relative levels of circulating sex hormones and their metabolites [127].

Turmeric (*Curcuma longa*), and specifically curcumin, is a biologically active phytochemical ingredient [128,129]. Curcumin seems to be an efficient reducer of oxidative-stress-related complications in patients with PCOS [130,131]. Moreover, curcumin attenuates proangiogenic and proinflammatory factors in human eutopic endometrial stromal cells through the NF-κB signaling pathway [132]. Nettle (*Urtica dioica*) is a multipurpose herb in medicine for which some antioxidative, anti-inflammatory, antimutation, and antitumor properties were identified [133,134]. The flavonoids are a family of compounds with antioxidant activities that can modify specific enzymes, so they can inactivate some agents such as nitrite peroxide and hydroxide radicals [135].

Ultimately, in advanced PCOS with accompanying disease associated with metabolic syndrome and the steatosis of internal organs (especially non-alcoholic fatty liver disease), herbs and their extracts with proven properties should be considered for their hepatoprotective activities [136]. These substances include the silymarin contained in milk thistle (*Silybum marianum*) [137,138] and sesquiterpenes and antioxidant-active ingredients in artichoke (*Cynara Cardunculus*) extract [139,140]. Dandelion (*Taraxacum officinale*) and its component taraxasterol may silence the gene of SIRT1, preventing the disruption of hepatic cells [141]. Black cumin (*Nigella sativa*) also has similar properties, which should be included in the diet of obese PCOS patients [142]. To summarize, herbs and the substances they contain offer many possibilities for interventions supporting the treatment of PCOS at various stages of disease. The selection of the appropriate mixture may be individualized depending on the occurrence of symptoms. Summary information has been added in Table 1.

Table 1. Table summarizing described interventions of herbs and their effects.

A Symptom Accompanying PCOS	Diet	Physical Activity	Sleep Regulation	Supplementation	Microbiota	Herbs
Hirsutism	reduced diet [26,44,45,54,58]			magnesium, zinc, calcium [89,108–111], and vitamin D [86–90], myo-inositol [93–96]		green mint [120,121], licorice smooth [122], *Serenoa repens*, *Camellia sinensis*, *Rosmarinus officinalis*, and *Glycyrrhiza glabra*
The androgens levels	diet with reduced GI and calorie [26,44,45,54,58], Ketogenic diet [64]			magnesium, zinc, calcium [89,108–111], and vitamin D [86–90], berberine [97–102], chromium [105–107], zinc [110]		green mint [120,121], licorice smooth [122], *Serenoa repens*, *Camellia sinensis*, *Rosmarinus officinalis*, and *Glycyrrhiza glabra* [124]
Ovulation disorders	diet with reduced GI and calorie [26,44,45,54,58], Ketogenic diet [64]			vitamin D [86–90], myo-inositol [97,98] berberine [99], zinc [108], PUFAs [112,113]		green mint [120,121], licorice smooth [121], *Vitex agnus-castus* [124], flax-seed [59,125,126]
Fat mass reduction	high-fiber diet with reduced GI and calorie [28,46,47,56,60], ketogenic diet [64] elimination SFA [22,58]	daily physical activity [68–71]	improving sleep [72–77]		microbiota and metabolites [46,47]	
Carbohydrate metabolism disorders	high-fiber diet with reduced GI and calorie [26,44,45,54,58], ketogenic diet [64]	daily physical activity [68–71]	improving sleep [72–77]	vitamin B1 [82–84], vitamin D [86–90], myo-inositol [91–96], berberine [97–102], chromium [105–107], zinc [109]	SCFA [47,52], microbiota and metabolites [50]	Aloe vera, cinnamon, green tea [115], chamomile and white mulberry [117]
Insulin resistance	high-fiber diet with reduced GI and calorie [26,44,45,54,58], elimination SFA [22,58]	daily physical activity [71–74]	improving sleep [72–77] melatonin [77]	vitamin D [86–90], myo-inositol [91–96], berberine [97–102]	Bifidobacteria [45,50]	Aloe vera, cinnamon, green tea, chamomile and white mulberry [117]
Lipids metabolism disorders	high-fiber diet with reduced GI and calorie [26,44,45,54,58], elimination SFA [25,60]	daily physical activity [68–71]		omega 3 [112,113], berberine [97–102], zinc [110]	SCFA [47,52]; microbiota and metabolites [50]	milk thistle [137,138] artichoke extract [139,140]. Dandelion [141], Black cumin [142]
Steatosis of organs-liver profile	high-fiber diet with reduced GI and calorie [46,47,56,60]			silymarin [137,138], sesquiterpenes [139,140], taraxasterol [141]		milk thistle [137,138] artichoke extract [139,140]. Dandelion [141], Black cumin [142]
Cardiovascular diseases	high-fiber diet with reduced GI and calorie [46,47,56,60]	intensity exercise [72]		α-linolenic acid [59], vitamin B3 [80,81], vitamin B1 [82–84], coenzyme Q10 [85]		
Intestinal dysbiosis	high-fiber diet [49,50]				Bifidobacteria [45,50]	

Table 1. Cont.

A Symptom Accompanying PCOS	Diet	Physical Activity	Sleep Regulation	Supplementation	Microbiota	Herbs
Chronic inflammation	high-fiber diet with reduced GI and calorie [28,46,47,56,60]		melatonin [79]	α-linolenic acid [59], vitamin B3 [80,81], coenzyme Q10 [85], vitamin D [88,89], selenium [112], flavonoids [135]	Bifidobacteria [45,50]	Green tea and Marjoram [117–119], Turmeric [128–131], Nettle [133,134], milk thistle [137,138] Artichoke extract [139,140]. Dandelion [141], Black cumin [142]
Limiting predisposition to cancer	elimination SFA [25,27]; high-fiber diet [49,50]			α-linolenic acid [59]		Turmeric [128–131], Nettle [133,134]
Mental health disorders		daily physical activity [71–74]	improving sleep [75]	vitamin D [86–90], omega 3 (fish oil) [72,90]		

SCFA—short-chain fatty acids; GI—glycemic index; SFA—saturated fat acids; PUFA—Polyunsaturated fatty acid.

3. Conclusions

The analysis of metabolic symptoms occurring in the course of PCOS points to the need for a multidirectional therapeutic approach. The metabolic pathways leading to the abnormalities are presented, which requires focusing on the improvement of parameters related to fertility, hirsutism, the occurrence of carbohydrate-lipid disturbances and the reduction of insulin resistance. One of the most important pathways for blocking carcinogenesis is presented. It has been shown that significant improvement of these parameters depends on modifiable factors related to the improvement of lifestyle, the introduction of a diet, especially a low-calorie diet with reduced GI, normalization of sleep and the introduction of daily physical activity. In addition, supplementing the diet with antioxidants and herbs seems to be highly effective in combating the chronic inflammation (*Curcuma longa*), improving liver steatosis (*Silybum marianum*, *Nigella sativa*) and the frequently occurring intestinal dysbiosis (probiotic therapy). Conducting our own research in this area, we examined how increasing the supply of vitamins and minerals with the diet affects the supply of these components in patients, so we also searched the literature and described suggested supplementation (inositol, thiamine, coenzyme Q10, vitamin D, zinc, selenium). Undoubtedly there is a need for further research to be undertaken to determine the efficacy and applicability of the ingredients described as a support for traditional PCOS management.

4. Methods of Searching

In this study, we reviewed the literature focused on PCOS therapy, unrelated to medical therapy, by searching the records of international PubMed and Embase (Elsevier) databases from the last 20 years.

All articles collected through the electronic search process used in this article were reviewed from the abstract. Articles unrelated to the main topic, duplicate papers in both databases (PubMed and Embase), and conference abstracts were excluded from the review process. Only articles published in English were considered.

The main core of the issue was the authors' own 10 years of experience and research in this patient group. From the authors' own studies, those that corresponded sequentially to the intervention steps discussed were selected. The physiological basis was discussed (searching the database for PCOS and insulin resistance or chronic inflammation or endocrine disorders or cancer or microbiota). Lifestyle changes were then discussed. Studies that examined the association between PCOS and diet or supplementation (pcos + inositol; PCOS + berberine; PCOS + vitamin D; PCOS + chromium; PCOS + zinc; PCOS + selenium; PCOS + melatonin) or adjunctive herbs were included in the review. In the case of duplication of information in publications, those that contribute most to the main topic were selected.

Author Contributions: Conceptualization, M.S.; Data curation: M.S., J.K., U.S.; Funding acquisition, M.S., I.S. and J.N.-R.; Methodology M.S., J.K., U.S., M.Z.; Visualization M.S. and L.S; Writing—original draft preparation, M.S., J.K., D.V.; Writing—review and editing, MS., J.K., I.S., J.N.-R., M.Z. and L.S.; Project administration, M.S.; Supervision, M.S. All authors have read and agreed to the published version of the manuscript.

Funding: This research received no external funding.

Institutional Review Board Statement: Does not apply to this study.

Informed Consent Statement: Informed consent was obtained from all subjects involved in the study.

Data Availability Statement: The study did not report any data.

Conflicts of Interest: The authors declare no conflict of interest.

References

1. Fauser, B.C.J.M.; Tarlatzis, B.C.; Rebar, R.W.; Legro, R.S.; Balen, A.H.; Lobo, R.; Carmina, E.; Chang, J.; Yildiz, B.O.; Laven, J.S.E.; et al. Consensus on Women's Health Aspects of Polycystic Ovary Syndrome (PCOS): The Amsterdam ESHRE/ASRM-Sponsored 3rd PCOS Consensus Workshop Group. *Fertil. Steril.* **2012**, *97*, 28–38.e25. [CrossRef]
2. Zuo, M.; Liao, G.; Zhang, W.; Xu, D.; Lu, J.; Tang, W.; Yan, Y.; Hong, C.; Wang, Y. Effects of Exogenous Adiponectin Supplementation in Early Pregnant PCOS Mice on the Metabolic Syndrome of Adult Female Offspring. *J. Ovarian Res.* **2021**, *14*, 15. [CrossRef]
3. Szczuko, M.; Zapałowska-Chwyć, M.; Maciejewska, D.; Drozd, A.; Starczewski, A.; Stachowska, E. Significant Improvement Selected Mediators of Inflammation in Phenotypes of Women with PCOS after Reduction and Low GI Diet. *Mediat. Inflamm.* **2017**, *2017*, 5489523. [CrossRef]
4. Ma, L.; Cao, Y.; Ma, Y.; Zhai, J. Association between hyperandrogenism and adverse pregnancy outcomes in patients with different polycystic ovary syndrome phenotypes undergoing in vitro fertilization/intracytoplasmic sperm injection: A systematic review and meta-analysis. *Gynecol. Endocrinol.* **2021**, 1–8. [CrossRef] [PubMed]
5. Martini, A.E.; Healy, M.W. Polycystic Ovarian Syndrome: Impact on Adult and Fetal Health. *Clin. Obs. Gynecol.* **2021**, *64*, 26–32. [CrossRef]
6. Hong, G.; Wu, H.; Ma, S.-T.; Su, Z. Catechins from Oolong Tea Improve Uterine Defects by Inhibiting STAT3 Signaling in Polycystic Ovary Syndrome Mice. *Chin. Med.* **2020**, *15*, 125. [CrossRef]
7. Del Pup, L.; Cagnacci, A. IMPROVE Lifestyle in Polycystic Ovary Syndrome: A Systematic Strategy. *Gynecol. Endocrinol.* **2021**, 1–4. [CrossRef]
8. Szczuko, M.; Skowronek, M.; Zapałowska-Chwyć, M.; Starczewski, A. Quantitative Assessment of Nutrition in Patients with Polycystic Ovary Syndrome (PCOS). *Rocz. Panstw. Zakl. Hig.* **2016**, *67*, 419–426. [PubMed]
9. Makki, K.; Froguel, P.; Wolowczuk, I. Adipose Tissue in Obesity-Related Inflammation and Insulin Resistance: Cells, Cytokines, and Chemokines. *ISRN Inflamm.* **2013**, *2013*, 139239. [CrossRef] [PubMed]
10. Dniak-Nikolajew, A. Zespół Policystycznych Jajników Jako Przyczyna Niepłodności Kobiecej [Polycystic Ovary Syndrome as a Cause of Female Infertility]. *Położna Nauka I Prakt.* **2012**, *17*, 14–17.
11. Panjeshahin, A.; Salehi-Abargouei, A.; Anari, A.G.; Mohammadi, M.; Hosseinzadeh, M. Association between Empirically Derived Dietary Patterns and Polycystic Ovary Syndrome: A Case-Control Study. *Nutrition* **2020**, *79–80*, 110987. [CrossRef]
12. Szczuko, M.; Zapalowska-Chwyć, M.; Drozd, R. A Low Glycemic Index Decreases Inflammation by Increasing the Concentration of Uric Acid and the Activity of Glutathione Peroxidase (GPx3) in Patients with Polycystic Ovary Syndrome (PCOS). *Molecules* **2019**, *24*, 1508. [CrossRef]
13. Di Meo, S.; Iossa, S.; Venditti, P. Skeletal Muscle Insulin Resistance: Role of Mitochondria and Other ROS Sources. *J. Endocrinol.* **2017**, *233*, R15–R42. [CrossRef]
14. Barber, T.M.; Kyrou, I.; Randeva, H.S.; Weickert, M.O. Mechanisms of Insulin Resistance at the Crossroad of Obesity with Associated Metabolic Abnormalities and Cognitive Dysfunction. *Int. J. Mol. Sci.* **2021**, *22*, 546. [CrossRef]
15. Kempegowda, P.; Melson, E.; Manolopoulos, K.N.; Arlt, W.; O'Reilly, M.W. Implicating Androgen Excess in Propagating Metabolic Disease in Polycystic Ovary Syndrome. *Adv. Endocrinol. Metab.* **2020**, *11*. [CrossRef]
16. Kauffman, R.P.; Baker, V.M.; Dimarino, P.; Gimpel, T.; Castracane, V.D. Polycystic Ovarian Syndrome and Insulin Resistance in White and Mexican American Women: A Comparison of Two Distinct Populations. *Am. J. Obs. Gynecol.* **2002**, *187*, 1362–1369. [CrossRef] [PubMed]
17. Shoelson, S.E.; Herrero, L.; Naaz, A. Obesity, Inflammation, and Insulin Resistance. *Gastroenterology* **2007**, *132*, 2169–2180. [CrossRef] [PubMed]

18. Fajstova, A.; Galanova, N.; Coufal, S.; Malkova, J.; Kostovcik, M.; Cermakova, M.; Pelantova, H.; Kuzma, M.; Sediva, B.; Hudcovic, T.; et al. Diet Rich in Simple Sugars Promotes Pro-Inflammatory Response via Gut Microbiota Alteration and TLR4 Signaling. *Cells* **2020**, *9*, 2701. [CrossRef]
19. González, F.; Considine, R.V.; Abdelhadi, O.A.; Acton, A.J. Oxidative Stress in Response to Saturated Fat Ingestion Is Linked to Insulin Resistance and Hyperandrogenism in Polycystic Ovary Syndrome. *J. Clin. Endocrinol. Metab.* **2019**, *104*, 5360–5371. [CrossRef]
20. Wang, H.; Wang, X.; Zhu, Y.; Chen, F.; Sun, Y.; Han, X. Increased Androgen Levels in Rats Impair Glucose-Stimulated Insulin Secretion through Disruption of Pancreatic Beta Cell Mitochondrial Function. *J. Steroid Biochem. Mol. Biol.* **2015**, *154*, 254–266. [CrossRef] [PubMed]
21. Liu, S.; Navarro, G.; Mauvais-Jarvis, F. Androgen Excess Produces Systemic Oxidative Stress and Predisposes to Beta-Cell Failure in Female Mice. *PLoS ONE* **2010**, *5*, e11302. [CrossRef]
22. Jiang, F.; Zhang, Y.; Dusting, G.J. NADPH Oxidase-Mediated Redox Signaling: Roles in Cellular Stress Response, Stress Tolerance, and Tissue Repair. *Pharm. Rev.* **2011**, *63*, 218–242. [CrossRef] [PubMed]
23. Bedard, K.; Krause, K.-H. The NOX Family of ROS-Generating NADPH Oxidases: Physiology and Pathophysiology. *Physiol. Rev.* **2007**, *87*, 245–313. [CrossRef] [PubMed]
24. Evans, J.L.; Goldfine, I.D.; Maddux, B.A.; Grodsky, G.M. Oxidative Stress and Stress-Activated Signaling Pathways: A Unifying Hypothesis of Type 2 Diabetes. *Endocr. Rev.* **2002**, *23*, 599–622. [CrossRef] [PubMed]
25. González, F.; Considine, R.V.; Abdelhadi, O.A.; Acton, A.J. Saturated Fat Ingestion Promotes Lipopolysaccharide-Mediated Inflammation and Insulin Resistance in Polycystic Ovary Syndrome. *J. Clin. Endocrinol. Metab.* **2018**, *104*, 934–946. [CrossRef] [PubMed]
26. Szczuko, M.; Zapałowska-Chwyć, M.; Maciejewska, D.; Drozd, A.; Starczewski, A.; Stachowska, E. High Glycemic Index Diet in PCOS Patients. The Analysis of IGF I and TNF-α Pathways in Metabolic Disorders. *Med. Hypotheses* **2016**, *96*, 42–47. [CrossRef]
27. Panieri, E.; Saso, L. Potential Applications of NRF2 Inhibitors in Cancer Therapy. *Oxidative Med. Cell. Longev.* **2019**, *2019*, e8592348. [CrossRef]
28. Panieri, E.; Buha, A.; Telkoparan-Akillilar, P.; Cevik, D.; Kouretas, D.; Veskoukis, A.; Skaperda, Z.; Tsatsakis, A.; Wallace, D.; Suzen, S.; et al. Potential Applications of NRF2 Modulators in Cancer Therapy. *Antioxidants* **2020**, *9*, 193. [CrossRef]
29. Panieri, E.; Telkoparan-Akillilar, P.; Suzen, S.; Saso, L. The NRF2/KEAP1 Axis in the Regulation of Tumor Metabolism: Mechanisms and Therapeutic Perspectives. *Biomolecules* **2020**, *10*, 791. [CrossRef] [PubMed]
30. Suzuki, T.; Yamamoto, M. Stress-Sensing Mechanisms and the Physiological Roles of the Keap1-Nrf2 System during Cellular Stress. *J. Biol. Chem.* **2017**, *292*, 16817–16824. [CrossRef]
31. Chowdhry, S.; Zhang, Y.; McMahon, M.; Sutherland, C.; Cuadrado, A.; Hayes, J.D. Nrf2 Is Controlled by Two Distinct β-TrCP Recognition Motifs in Its Neh6 Domain, One of Which Can Be Modulated by GSK-3 Activity. *Oncogene* **2013**, *32*, 3765–3781. [CrossRef]
32. Wu, T.; Zhao, F.; Gao, B.; Tan, C.; Yagishita, N.; Nakajima, T.; Wong, P.K.; Chapman, E.; Fang, D.; Zhang, D.D. Hrd1 Suppresses Nrf2-Mediated Cellular Protection during Liver Cirrhosis. *Genes Dev.* **2014**, *28*, 708–722. [CrossRef]
33. Rojo, A.I.; Rada, P.; Mendiola, M.; Ortega-Molina, A.; Wojdyla, K.; Rogowska-Wrzesinska, A.; Hardisson, D.; Serrano, M.; Cuadrado, A. The PTEN/NRF2 Axis Promotes Human Carcinogenesis. *Antioxid. Redox. Signal.* **2014**, *21*, 2498–2514. [CrossRef] [PubMed]
34. Zhang, C.; Wang, H.-J.; Bao, Q.-C.; Wang, L.; Guo, T.-K.; Chen, W.-L.; Xu, L.-L.; Zhou, H.-S.; Bian, J.-L.; Yang, Y.-R.; et al. NRF2 Promotes Breast Cancer Cell Proliferation and Metastasis by Increasing RhoA/ROCK Pathway Signal Transduction. *Oncotarget* **2016**, *7*, 73593–73606. [CrossRef] [PubMed]
35. Bao, L.; Wu, J.; Dodson, M.; Rojo de la Vega, E.M.; Ning, Y.; Zhang, Z.; Yao, M.; Zhang, D.D.; Xu, C.; Yi, X. ABCF2, an Nrf2 Target Gene, Contributes to Cisplatin Resistance in Ovarian Cancer Cells. *Mol. Carcinog.* **2017**, *56*, 1543–1553. [CrossRef]
36. Wong, T.F.; Yoshinaga, K.; Monma, Y.; Ito, K.; Niikura, H.; Nagase, S.; Yamamoto, M.; Yaegashi, N. Association of Keap1 and Nrf2 Genetic Mutations and Polymorphisms with Endometrioid Endometrial Adenocarcinoma Survival. *Int. J. Gynecol. Cancer* **2011**, *21*, 1428–1435. [CrossRef] [PubMed]
37. Shibata, T.; Kokubu, A.; Gotoh, M.; Ojima, H.; Ohta, T.; Yamamoto, M.; Hirohashi, S. Genetic Alteration of Keap1 Confers Constitutive Nrf2 Activation and Resistance to Chemotherapy in Gallbladder Cancer. *Gastroenterology* **2008**, *135*, 1358–1368. e4. [CrossRef]
38. Nioi, P.; Nguyen, T. A Mutation of Keap1 Found in Breast Cancer Impairs Its Ability to Repress Nrf2 Activity. *Biochem. Biophys. Res. Commun* **2007**, *362*, 816–821. [CrossRef]
39. Sjöblom, T.; Jones, S.; Wood, L.D.; Parsons, D.W.; Lin, J.; Barber, T.D.; Mandelker, D.; Leary, R.J.; Ptak, J.; Silliman, N.; et al. The Consensus Coding Sequences of Human Breast and Colorectal Cancers. *Science* **2006**, *314*, 268–274. [CrossRef] [PubMed]
40. Chu, X.-Y.; Li, Z.-J.; Zheng, Z.-W.; Tao, Y.-L.; Zou, F.-X.; Yang, X.-F. KEAP1/NRF2 Signaling Pathway Mutations in Cervical Cancer. *Eur. Rev. Med. Pharm. Sci.* **2018**, *22*, 4458–4466. [CrossRef]
41. Konstantinopoulos, P.A.; Spentzos, D.; Fountzilas, E.; Francoeur, N.; Sanisetty, S.; Grammatikos, A.P.; Hecht, J.L.; Cannistra, S.A. Keap1 Mutations and Nrf2 Pathway Activation in Epithelial Ovarian Cancer. *Cancer Res.* **2011**, *71*, 5081–5089. [CrossRef]

42. Martinez, V.D.; Vucic, E.A.; Thu, K.L.; Hubaux, R.; Enfield, K.S.S.; Pikor, L.A.; Becker-Santos, D.D.; Brown, C.J.; Lam, S.; Lam, W.L. Unique Somatic and Malignant Expression Patterns Implicate PIWI-Interacting RNAs in Cancer-Type Specific Biology. *Sci Rep.* **2015**, *5*. [CrossRef]
43. Yamamoto, S.; Inoue, J.; Kawano, T.; Kozaki, K.; Omura, K.; Inazawa, J. The Impact of MiRNA-Based Molecular Diagnostics and Treatment of NRF2-Stabilized Tumors. *Mol. Cancer Res.* **2014**, *12*, 58–68. [CrossRef] [PubMed]
44. Jiao, N.; Baker, S.S.; Nugent, C.A.; Tsompana, M.; Cai, L.; Wang, Y.; Buck, M.J.; Genco, R.J.; Baker, R.D.; Zhu, R.; et al. Gut Microbiome May Contribute to Insulin Resistance and Systemic Inflammation in Obese Rodents: A Meta-Analysis. *Physiol Genom.* **2018**, *50*, 244–254. [CrossRef]
45. Zhang, Z.; Bai, L.; Guan, M.; Zhou, X.; Liang, X.; Lv, Y.; Yi, H.; Zhou, H.; Liu, T.; Gong, P.; et al. Potential probiotics Lactobacillus casei K11 combined with plant extracts reduce markers of type 2 diabetes mellitus in mice. *J. Appl. Microbiol.* **2021**. [CrossRef]
46. Bamberger, C.; Rossmeier, A.; Lechner, K.; Wu, L.; Waldmann, E.; Fischer, S.; Stark, R.G.; Altenhofer, J.; Henze, K.; Parhofer, K.G. A Walnut-Enriched Diet Affects Gut Microbiome in Healthy Caucasian Subjects: A Randomized, Controlled Trial. *Nutrients* **2018**, *10*, 244. [CrossRef] [PubMed]
47. Gomez-Arango, L.F.; Barrett, H.L.; Wilkinson, S.A.; Callaway, L.K.; McIntyre, H.D.; Morrison, M.; Dekker Nitert, M. Low Dietary Fiber Intake Increases Collinsella Abundance in the Gut Microbiota of Overweight and Obese Pregnant Women. *Gut Microbes* **2018**, *9*, 189–201. [CrossRef] [PubMed]
48. Ojo, O.; Feng, Q.-Q.; Ojo, O.O.; Wang, X.-H. The Role of Dietary Fibre in Modulating Gut Microbiota Dysbiosis in Patients with Type 2 Diabetes: A Systematic Review and Meta-Analysis of Randomised Controlled Trials. *Nutrients* **2020**, *12*, 3239. [CrossRef] [PubMed]
49. den Besten, G.; van Eunen, K.; Groen, A.K.; Venema, K.; Reijngoud, D.-J.; Bakker, B.M. The Role of Short-Chain Fatty Acids in the Interplay between Diet, Gut Microbiota, and Host Energy Metabolism. *J. Lipid Res.* **2013**, *54*, 2325–2340. [CrossRef]
50. Heimann, E.; Nyman, M.; Pålbrink, A.-K.; Lindkvist-Petersson, K.; Degerman, E. Branched Short-Chain Fatty Acids Modulate Glucose and Lipid Metabolism in Primary Adipocytes. *Adipocyte* **2016**, *5*, 359–368. [CrossRef]
51. Matijašić, M.; Meštrović, T.; Perić, M.; Čipčić Paljetak, H.; Panek, M.; Vranešić Bender, D.; Ljubas Kelečić, D.; Krznarić, Ž.; Verbanac, D. Modulating Composition and Metabolic Activity of the Gut Microbiota in IBD Patients. *Int. J. Mol. Sci* **2016**, *17*, 578. [CrossRef]
52. Meštrović, T.; Matijašić, M.; Perić, M.; Čipčić Paljetak, H.; Barešić, A.; Verbanac, D. The Role of Gut, Vaginal, and Urinary Microbiome in Urinary Tract Infections: From Bench to Bedside. *Diagnostics* **2020**, *11*, 7. [CrossRef]
53. Franks, S.; Kiddy, D.S.; Hamilton-Fairley, D.; Bush, A.; Sharp, P.S.; Reed, M.J. The Role of Nutrition and Insulin in the Regulation of Sex Hormone Binding Globulin. *J. Steroid Biochem. Mol. Biol.* **1991**, *39*, 835–838. [CrossRef]
54. Tymchuk, C.N.; Tessler, S.B.; Barnard, R.J. Changes in Sex Hormone-Binding Globulin, Insulin, and Serum Lipids in Postmenopausal Women on a Low-Fat, High-Fiber Diet Combined with Exercise. *Nutr. Cancer* **2000**, *38*, 158–162. [CrossRef] [PubMed]
55. Gann, P.H.; Chatterton, R.T.; Gapstur, S.M.; Liu, K.; Garside, D.; Giovanazzi, S.; Thedford, K.; Van Horn, L. The Effects of a Low-Fat/High-Fiber Diet on Sex Hormone Levels and Menstrual Cycling in Premenopausal Women: A 12-Month Randomized Trial (the Diet and Hormone Study). *Cancer* **2003**, *98*, 1870–1879. [CrossRef]
56. Moran, L.J.; Noakes, M.; Clifton, P.M.; Tomlinson, L.; Galletly, C.; Norman, R.J. Dietary Composition in Restoring Reproductive and Metabolic Physiology in Overweight Women with Polycystic Ovary Syndrome. *J. Clin. Endocrinol. Metab.* **2003**, *88*, 812–819. [CrossRef]
57. Szczuko, M.; Zapałowska-Chwyć, M.; Drozd, A.; Maciejewska, D.; Starczewski, A.; Wysokiński, P.; Stachowska, E. Changes in the IGF-1 and TNF-α Synthesis Pathways before and after Three-Month Reduction Diet with Low Glicemic Index in Women with PCOS. *Ginekol. Pol.* **2018**, *89*, 295–303. [CrossRef]
58. Kazemi, M.; Hadi, A.; Pierson, R.A.; Lujan, M.E.; Zello, G.A.; Chilibeck, P.D. Effects of Dietary Glycemic Index and Glycemic Load on Cardiometabolic and Reproductive Profiles in Women with Polycystic Ovary Syndrome: A Systematic Review and Meta-Analysis of Randomized Controlled Trials. *Adv. Nutr.* **2021**, *12*, 161–178. [CrossRef]
59. Wang, T.; Sha, L.; Li, Y.; Zhu, L.; Wang, Z.; Li, K.; Lu, H.; Bao, T.; Guo, L.; Zhang, X.; et al. Dietary α-Linolenic Acid-Rich Flaxseed Oil Exerts Beneficial Effects on Polycystic Ovary Syndrome Through Sex Steroid Hormones-Microbiota-Inflammation Axis in Rats. *Front. Endocrinol.* **2020**, *11*, 284. [CrossRef]
60. Barber, T.M.; Kabisch, S.; Pfeiffer, A.F.H.; Weickert, M.O. The Health Benefits of Dietary Fibre. *Nutrients* **2020**, *12*, 3209. [CrossRef]
61. Hoover, S.E.; Gower, B.A.; Cedillo, Y.E.; Chandler-Laney, P.C.; Deemer, S.E.; Goss, A.M. Changes in Ghrelin and Glucagon Following a Low Glycemic Load Diet in Women with PCOS. *J. Clin. Endocrinol. Metab.* **2021**. [CrossRef]
62. Akintayo, C.O.; Johnson, A.D.; Badejogbin, O.C.; Olaniyi, K.S.; Oniyide, A.A.; Ajadi, I.O.; Ojewale, A.O.; Adeyomoye, O.I.; Kayode, A.B. High Fructose-Enriched Diet Synergistically Exacerbates Endocrine but Not Metabolic Changes in Letrozole-Induced Polycystic Ovarian Syndrome in Wistar Rats. *Heliyon* **2021**, *7*, e05890. [CrossRef]
63. Shang, Y.; Zhou, H.; Hu, M.; Feng, H. Effect of Diet on Insulin Resistance in Polycystic Ovary Syndrome. *J. Clin. Endocrinol. Metab.* **2020**, *105*. [CrossRef]
64. Porchia, L.M.; Hernandez-Garcia, S.C.; Gonzalez-Mejia, M.E.; López-Bayghen, E. Diets with Lower Carbohydrate Concentrations Improve Insulin Sensitivity in Women with Polycystic Ovary Syndrome: A Meta-Analysis. *Eur. J. Obs. Gynecol. Reprod. Biol.* **2020**, *248*, 110–117. [CrossRef] [PubMed]

65. Shishehgar, F.; Mirmiran, P.; Rahmati, M.; Tohidi, M.; Ramezani Tehrani, F. Does a Restricted Energy Low Glycemic Index Diet Have a Different Effect on Overweight Women with or without Polycystic Ovary Syndrome? *BMC Endocr. Disord.* **2019**, *19*, 93. [CrossRef] [PubMed]
66. Paoli, A.; Mancin, L.; Giacona, M.C.; Bianco, A.; Caprio, M. Effects of a Ketogenic Diet in Overweight Women with Polycystic Ovary Syndrome. *J. Transl. Med.* **2020**, *18*, 104. [CrossRef] [PubMed]
67. Fonseka, S.; Subhani, B.; Wijeyaratne, C.N.; Gawarammana, I.B.; Kalupahana, N.S.; Ratnatunga, N.; Rosairo, S.; Vithane, K.P. Association between Visceral Adiposity Index, Hirsutism and Cardiometabolic Risk Factors in Women with Polycystic Ovarian Syndrome: A Cross-Sectional Study. *Ceylon Med. J.* **2019**, *64*, 111–117. [CrossRef]
68. Marson, E.C.; Delevatti, R.S.; Prado, A.K.G.; Netto, N.; Kruel, L.F.M. Effects of Aerobic, Resistance, and Combined Exercise Training on Insulin Resistance Markers in Overweight or Obese Children and Adolescents: A Systematic Review and Meta-Analysis. *Prev. Med.* **2016**, *93*, 211–218. [CrossRef]
69. Patten, R.K.; Boyle, R.A.; Moholdt, T.; Kiel, I.; Hopkins, W.G.; Harrison, C.L.; Stepto, N.K. Exercise Interventions in Polycystic Ovary Syndrome: A Systematic Review and Meta-Analysis. *Front. Physiol.* **2020**, *11*, 606. [CrossRef]
70. Santos, I.K.D.; Nunes, F.A.S.d.S.; Queiros, V.S.; Cobucci, R.N.; Dantas, P.B.; Soares, G.M.; Cabral, B.G.d.A.T.; Maranhão, T.M.d.O.; Dantas, P.M.S. Effect of High-Intensity Interval Training on Metabolic Parameters in Women with Polycystic Ovary Syndrome: A Systematic Review and Meta-Analysis of Randomized Controlled Trials. *PLoS ONE* **2021**, *16*, e0245023. [CrossRef]
71. Shele, G.; Genkil, J.; Speelman, D. A Systematic Review of the Effects of Exercise on Hormones in Women with Polycystic Ovary Syndrome. *J. Funct. Morphol. Kinesiol.* **2020**, *5*, 35. [CrossRef]
72. Yang, Y.; Deng, H.; Li, T.; Xia, M.; Liu, C.; Bu, X.-Q.; Li, H.; Fu, L.-J.; Zhong, Z.-H. The Mental Health of Chinese Women with Polycystic Ovary Syndrome Is Related to Sleep Disorders, Not Disease Status. *J. Affect. Disord.* **2021**, *282*, 51–57. [CrossRef]
73. Leproult, R.; Van Cauter, E. Role of Sleep and Sleep Loss in Hormonal Release and Metabolism. *Endocr. Dev.* **2010**, *17*, 11–21. [CrossRef]
74. Donga, E.; Romijn, J.A. Sleep Characteristics and Insulin Sensitivity in Humans. *Handb. Clin. Neurol.* **2014**, *124*, 107–114. [CrossRef]
75. Reutrakul, S.; Van Cauter, E. Sleep Influences on Obesity, Insulin Resistance, and Risk of Type 2 Diabetes. *Metabolism* **2018**, *84*, 56–66. [CrossRef]
76. Poroyko, V.A.; Carreras, A.; Khalyfa, A.; Khalyfa, A.A.; Leone, V.; Peris, E.; Almendros, I.; Gileles-Hillel, A.; Qiao, Z.; Hubert, N.; et al. Chronic Sleep Disruption Alters Gut Microbiota, Induces Systemic and Adipose Tissue Inflammation and Insulin Resistance in Mice. *Sci. Rep.* **2016**, *6*, 35405. [CrossRef]
77. Mojaverrostami, S.; Asghari, N.; Khamisabadi, M.; Heidari Khoei, H. The Role of Melatonin in Polycystic Ovary Syndrome: A Review. *Int. J. Reprod. Biomed.* **2019**, *17*, 865–882. [CrossRef] [PubMed]
78. Szczuko, M.; Hawryłkowicz, V.; Kikut, J.; Drozd, A. The Implications of Vitamin Content in the Plasma in Reference to the Parameters of Carbohydrate Metabolism and Hormone and Lipid Profiles in PCOS. *J. Steroid Biochem. Mol. Biol.* **2020**, *198*, 105570. [CrossRef]
79. Szczuko, M.; Szydłowska, I.; Nawrocka-Rutkowska, J. A Properly Balanced Reduction Diet and/or Supplementation Solve the Problem with the Deficiency of These Vitamins Soluble in Water in Patients with PCOS. *Nutrients* **2021**, *13*, 746. [CrossRef] [PubMed]
80. Suzuki, H.; Kunisawa, J. Vitamin-Mediated Immune Regulation in the Development of Inflammatory Diseases. *Endocr. Metab. Immune Disord. Drug Targets* **2015**, *15*, 212–215. [CrossRef] [PubMed]
81. Wanders, D.; Graff, E.C.; White, B.D.; Judd, R.L. Niacin Increases Adiponectin and Decreases Adipose Tissue Inflammation in High Fat Diet-Fed Mice. *PLoS ONE* **2013**, *8*, e71285. [CrossRef]
82. Esmaeilzadeh, S.; Gholinezhad-Chari, M.; Ghadimi, R. The Effect of Metformin Treatment on the Serum Levels of Homocysteine, Folic Acid, and Vitamin B12 in Patients with Polycystic Ovary Syndrome. *J. Hum. Reprod. Sci.* **2017**, *10*, 95–101. [CrossRef] [PubMed]
83. DiNicolantonio, J.J.; Liu, J.; O'Keefe, J.H. Thiamine and Cardiovascular Disease: A Literature Review. *Prog. Cardiovasc. Dis.* **2018**, *61*, 27–32. [CrossRef] [PubMed]
84. Eshak, E.S.; Arafa, A.E. Thiamine Deficiency and Cardiovascular Disorders. *Nutr. Metab. Cardiovasc. Dis.* **2018**, *28*, 965–972. [CrossRef] [PubMed]
85. Taghizadeh, S.; Izadi, A.; Shirazi, S.; Parizad, M.; Pourghassem Gargari, B. The Effect of Coenzyme Q10 Supplementation on Inflammatory and Endothelial Dysfunction Markers in Overweight/Obese Polycystic Ovary Syndrome Patients. *Gynecol. Endocrinol.* **2021**, *37*, 26–30. [CrossRef]
86. Teegarden, D.; Donkin, S.S. Vitamin D: Emerging New Roles in Insulin Sensitivity. *Nutr. Res. Rev.* **2009**, *22*, 82–92. [CrossRef] [PubMed]
87. He, C.; Lin, Z.; Robb, S.W.; Ezeamama, A.E. Serum Vitamin D Levels and Polycystic Ovary Syndrome: A Systematic Review and Meta-Analysis. *Nutrients* **2015**, *7*, 4555–4577. [CrossRef]
88. Wehr, E.; Pieber, T.R.; Obermayer-Pietsch, B. Effect of Vitamin D3 Treatment on Glucose Metabolism and Menstrual Frequency in Polycystic Ovary Syndrome Women: A Pilot Study. *J. Endocrinol. Investig.* **2011**, *34*, 757–763. [CrossRef]

89. Maktabi, M.; Jamilian, M.; Asemi, Z. Magnesium-Zinc-Calcium-Vitamin D Co-Supplementation Improves Hormonal Profiles, Biomarkers of Inflammation and Oxidative Stress in Women with Polycystic Ovary Syndrome: A Randomized, Double-Blind, Placebo-Controlled Trial. *Biol. Trace Elem. Res.* **2018**, *182*, 21–28. [CrossRef]
90. Jamilian, M.; Samimi, M.; Mirhosseini, N.; Afshar Ebrahimi, F.; Aghadavod, E.; Talaee, R.; Jafarnejad, S.; Hashemi Dizaji, S.; Asemi, Z. The Influences of Vitamin D and Omega-3 Co-Supplementation on Clinical, Metabolic and Genetic Parameters in Women with Polycystic Ovary Syndrome. *J. Affect. Disord.* **2018**, *238*, 32–38. [CrossRef]
91. Formuso, C.; Stracquadanio, M.; Ciotta, L. Myo-Inositol vs. D-Chiro Inositol in PCOS Treatment. *Minerva Ginecol.* **2015**, *67*, 321–325. [PubMed]
92. Fruzzetti, F.; Perini, D.; Russo, M.; Bucci, F.; Gadducci, A. Comparison of Two Insulin Sensitizers, Metformin and Myo-Inositol, in Women with Polycystic Ovary Syndrome (PCOS). *Gynecol. Endocrinol.* **2017**, *33*, 39–42. [CrossRef] [PubMed]
93. Saleem, F.; Rizvi, S.W. New Therapeutic Approaches in Obesity and Metabolic Syndrome Associated with Polycystic Ovary Syndrome. *Cureus* **2017**, *9*, e1844. [CrossRef] [PubMed]
94. Genazzani, A.D.; Santagni, S.; Ricchieri, F.; Campedelli, A.; Rattighieri, E.; Chierchia, E.; Marini, G.; Despini, G.; Prati, A.; Simoncini, T. Myo-Inositol Modulates Insulin and Luteinizing Hormone Secretion in Normal Weight Patients with Polycystic Ovary Syndrome. *J. Obs. Gynaecol. Res.* **2014**, *40*, 1353–1360. [CrossRef] [PubMed]
95. Facchinetti, F.; Bizzarri, M.; Benvenga, S.; D'Anna, R.; Lanzone, A.; Soulage, C.; Di Renzo, G.C.; Hod, M.; Cavalli, P.; Chiu, T.T.; et al. Results from the International Consensus Conference on Myo-Inositol and d-Chiro-Inositol in Obstetrics and Gynecology: The Link between Metabolic Syndrome and PCOS. *Eur. J. Obs. Gynecol. Reprod. Biol.* **2015**, *195*, 72–76. [CrossRef] [PubMed]
96. Unfer, V.; Nestler, J.E.; Kamenov, Z.A.; Prapas, N.; Facchinetti, F. Effects of Inositol(s) in Women with PCOS: A Systematic Review of Randomized Controlled Trials. *Int. J. Endocrinol.* **2016**, *2016*, 1849162. [CrossRef]
97. Li, Y.; Ma, H.; Zhang, Y.; Kuang, H.; Ng, E.H.Y.; Hou, L.; Wu, X. Effect of Berberine on Insulin Resistance in Women with Polycystic Ovary Syndrome: Study Protocol for a Randomized Multicenter Controlled Trial. *Trials* **2013**, *14*, 226. [CrossRef]
98. Rondanelli, M.; Infantino, V.; Riva, A.; Petrangolini, G.; Faliva, M.A.; Peroni, G.; Naso, M.; Nichetti, M.; Spadaccini, D.; Gasparri, C.; et al. Polycystic Ovary Syndrome Management: A Review of the Possible Amazing Role of Berberine. *Arch. Gynecol. Obs.* **2020**, *301*, 53–60. [CrossRef]
99. Xiang, D.; Lu, J.; Wei, C.; Cai, X.; Wang, Y.; Liang, Y.; Xu, M.; Wang, Z.; Liu, M.; Wang, M.; et al. Berberine Ameliorates Prenatal Dihydrotestosterone Exposure-Induced Autism-Like Behavior by Suppression of Androgen Receptor. *Front. Cell Neurosci.* **2020**, *14*. [CrossRef] [PubMed]
100. Bertuccioli, A.; Moricoli, S.; Amatori, S.; Rocchi, M.B.L.; Vici, G.; Sisti, D. Berberine and Dyslipidemia: Different Applications and Biopharmaceutical Formulations Without Statin-Like Molecules-A Meta-Analysis. *J. Med. Food* **2020**, *23*, 101–113. [CrossRef] [PubMed]
101. Wei, W.; Zhao, H.; Wang, A.; Sui, M.; Liang, K.; Deng, H.; Ma, Y.; Zhang, Y.; Zhang, H.; Guan, Y. A Clinical Study on the Short-Term Effect of Berberine in Comparison to Metformin on the Metabolic Characteristics of Women with Polycystic Ovary Syndrome. *Eur. J. Endocrinol.* **2012**, *166*, 99–105. [CrossRef] [PubMed]
102. Kuang, H.; Duan, Y.; Li, D.; Xu, Y.; Ai, W.; Li, W.; Wang, Y.; Liu, S.; Li, M.; Liu, X.; et al. The Role of Serum Inflammatory Cytokines and Berberine in the Insulin Signaling Pathway among Women with Polycystic Ovary Syndrome. *PLoS ONE* **2020**, *15*. [CrossRef] [PubMed]
103. Lucidi, R.S.; Thyer, A.C.; Easton, C.A.; Holden, A.E.C.; Schenken, R.S.; Brzyski, R.G. Effect of Chromium Supplementation on Insulin Resistance and Ovarian and Menstrual Cyclicity in Women with Polycystic Ovary Syndrome. *Fertil. Steril.* **2005**, *84*, 1755–1757. [CrossRef] [PubMed]
104. Tang, X.-L.; Sun, Z.; Gong, L. Chromium Supplementation in Women with Polycystic Ovary Syndrome: Systematic Review and Meta-Analysis. *J. Obs. Gynaecol. Res.* **2018**, *44*, 134–143. [CrossRef]
105. Fazelian, S.; Rouhani, M.H.; Bank, S.S.; Amani, R. Chromium Supplementation and Polycystic Ovary Syndrome: A Systematic Review and Meta-Analysis. *J. Trace Elem. Med. Biol.* **2017**, *42*, 92–96. [CrossRef] [PubMed]
106. Ashoush, S.; Abou-Gamrah, A.; Bayoumy, H.; Othman, N. Chromium Picolinate Reduces Insulin Resistance in Polycystic Ovary Syndrome: Randomized Controlled Trial. *J. Obs. Gynaecol. Res.* **2016**, *42*, 279–285. [CrossRef]
107. Piotrowska, A.; Pilch, W.; Czerwińska-Ledwig, O.; Zuziak, R.; Siwek, A.; Wolak, M.; Nowak, G. The Possibilities of Using Chromium Salts as an Agent Supporting Treatment of Polycystic Ovary Syndrome. *Biol. Trace Elem. Res.* **2019**, *192*, 91–97. [CrossRef]
108. Maxel, T.; Svendsen, P.F.; Smidt, K.; Lauridsen, J.K.; Brock, B.; Pedersen, S.B.; Rungby, J.; Larsen, A. Expression Patterns and Correlations with Metabolic Markers of Zinc Transporters ZIP14 and ZNT1 in Obesity and Polycystic Ovary Syndrome. *Front. Endocrinol.* **2017**, *8*. [CrossRef]
109. Nasiadek, M.; Stragierowicz, J.; Klimczak, M.; Kilanowicz, A. The Role of Zinc in Selected Female Reproductive System Disorders. *Nutrients* **2020**, *12*, 2464. [CrossRef]
110. Guler, I.; Himmetoglu, O.; Turp, A.; Erdem, A.; Erdem, M.; Onan, M.A.; Taskiran, C.; Taslipinar, M.Y.; Guner, H. Zinc and Homocysteine Levels in Polycystic Ovarian Syndrome Patients with Insulin Resistance. *Biol. Trace Elem. Res.* **2014**, *158*, 297–304. [CrossRef]
111. Coskun, A.; Arikan, T.; Kilinc, M.; Arikan, D.C.; Ekerbiçer, H.Ç. Plasma Selenium Levels in Turkish Women with Polycystic Ovary Syndrome. *Eur. J. Obs. Gynecol. Reprod. Biol.* **2013**, *168*, 183–186. [CrossRef] [PubMed]

112. Michael, P.J.; Stepanić, V.; Nadja, T.; Panek, M.; Verbanac, D. Mild Plant and Dietary Immunomodulators. *Nijkamp Parnham's Princ. Immunopharmacol.* **2019**, 561–587. [CrossRef]
113. Ma, X.; Weng, X.; Hu, X.; Wang, Q.; Tian, Y.; Ding, Y.; Zhang, C. Roles of Different N-3/n-6 PUFA Ratios in Ovarian Cell Development and Steroidogenesis in PCOS Rats. *Food. Funct.* **2019**, *10*, 7397–7406. [CrossRef]
114. Popova, A.; Mihaylova, D. A Review of the Medicinal Plants in Bulgaria: Collection, Storage, And Extraction Techniques. *Asian J. Pharm. Clin. Res.* **2018**, *28*–35. [CrossRef]
115. Ashkar, F.; Rezaei, S.; Salahshoornezhad, S.; Vahid, F.; Gholamalizadeh, M.; Dahka, S.M.; Doaei, S. The Role of Medicinal Herbs in Treatment of Insulin Resistance in Patients with Polycystic Ovary Syndrome: A Literature Review. *Biomol. Concepts* **2020**, *11*, 57–75. [CrossRef]
116. Tehrani, H.G.; Allahdadian, M.; Zarre, F.; Ranjbar, H.; Allahdadian, F. Effect of Green Tea on Metabolic and Hormonal Aspect of Polycystic Ovarian Syndrome in Overweight and Obese Women Suffering from Polycystic Ovarian Syndrome: A Clinical Trial. *J. Educ. Health Promot.* **2017**, *6*, 36. [CrossRef]
117. Haj-Husein, I.; Tukan, S.; Alkazaleh, F. The Effect of Marjoram (Origanum Majorana) Tea on the Hormonal Profile of Women with Polycystic Ovary Syndrome: A Randomised Controlled Pilot Study. *J. Hum. Nutr. Diet.* **2016**, *29*, 105–111. [CrossRef]
118. Rababa'h, A.M.; Matani, B.R.; Ababneh, M.A. The Ameliorative Effects of Marjoram in Dehydroepiandrosterone Induced Polycystic Ovary Syndrome in Rats. *Life Sci.* **2020**, *261*, 118353. [CrossRef] [PubMed]
119. Grant, P. Spearmint Herbal Tea Has Significant Anti-Androgen Effects in Polycystic Ovarian Syndrome. A Randomized Controlled Trial. *Phytother. Res.* **2010**, *24*, 186–188. [CrossRef]
120. Sadeghi Ataabadi, M.; Alaee, S.; Bagheri, M.J.; Bahmanpoor, S. Role of Essential Oil of Mentha Spicata (Spearmint) in Addressing Reverse Hormonal and Folliculogenesis Disturbances in a Polycystic Ovarian Syndrome in a Rat Model. *Adv. Pharm. Bull.* **2017**, *7*, 651–654. [CrossRef]
121. Sabbadin, C.; Bordin, L.; Donà, G.; Manso, J.; Avruscio, G.; Armanini, D. Licorice: From Pseudohyperaldosteronism to Therapeutic Uses. *Front. Endocrinol.* **2019**, *10*, 484. [CrossRef] [PubMed]
122. Arentz, S.; Abbott, J.A.; Smith, C.A.; Bensoussan, A. Herbal Medicine for the Management of Polycystic Ovary Syndrome (PCOS) and Associated Oligo/Amenorrhoea and Hyperandrogenism; a Review of the Laboratory Evidence for Effects with Corroborative Clinical Findings. *BMC Complement. Altern Med.* **2014**, *14*, 511. [CrossRef] [PubMed]
123. Adamczak, M.; Wiecek, A. Food Products That May Cause an Increase in Blood Pressure. *Curr. Hypertens. Rep.* **2020**, *22*, 2. [CrossRef] [PubMed]
124. Dhariwala, M.Y.; Ravikumar, P. An Overview of Herbal Alternatives in Androgenetic Alopecia. *J. Cosmet Derm.* **2019**, *18*, 966–975. [CrossRef] [PubMed]
125. Kakadia, N.; Patel, P.; Deshpande, S.; Shah, G. Effect of Vitex Negundo L. Seeds in Letrozole Induced Polycystic Ovarian Syndrome. *J. Tradit Complement. Med.* **2019**, *9*, 336–345. [CrossRef]
126. Mehraban, M.; Jelodar, G.; Rahmanifar, F. A Combination of Spearmint and Flaxseed Extract Improved Endocrine and Histomorphology of Ovary in Experimental PCOS. *J. Ovarian Res.* **2020**, *13*, 32. [CrossRef]
127. Brooks, J.D.; Thompson, L.U. Mammalian Lignans and Genistein Decrease the Activities of Aromatase and 17beta-Hydroxysteroid Dehydrogenase in MCF-7 Cells. *J. Steroid Biochem. Mol. Biol.* **2005**, *94*, 461–467. [CrossRef]
128. Heshmati, J.; Moini, A.; Sepidarkish, M.; Morvaridzadeh, M.; Salehi, M.; Palmowski, A.; Mojtahedi, M.F.; Shidfar, F. Effects of Curcumin Supplementation on Blood Glucose, Insulin Resistance and Androgens in Patients with Polycystic Ovary Syndrome: A Randomized Double-Blind Placebo-Controlled Clinical Trial. *Phytomedicine* **2021**, *80*, 153395. [CrossRef]
129. Marmitt, D.J.; Shahrajabian, M.H.; Goettert, M.I.; Rempel, C. Clinical Trials with Plants in Diabetes Mellitus Therapy: A Systematic Review. *Expert Rev. Clin. Pharm.* **2021**, 1–13. [CrossRef]
130. Heshmati, J.; Golab, F.; Morvaridzadeh, M.; Potter, E.; Akbari-Fakhrabadi, M.; Farsi, F.; Tanbakooei, S.; Shidfar, F. The Effects of Curcumin Supplementation on Oxidative Stress, Sirtuin-1 and Peroxisome Proliferator Activated Receptor γ Coactivator 1α Gene Expression in Polycystic Ovarian Syndrome (PCOS) Patients: A Randomized Placebo-Controlled Clinical Trial. *Diabetes Metab. Syndr.* **2020**, *14*, 77–82. [CrossRef]
131. Yuandani, I.J.; Rohani, A.S.; Sumantri, I.B. Immunomodulatory Effects and Mechanisms of Curcuma Species and Their Bioactive Compounds: A Review. *Front. Pharm.* **2021**, *12*, 643119. [CrossRef]
132. Chowdhury, I.; Banerjee, S.; Driss, A.; Xu, W.; Mehrabi, S.; Nezhat, C.; Sidell, N.; Taylor, R.N.; Thompson, W.E. Curcumin Attenuates Proangiogenic and Proinflammatory Factors in Human Eutopic Endometrial Stromal Cells through the NF-KB Signaling Pathway. *J. Cell Physiol* **2019**, *234*, 6298–6312. [CrossRef]
133. İşler, S.C.; Demircan, S.; Çakarer, S.; Çebi, Z.; Keskin, C.; Soluk, M.; Yüzbaşıoğlu, E. Effects of Folk Medicinal Plant Extract Ankaferd Blood Stopper®on Early Bone Healing. *J. Appl. Oral Sci.* **2010**, *18*, 409–414. [CrossRef] [PubMed]
134. Ziaei, R.; Foshati, S.; Hadi, A.; Kermani, M.A.H.; Ghavami, A.; Clark, C.C.T.; Tarrahi, M.J. The Effect of Nettle (Urtica Dioica) Supplementation on the Glycemic Control of Patients with Type 2 Diabetes Mellitus: A Systematic Review and Meta-Analysis. *Phytother. Res.* **2020**, *34*, 282–294. [CrossRef] [PubMed]
135. Sarma Kataki, M.; Murugamani, V.; Rajkumari, A.; Singh Mehra, P.; Awasthi, D.; Shankar Yadav, R. Antioxidant, Hepatoprotective, and Anthelmintic Activities of Methanol Extract of Urtica Dioica L. Leaves. *Pharm. Crop.* **2012**, *3*, 38–46. [CrossRef]
136. Ferro, D.; Baratta, F.; Pastori, D.; Cocomello, N.; Colantoni, A.; Angelico, F.; Del Ben, M. New Insights into the Pathogenesis of Non-Alcoholic Fatty Liver Disease: Gut-Derived Lipopolysaccharides and Oxidative Stress. *Nutrients* **2020**, *12*, 2762. [CrossRef]

137. Wat, E.; Wang, Y.; Chan, K.; Law, H.W.; Koon, C.M.; Lau, K.M.; Leung, P.C.; Yan, C.; Lau, C.B.S. An in Vitro and in Vivo Study of a 4-Herb Formula on the Management of Diet-Induced Metabolic Syndrome. *Phytomedicine* **2018**, *42*, 112–125. [CrossRef]
138. MacDonald-Ramos, K.; Michán, L.; Martínez-Ibarra, A.; Cerbón, M. Silymarin Is an Ally against Insulin Resistance: A Review. *Ann. Hepatol.* **2020**, *23*, 100255. [CrossRef]
139. Oppedisano, F.; Muscoli, C.; Musolino, V.; Carresi, C.; Macrì, R.; Giancotta, C.; Bosco, F.; Maiuolo, J.; Scarano, F.; Paone, S.; et al. The Protective Effect of Cynara Cardunculus Extract in Diet-Induced NAFLD: Involvement of OCTN1 and OCTN2 Transporter Subfamily. *Nutrients* **2020**, *12*, 1435. [CrossRef]
140. Zhao, Y.-M.; Wang, C.; Zhang, R.; Hou, X.-J.; Zhao, F.; Zhang, J.-J.; Wang, C. [Study on literature of artichoke and properties of traditional Chinese medicine]. *Zhongguo Zhong Yao Za Zhi* **2020**, *45*, 3481–3488. [CrossRef] [PubMed]
141. Park, S.; Kim, D.S.; Wu, X.; J Yi, Q. Mulberry and Dandelion Water Extracts Prevent Alcohol-Induced Steatosis with Alleviating Gut Microbiome Dysbiosis. *Exp. Biol. Med.* **2018**, *243*, 882–894. [CrossRef] [PubMed]
142. Azizi, N.; Amini, M.R.; Djafarian, K.; Shab-Bidar, S. The Effects of Nigella Sativa Supplementation on Liver Enzymes Levels: A Systematic Review and Meta-Analysis of Randomized Controlled Trials. *Clin. Nutr. Res.* **2021**, *10*, 72–82. [CrossRef] [PubMed]

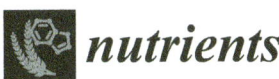

Systematic Review

Endometriosis and Phytoestrogens: Friends or Foes? A Systematic Review

Ludovica Bartiromo [1,†], Matteo Schimberni [1,†], Roberta Villanacci [1], Jessica Ottolina [1], Carolina Dolci [1], Noemi Salmeri [1], Paola Viganò [2,*] and Massimo Candiani [1]

[1] Gynecology/Obstetrics Unit, IRCCS San Raffaele Scientific Institute, 20132 Milan, Italy; bartiromo.ludovica@hsr.it (L.B.); schimberni.matteo@hsr.it (M.S.); villanacci.roberta@hsr.it (R.V.); ottolina.jessica@hsr.it (J.O.); dolci.carolina@hsr.it (C.D.); salmeri.noemi@hsr.it (N.S.); candiani.massimo@hsr.it (M.C.)
[2] Fondazione IRCCS Ca' Granda Ospedale Maggiore Policlinico, 20122 Milan, Italy
* Correspondence: paola.vigano@policlinico.mi.it; Tel.: +39-02-550-343-02
† These authors contributed equally to this work.

Citation: Bartiromo, L.; Schimberni, M.; Villanacci, R.; Ottolina, J.; Dolci, C.; Salmeri, N.; Viganò, P.; Candiani, M. Endometriosis and Phytoestrogens: Friends or Foes? A Systematic Review. *Nutrients* **2021**, *13*, 2532. https://doi.org/10.3390/nu13082532

Academic Editor: Pasquapina Ciarmela

Received: 16 June 2021
Accepted: 23 July 2021
Published: 24 July 2021

Publisher's Note: MDPI stays neutral with regard to jurisdictional claims in published maps and institutional affiliations.

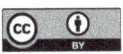

Copyright: © 2021 by the authors. Licensee MDPI, Basel, Switzerland. This article is an open access article distributed under the terms and conditions of the Creative Commons Attribution (CC BY) license (https:// creativecommons.org/licenses/by/ 4.0/).

Abstract: The aim of this systematic review was to provide comprehensive and available data on the possible role of phytoestrogens (PE) for the treatment of endometriosis. We conducted an advanced, systematic search of online medical databases PubMed and Medline. Only full-length manuscripts written in English up to September 2020 were considered. A total of 60 studies were included in the systematic review. According to in vitro findings, 19 out of 22 studies reported the ability of PE in inducing anti-proliferative, anti-inflammatory and proapoptotic effects on cultured cells. Various mechanisms have been proposed to explain this in vitro action including the alteration of cell cycle proteins, the activation/inactivation of regulatory pathways, and modification of radical oxidative species levels. Thirty-eight articles on the effects of phytoestrogens on the development of endometriotic lesions in in vivo experimental animal models of endometriosis have been included. In line with in vitro findings, results also derived from animal models of endometriosis generally supported a beneficial effect of the compounds in reducing lesion growth and development. Finally, only seven studies investigated the effects of phytoestrogens intake on endometriosis in humans. The huge amount of in vitro and in vivo animal findings did not correspond to a consistent literature in the women affected. Therefore, whether the experimental findings can be translated in women is currently unknown.

Keywords: phytoestrogens; endometriosis; lignan; resveratrol; flavonoid

1. Introduction

Endometriosis is a common benign chronic disease affecting reproductive-age women [1]. It is defined as the presence of endometrial tissue and fibrosis located outside the uterus and is frequently associated with pelvic pain, infertility, urinary and bowel dysfunction [2–4]. As a hormonal disease characterized by features of a chronic inflammatory condition, various theories on its development based on an uncontrolled hormonal response and immune-mediated dysfunctions have been proposed [5,6]. Estrogens are key promoters of endometrial cellular growth. Any insult that affects estradiol biosynthesis and catabolism in women with endometriosis have been proposed to play a part in aberrant cell growth. Levels of peripheral estrogens do not seem however altered in women with endometriosis. On the other hand, estrogens are both endocrine and paracrine agents and one may speculate that even a modest variation of estrogen production may be somehow detrimental locally. Indeed, locally accumulated estradiol can create an estrogenic microenvironment around endometriotic lesions. High local concentrations of estradiol and alterations in estrogen receptor (ER) α and ERβ receptor expression may activate a network of genes regulating cell proliferation [7,8]. In line with these observations, medical treatment for endometriosis is still focused on pain and lesion size control with hormonal therapies able to establish either a hypo-estrogenic or a hyper-progestogenic milieu [9,10]. In this context, a role of diet has been postulated based on the idea that estrogen activity can be influenced by nutrition [11,12]. In other conditions in which hormones exert a specific role, such as breast and endometrial carcinogenesis, research has demonstrated that diet may strongly affect incidence [13].

Phytoestrogens (PE) have been identified in various types of food stuffs including fruits, vegetables, sprouts, beans, cabbage, soybean, grains, tea and oilseeds. Based on their structure, the main classes of PE consist of flavonoids (i.e., puerarin, genistein, coumestrol, epicatechin and naringenin), lignans (i.e., enterolactone), and stilbenes (i.e., resveratrol). Classified into three main classes, PE include flavonoids (i.e., puerarin, genistein, coumestrol, epigallocatechin gallate (EGCG), naringenin, quercetin), lignans (i.e., enetrolactone), and stilbenes (i.e., resveratrol). [14]. Their close structural similarity to estrogens, characterized by a phenolic ring and two hydroxyl groups, allows them to act as weak estrogenic factors and to interfere with hormonal and molecular signaling, having positive effects including the prevention of menopausal symptoms, type 2 diabetes, cardiovascular disease, obesity and cancer [15]. Moreover, PE may have poor estrogenic activity in low-estrogen environments such as in menopause and have antiestrogenic activity in high-estrogen environments such as those observed in endometriosis or endometrial cancer [16,17]. Several studies have evaluated the associations between PE and endometriosis risk in animal and human models but the data obtained are quite inconsistent or conflicting [18–77].

The aim of this systematic review was to gain insight into the mechanisms of action of PE in endometriosis and to offer a general view of available data on their possible role for the treatment of endometriosis.

2. Materials and Methods

The study protocol was registered "a priori" and accepted for inclusion in PROSPERO (PROSPERO ID CRD42020220847). The methods for this systematic review were developed in accordance with the Preferred Reporting Item for Systematic Reviews and Meta-analysis (PRISMA) guidelines [78]. No Institutional Review Board Approval was needed. We performed an advanced, systematic search of online medical databases PubMed and Medline using the following keywords: "endometriosis" in combination with "phytoestrogen", "flavonoid", "non-flavonoid", "isoflavone", "coumestan", "lignan" and "resveratrol". To optimize search output, we used specific tools available in each database, such as Medical Subject Headings (MeSH) terms (PubMed/Medline). The EndNote software (available online: https://endnote.com, accessed on 19 September 2020) was used to remove duplicate articles. Only full-length manuscripts written in English up to September 2020 were considered. We checked all citations found by title and abstract to establish the eligibility of the source and obtained the full text of eligible articles. We also performed a manual scan of the references list of the review articles to identify any additional relevant citations. Three review authors (R.V., M.S. and L.B.) independently assessed the risk of bias for each study using the risk-of-bias tool for case–control studies developed by clarity group [79]. We assessed the risk of bias according to the following domains: (i) Can we be confident in the assessment of exposure?; (ii) Can we be confident that cases had developed the outcome of interest and controls had not?; (iii) Were the cases properly selected?; (iv) Were the controls properly selected?; (v) Were cases and controls matched according to important prognostic variables or was statistical adjustment carried out for those variables? We graded each potential source of bias as Definitely yes (low risk of bias), Probably yes (Moderate risk of bias), Probably no (Serious risk of bias), or Definitely no (Critical, high risk of bias). We summarized the risk of bias judgments across different studies for each of the domains listed.

3. Results

A total of 286 studies were initially identified by the search criteria. After applying the selection criteria, a total of 60 trials were included in the systematic review [18–77]. A flow diagram of the systematic review is shown in Figure 1 (PRISMA template). The risks of bias of the included studies are summarized in Supplementary Figure S1. Findings derived from the studies are herein presented based on in vitro results, evidence in in vivo animal models and finally in humans.

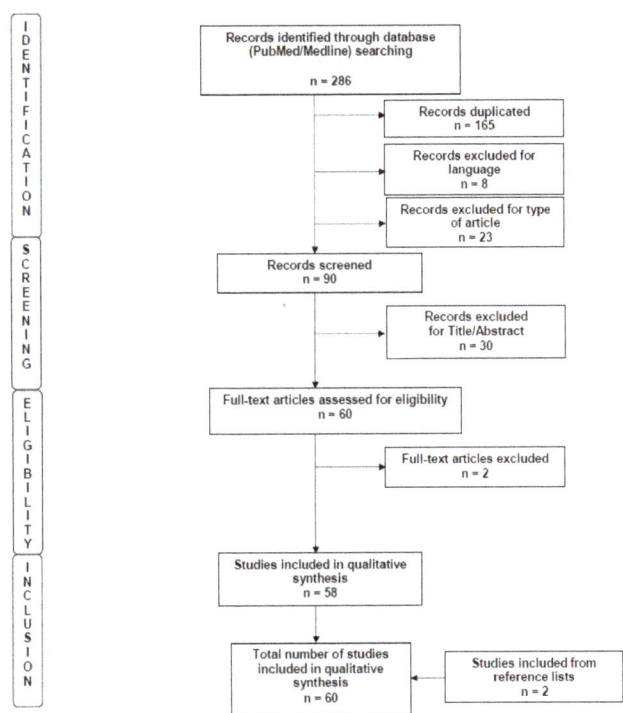

Figure 1. Flow diagram of the search strategy, screening, eligibility and inclusion criteria.

3.1. Studies Included

3.1.1. Phytoestrogens and Endometriosis: In Vitro Experimental Human Models

Several studies tried to assess PE effect on human endometrial/endometriotic cells. The results from 22 studies are summarized in Table 1. What is surprising is the heterogeneity of the substances studied and their respective biological effects, although for some of them it is possible to designate common actions.

Table 1. Studies investigating phytoestrogen effect on endometriosis in experimental in vitro in human models.

Authors	Date	Substance	Cases	Controls	Results	Adverse Events
Edmunds et al. [20]	2005	Genistein, Daidzein, Naringenin or Chrysin (10^{-4}–10^{-9} M)	EuSC from 11 women with endometriosis	EuSC from 7 women without endometriosis	- PE treatment did not attenuate aromatase activity in EuSC cultures from cases and controls - Genistein (10^{-9}–10^{-6} M) increased aromatase activity in controls - Naringenin and Chrysin were potent inhibitors of aromatase in FCA - Genistein was inactive in FCA	Genistein consumption in reproductive age may have health risks
Wang et al. [28]	2011	Puerarin (10^{-9} M)	EcSC treated with Puerarin	EcSC treated with E2 (10^{-8} M) Untreated EcSC	- E2 showed a stimulatory effect on EcSC invasion compared with the untreated cells, but the combination of E2 with Puerarin reduced this effect - E2 treatment determined MMP-9 increase and TIMP-1 decrease, but the combination with Puerarin reversed this effect	NR
Cheng et al. [30]	2012	Puerarin (10^{-9} M)	EcSC treated with Puerarin +/− E2-BSA	EcSC treated with E2-BSA	- ERK1/2 (MAPK signaling) was highly activated by E2-BSA, which was reversed by Puerarin - E2-BSA induced the proliferation of EcSCs, which was reversed by Puerarin - Puerarin suppressed gene expression of Cyclin D1, COX-2 and cyp19	NR
Ji et al. [34]	2013	Puerarin (10^{-9} M)	EcSC treated with Puerarin +/− E2	EcSC treated with E2 +/− fulvestrant (anti-E2)	- Puerarin: • suppressed proliferation of E2-stimulated EcSCs by increasing G1 phase of the cell cycle and down-regulating cyclin D1 and cdc25A expression • changed recruitment pattern of nuclear receptor coregulators to estrogen receptor (less SRC-1 and SRC-3 coactivators but more NCoR and SMRT corepressors)	NR
Ricci et al. [35]	2013	Resveratrol (0, 25, 50 and 100 mM) EGCG (0, 20, 40, 80 and 100 mM).	EuEC from women with endometriosis	EuEC from women without endometriosis	- Both compounds induced reduction in EuEC proliferation and increased apoptosis in both groups - No significant difference in cell proliferation and apoptosis between cases and controls	NR

Table 1. Cont.

Authors	Date	Substance	Cases	Controls	Results	Adverse Events
Matsuzaki et al. [40]	2014	EGCG (10^{-9} M)	EcSC and EuSC treated with EGCG (from 45 women with endometriosis)	EuSC and EuSC vehicle-treated or treated with NAC(10 mM) (from 45 patients with endometriosis)	- EGCG: • significantly inhibited cell proliferation, migration and invasion of both EuSC and EcSC • significantly decreased the TGF-b1-dependent increase in the mRNA expression of fibrotic markers in both EuSC and EcSC • Both EuSC and EcSC-mediated contraction of collagen gels were significantly attenuated at 8, 12 and 24 h after treatment with EGCG • significantly inhibited TGF-β1-stimulated activation of MAPK and Smad signaling pathways in both cells.	NR
Taguchi et al. [41]	2014	Resveratrol (10, 20 or 40 μM) (SIRT-1 activator) Sirtinol at 20 μM (SIRT-1 inhibitor)	EcSC	EuSC from patients without endometriosis	- No difference in the basal expression level of SIRT1 mRNA between EcSC and EuSC - Resveratrol: • suppressed TNF-α-induced IL-8 release from EcSC in a dose-dependent manner while Sirtinol increased IL-8 release • had increased anti-inflammatory effects on EcSC than on EuSC	NR
Taguchi et al. [47]	2016	Resveratrol (40–120 mM) TRAIL 100 ng/mL	EcSC treated with resveratrol and TRAIL	EcSC treated with TRAIL	- Resveratrol: • alone did not induce apoptosis in EcSC, but significantly reduced survivin mRNA expression • enhanced TRAIL-induced apoptosis	NR

Table 1. *Cont.*

Authors	Date	Substance	Cases	Controls	Results	Adverse Events
Kim et al. [48]	2017	PFE (25, 50, and 100 µg/mL) containing Genistein, Daidzein, Kakkalide, Puerarin, Tectoridin	Human endometriotic (11Z and 12Z) and mesothelial (Met5A) cells treated with PFE	Human endometriotic (11Z and 12Z) and mesothelial (Met5A) cells not treated with PFE	- PFE: • inhibited endometriotic cell adhesion to mesothelial cells • inhibited endometriotic cell migration at 100 µg/mL • inhibited RNA and protein expression of MMP-2 and MMP-9 and increased the phosphorylation of ERK1/2 in endometriotic cells	NR
Park et al. [50]	2017	Narigenin (100 µM)	VK2/E6E7 and End1/E6E7 cells treated with Narigenin	VK2/E6E7 and End1/E6E7 cells not treated with Narigenin	- Narigenin: • decreased proliferation and increased apoptosis • increased ROS production • increased apoptosis through generation of ER stress regulatory genes, activation of MAPK signaling and inactivation of PI3K pathway	NR
Park et al. [55]	2018	Apigenin (20 µM)	VK2/E6E7 and End1/E6E7 cells treated with Apigenin	VK2/E6E7 and End1/E6E7 cells not treated with Apigenin	- Apigenin: • decreased cell proliferation, reduced MMP expression • increased apoptosis inducing mitochondrial pro-apoptotic proteins, Bax, Bak and Cyt c in End1/E6E7 cells • increased concentrations of calcium ions in the cytosol and ROS generation with lipid peroxidation • induced ER stress by increasing phosphorylation of unfolded proteins • inhibited the phosphorylation of ERK1/2 in both cell lines, but the phosphorylation of AKT increased only in End1/E6E7 cells	NR

Table 1. *Cont.*

Authors	Date	Substance	Cases	Controls	Results	Adverse Events
Takaoka et al. [57]	2018	DRIAs (0.2, 2, 20 μM)	EcSC from 24 patients with endometriosis	EuSC from 12 patients without endometriosis	- DRIAs: • inhibited proliferation of EcSCs in a concentration-dependent manner, but not of EuSCs • decreased IL-6, IL-8, COX-2 and aromatase mRNA levels, PGE2 protein levels and aromatase enzyme activity • suppressed TNF-α-induced IκB expression, the NF-kB-ikb complex formation, and the uptake of p65 into the nucleus	NR
Arablou et al. [59]	2019	Resveratrol (100 μM)	13 EuSC 8 EcSC from 40 women with endometriosis	11 EuSC from 15 women without endometriosis	- Basal expression of IGF-1 and HGF gene were significantly higher in EcSC - Resveratrol: • decreased IGF-1 and HGF gene expression more in EuSC from control women than in EcSC and EuSC from women without endometriosis • decreased IGF-1 and HGF protein production in EuSC from women with endometriosis and EcSC	Resveratrol at 200- and 400-μM concentrations

Table 1. *Cont.*

Authors	Date	Substance	Cases	Controls	Results	Adverse Events
Ham et al. [61]	2019	Silibinin (0.2, 5, 10, 25, 50 μM)	VK2/E6E7 and End1/E6E7 cells treated with Silibinin	EuSC treated with Silibinin	- Silibinin: • decreased proliferation of endometriotic cells but not of EuSC • induced cell cycle arrest and apoptosis in endometriotic cells with an increase of the sub-G1 population in a dose-dependent manner • increased ROS levels and lipid peroxidation in endometriotic cells • stimulated ER stress through the disruption of calcium homeostasis in cytosol and mitochondrial matrix in endometriotic cells causing cell death • induced changes in the MAPK signaling pathway in VK2-End1cells	NR
Ryu et al. [66]	2019	Chyrisin (0.5, 10, 20, 50, 100 μM)	VK2/E6E7 and End1/E6E7 cells treated with Chyrisin	VK2/E6E7 and End1/E6E7 cells not treated with Chyrisin EuC	- Chyrisin: • decreased proliferation and stimulated apoptosis and cell cycle arrest in the sub-G1 phase • increased cytosolic calcium levels and ROS production • activated ER stress by stimulating the unfolded protein response proteins • inactivated PI3K/PKB signaling pathway in a dose-dependent manner	NR

Table 1. Cont.

Authors	Date	Substance	Cases	Controls	Results	Adverse Events
Park et al. [67]	2019	Delphinidin (0, 5, 10, 20, 50, 100 μM)	VK2/E6E7 and End1/E6E7 cells treated with Delphinidin	VK2/E6E7 and End1/E6E7 cells not treated with Delphinidin	- Delphinidin: • decreased cell proliferation at 100 μM. In both cell lines, the percentage of cells in the sub G0/G1 stage gradually increased with increase of Delphinidin concentration • increased levels of cytosolic calcium ions and mitochondrial depolarization • inactivated PI3K/AKT and ERK1/2 and increased the phosphorylation of P38 MAPK and P90RSK proteins in both cell lines- Cells in late apoptosis increased by 1016%	NR
Park et al. [68]	2019	Quercetin (0, 2, 5, 10, 20, 50 μM)	VK2/E6E7 and End1/E6E7 cells treated with Quercetin	VK2/E6E7 and End1/E6E7 cells not treated with Quercetin	- Quercetin: • decreased cell proliferation at 20 μM. The percentage of G0/G1 stage cells increased in VK2/E6E7 cells although there was a decrease in End1/E6E7 cells • increased ROS production in both cell types • decreased phosphorylation of ERK1/2, P90RSK, P38, AKT, P70S6K, and S6 proteins - Cells in late apoptosis increased for both cell lines - The loss of MMP increased to 2300% in VK2/E6E7 cells and 670% in End1/E6E7 cells at 20 μM	NR
Park et al. [69]	2019	Luteolin (0, 5, 10, 20, 50 and 100 μM)	VK2/E6E7 and End1/E6E7 cells treated with luteolin	VK2/E6E7 and End1/E6E7 cells not treated with luteolin	- Luteolin: • decreased proliferation in a dose-dependent manner. • induced cell cycle arrest in the sub-G0/G1 stage and decreased the cell percentage in the G0/G1 stage in both cell lines • increased cell apoptosis through cytosolic calcium regulation and ROS accumulation • inhibited the phosphorylation of ERK1/2, JNK and PI3K/AKT signal proteins while activating P38 MAPK proteins	NR

Table 1. Cont.

Authors	Date	Substance	Cases	Controls	Results	Adverse Events
Hernandes et al. [71]	2020	Rutin and extract of Uncaria guianensis	EuSC and EcSC from 4 women with endometriosis	EuSC from 2 women without endometriosis	- Increased ROS levels in EuC from controls treated with ALE, ABE, and ARE and in EuC of patients with endometriosis treated with Rutin, ARE, Rutin + ALE, and Rutin + ARE - Increased ROS levels in EcC treated with ALE - Increased IL-15, IL-17A, IL-4, IL-6, TNF-alfa and VEGF levels in EuC from controls treated with ABE - Increased EGF in EcC treated with ALE	NR
Khazaei et al. [74]	2020	Resveratrol (0, 10, 50, 100, 200 µM)	EcSC from 9 patients with endometriosis	EuSC from 9 patients without endometriosis	- Resveratrol (200 µM) completely inhibited growth and angiogenesis in both cells types in a dose-dependent manner - NO level was higher in endometriotic cells. Resveratrol reduced NO level in both endometriotic and endometrial cells - Effect on apoptotic genes (P53, Bax, Bcl2 and caspase 3) and SIRT1	
Park et al. [75]	2020	DMF (Chyrisin) (0, 20, 50, 100 µM)	VK2/E6E7 and End1/E6E7 cells treated with DMF	VK2/E6E7 and End1/E6E7 cells not treated with DMF	- DMF: • induced sub-G1 cell cycle arrest in VK2/E6E7 cell, while End1/E6E7 cells were arrested at the G2/M phase • decreased proliferation and induced apoptosis in both cell lines • disrupted mitochondrial regulation and increased ROS production and lipid peroxidation in both cell lines, increasing ER stress-response pathways • down-regulated ERK1/2 pathway in End1/E6E7 cells but upregulated it in VK2/E6E7 cells • inhibited PI3K/AKT pathway in both cell lines	

Table 1. Cont.

Authors	Date	Substance	Cases	Controls	Results	Adverse Events
Park et al. [76]	2020	Myricetin (0, 5, 10, 20, 50, 100 μM)	VK2/E6E7 and End1/E6E7 cells treated with Myricetin	VK2/E6E7 and End1/E6E7 cells not treated with Myricetin	- Myricetin • decreased proliferation in a dose-dependent manner, caused by cycle arrest at the sub G0/G1 phase and increased late apoptosis • induced depolarization of the mitochondrial membrane, increased level of cytosolic calcium ions in the cells and ROS generation and accumulation in the cytoplasm • down-regulated the phosphorylated ERK1/2 and PI3K/AKT signal proteins, induced p38 protein activation in a dose-dependent manner	NR

Only p-values statistically significant ($p < 0.05$) were reported. *Legend*: EuSC = eutopic endometrial stromal cells; PE = phytoestrogen; FCA = free cell assay; EcSC = ectopic endometrial stromal cells; E2 = 17 beta-estradiol; MMP = matrix metalloproteinase; TIMP = tissue inhibitors of metalloproteinases; NR = not reported; BSA = bovine serum albumin; ERK = extracellular signal-regulated kinases; MAPK = mitogen-activated protein kinase; COX-2 = cyclooxygenase-2; cyp19 = cytochrome P450 19; EGCG = epigallocatechin gallate; EuEC = eutopic endometrial epithelial cells; cdc25a = cell division cycle 25 homolog A; SRC = steroid receptor coactivator; NCoR = nuclear receptor corepressor; SMRT = silencing mediator for retinoid or thyroid-hormone receptors; SIRT-1 = sirtuin 1; TNF alfa = tumor necrosis factor alfa; IL = interleukin; TRAIL = TNF alfa related-apoptosis-inducing ligand; PFE = Pueraria lowers extract; VK2 = vaginal mucosa-derived epithelial endometriotic cell; End1/E6E7 = endocervix epithelial-derived endometriotic cell line; ROS = reactive oxygen species; ER = endoplasmic reticulum; GADD153 = G1 arrest and DNA damage 153; IRE1α = inositol-requiring protein 1α; GRP78: the 78-kDa glucose-regulated protein; PI3K = phosphatidylinositol 3-kinase; DRIA: daidzein-rich isoflavone aglycones; Bax = Bcl-2-associated X protein; Bak = Bcl-2-antagonist/killer; Cyt C = cytochrome complex; PERK = PRKR-like ER kinase; eIF2α: eukaryotic translation initiation factor 2α; PG = prostaglandin; NF-kB-ikb = nuclear factor-κB-IKB-inhibitory proteins; EuC = eutopic endometrial cells; IGF-1: insulin-like growth factor-1; HGF: hepatocyte growth factor; NO = nitric oxide; Bcl 2 = B-cell lymphoma 2; DMF: 5,7-dimethoxyflavone; EcC = ectopic endometrial cells; ABE = aqueous bark extract of U. guianensis; ALE = aqueous leaf extract of U. guianensis; ARE = aqueous root extract of U. guianensis; EGF = epidermal growth factor; NAC = N-acetyl-L-cysteine; TGF-b1 = tumor growth factor-b1; Smad protein = small mother against decapentaplegic protein.

Resveratrol was the most studied substance whose effects have been investigated in 5 out of 22 studies with significant findings in all of them [35,41,47,59,74]. According to Ricci and coworkers [35], resveratrol could induce significant changes in cell proliferation and apoptosis of eutopic endometrial epithelial cell cultures although without significant differences between endometriosis patients and control women. In line, Khazei et al. have recently reported that the anti-proliferative, proapoptotic and anti-angiogenetic effect of this substance was not specific for ectopic endometrial cells [74].

They claimed a role for the treatment in reducing nitric oxide (NO) levels, found to be higher in endometriotic cells, and in increasing significantly the expression of apoptotic genes (P53, Bax, Bcl2 and caspase 3) and of sirtuin 1 (SIRT1) in both eutopic and ectopic cells. A relationship between activation of SIRT1 by resveratrol and interleukin (IL)-8 was investigated by Taguchi et al. [41] who, conversely, demonstrated that the anti-inflammatory effects of the compound were more prominent in endometriotic cells than in eutopic cells from controls. The same group, one year later, reported that, even if resveratrol alone was not capable of inducing apoptosis in endometriotic cells, it determined an altered expression of some key molecules involved in apoptosis such as survivin or TNF-α-related-apoptosis-inducing ligand (TRAIL), favoring cell death in ectopic lesions [47]. Finally, a higher insulin-like growth factor-1 (IGF-1) and hepatocyte growth factor (HGF) gene expression in ectopic endometrial cells has been demonstrated by Arablou and coworkers [59]. In this case, resveratrol biological effect in terms of decrease in IGF-1 and HGF protein production was reported for both eutopic and ectopic endometrial stromal cells from women with endometriosis but not for cells from controls. Resveratrol was also shown to inhibit IGF-1/ERK and HGF/MAPK signal transduction pathways in a dose-dependent manner, thus resulting in anti-inflammatory and anti-proliferative effects. Therefore, although the exact mechanism involved is still poorly defined, all the papers supported some in vitro benefit of resveratrol.

Three studies investigated the effects of puerarin (10^{-9} M), a major isoflavonoid compound extracted from the Chinese medicinal herb, *Radix puerariae* [28,30,34]. Studies were concordant in demonstrating that puerarin treatment in combination with ethinylestradiol (E2) significantly suppressed the E2-mediated proliferation of stromal cells from endometriotic lesions. Moreover, treating ectopic stromal cells with Puerarin abrogated ERK phosphorylation through a competition with estrogen for the binding to membrane receptors of MAPK signaling, thus significantly decreasing cell proliferation, as well as gene expression levels of cyclin D1, cyclo-oxygenase (COX) 2 and cyp19 involved in this process [30,34]. Finally, Ji and coworkers demonstrated that puerarin can partly suppress estrogen-stimulated proliferation by promoting the recruitment of corepressors to estrogen receptor, as well as limiting that of coactivators, in order to arrest ectopic stromal cells in the G1 phase [34]. Three studies out of 22 investigated the biological effect of chyrisin, a natural compound derived from honey, propolis, or passion flowers, on human endometrial cells [20,66,75]. Although shown to be potent inhibitor of aromatase activity in a free cell assay, chyrisin, daidzein or naringenin could not attenuate aromatase activity in endometrial stromal cells in women with and without endometriosis at any concentration tested. Only genistein (10^{-9}–10^{-6} M) indirectly increased aromatase activity in endometrial stromal cells from controls. On the other hand, in both VK2/E6E7 and End1/E6E7 endometriotic cell lines, chyrisin was shown to suppress cell proliferation and induced the programmed cell death through changing the cell cycle proportion, increasing the cytosolic calcium level and generating reactive oxygen species (ROS) [66]. In addition, Chrysin activated endoplasmic reticulum (ER) stress by stimulating the unfolded protein response proteins, especially the 78-kDa glucose-regulated protein, GRP78, the PRKR-like ER kinase (PERK) and the eukaryotic translation initiation factor 2α (eIF2α). Finally, the compound was shown to inactivate the intracellular phosphatidylinositol 3-kinase (PI3K)/protein kinase B signaling pathway in a dose-dependent manner from 5 to 100 μM. Similar results and the same biological mechanisms were reported for chyrisin by Park et al. [75], actually testing 5,7-Dimethoxyflavone (DMF), a methylated form of chrysin extracted from *Kaempferia parviflora* (KP). The methylation of flavonoids has been demonstrated to greatly increase their absorption and bioavailability. A similar biological effect was demonstrated for naringenin by the same authors [50]. Indeed, naringenin (100 μM) decreased the proliferation and increased apoptosis of VK2/E6E7 and End1/E6E7 cells. In the same cells, it also increased the production of ROS 3-fold, induced mitochondrial pro-apoptotic proteins (Bax and Bak), in VK2/E6E7 cells by ~7-fold and in End1/E6E7 cells by 2-fold. Finally, naringenin significantly increased apoptosis through generation of ER stress regulatory genes, in particular G1 arrest and DNA damage 153 (GADD153), inositol-requiring protein 1α (IRE1α) and GRP78, and through activation of MAPK signaling and inactivation of PI3K pathway. It is interesting to note that the same group of authors investigated these same biological mechanisms highlighted for chirisin, narigenin for other substances, such as apigenin, delphinidin, luteolin, quercetin, silibinin and myricetin in VK2/E6E7 and End1/E6E7 endometriotic cells lines [50,55,61,67–69]. All these studies are summarized in Table 1. Overall, they demonstrated that the PE effect on endometriosis is always antiproliferative and proapoptic through the activation of intracellular signals of calcium, ER stress and ROS production and through the activation of the MAPK pathway and a decreased phosphorylation of ERK1/2 and PI3K/AKT signaling proteins.

Two studies out of 22 investigated the biological effect of EGCG in eutopic endometrial stromal cells (EuSC) from women with or without endometriosis [35] or in EuSC and ectopic endometrial stromal cells (EcSC) from women affected by endometriosis [40]. The results from these studies were contradictory: while Ricci and coworkers showed no significant difference in cell proliferation and apoptosis between cases and controls [35], Matsuzaki et al. demonstrated an inhibited cell proliferation, migration and invasion of both EuSC and EcSC after EGCG treatment. Moreover, EGCG significantly decreased the Tumor growth factor b-1 (TGF-b1)-dependent increase in the mRNA expression of fibrotic markers and significantly inhibited TGF-b1-stimulated activation of the MAPK and Smad signaling pathways in both cells [40].

Kim et al. [48] examined the effect of Pueraria flowers extract (PFE), a rich source of isoflavones such as genistein, daidzein, kakkalide, puerarin, and tectoridin, on immortalised human endometriotic cells, 11Z and 12Z. Mesothelial Met5A cells were used for adhesion assessment after PFE treatment. They concluded that PFE significantly inhibited adhesion and migration of endometriotic cells to mesothelial cells, suppressing the mRNA and protein expressions of matrix metalloproteinases (MMP)-2 and MMP-9 and increasing the phosphorylation of ERK1/2 in endometriotic cells. A decreased MMP expression was also reported for apigenin [55] and for quercetin [68].

Takaoka and coworkers showed that Daidzein-rich isoflavone aglycones (DRIAs) significantly inhibited the proliferation of ectopic cells in a concentration dependent manner [57]. It also decreased IL-6, IL-8, COX-2 and aromatase mRNA levels, prostaglandin E2 (PGE2) protein levels, and aromatase enzyme activity. DRIAs suppressed the Tumor necrosis factor-α (TNF-α) induced IκB expression, the nuclear factor-κB-IKB-inhibitory proteins (NF-kB-ikb) complex formation, and the uptake of p65 into the nucleus.

In contrast to all this evidence, Hernandes and colleagues have shown that rutin, a glycosylated flavonoid and extract of *Uncaria guianensis,* or a combination of both, was not able to reduce cellular viability, although ROS production did increase in both eutopic and ectopic cells [71]. In addition, significant increases levels of interleukin (IL)-15, IL-17A, IL-4, IL-6, TNF-α, and vascular endothelium growth factor (VEGF) were observed when eutopic endometrial cells were treated with aqueous bark extract of *U. guianensis* (ABE), while exposure to aqueous bark leaf of *U. guianensis* (ALE) induced significant increases in epidermal growth factor in lesion cells.

3.1.2. Phytoestrogens and Endometriosis: In Vivo Experimental Animal Models

Thirty-eight articles on the effects of PE on the development of endometriotic lesions in in vivo experimental animal models of endometriosis have been included in this systematic review. Among them, PE were administered non orally (18 studies, Table 2), orally (18 studies, Table 3) or both (2 studies, reported in both tables). Seven studies investigated the effects of EGCG on endometriosis development, five in mice and one in hamsters. ECGC was administered either orally [35] or through an intraperitoneal injection [23,24,29,35,37,40,45]. In all the studies in which endometriotic lesions were measured, ECGC induced the regression of lesions.

The compound could suppress E2-stimulated activation, proliferation and VEGF expression of endometrial cells in vitro isolated from hamsters. When evaluated by intravital fluorescence microscopy and histology, in vivo treatment with ECGC mediated a selective inhibition of angiogenesis and blood perfusion of endometriotic lesions without affecting blood vessel development in ovarian follicles [23,24,35,37]. Moreover, EGCG showed to increase total apoptotic cell numbers in the lesions [24,35,37]. Molecular mechanisms put forward to explain these phenomena in the lesions include: selective inhibition of VEGFC expression; down-regulation of MMP-9, chemokine (C-X-C motif) ligand 3 (CXCL3), c-JUN, and interferon-γ expression, decreased ROS generation and lipid peroxidation and reduced MMP-2 and MMP-9 activity [29,45]. Matsuzaki and colleagues observed significantly lower scores for both Sirius red and Masson trichrome staining in EGCG-treated mice suggesting that this treatment may prevent the progression of fibrosis [40].

Eight studies investigated the effects of resveratrol on endometriosis development, three in rats and five in mice. Resveratrol was administered either orally [26,36,44], or through an intramuscular [33,43], subcutaneous [38] or intraperitoneal [35,42] injection. The administration of resveratrol showed a marked reduction in endometriotic implants when they were measured. Histological evaluations of tissue sections revealed that both the dimensions and the vascularization of the implants were diminished in the resveratrol-treated animal model. Molecular mechanisms proposed to explain this finding include: decreased levels of VEGF, monocyte chemotactic protein 1 (MCP-1), IL-6, IL-8 and TNF-α in the peritoneal fluid and lower presence of lesional MMP-2, MMP-9 and VEGF [33,35,36,43,44]. Investigating the effects of resveratrol on the expression of estrogen receptor α (ER-α), the proliferative marker Ki-67, aryl hydrocarbon receptor (AhR) and members of the cytochrome P450 superfamily of enzymes, Amaya and colleagues found that mice treated with estradiol (E2) plus progesterone or E2 plus the highest dose (60 mg) of resveratrol exhibited a reduction in both ER-α and Ki-67 in eutopic endometrial epithelial cells. In stromal cells, ER-α levels were reduced by E2 plus P, but not by resveratrol while Ki-67 expression was reduced in presence of 60 mg/day of resveratrol suggesting the potential benefit of high doses of the compound in reducing the proliferation of human endometrium [38]. Bruner-Tran and colleagues have demonstrated that oral administration of resveratrol at dose of 6 mg either for 10–12 days or 18–20 days decreased number of endometrial implants per mouse by 60% and the total volume of lesions per mouse by 80% [26]. Moreover, the authors studied the effect of resveratrol on EcSC in vitro invasiveness, finding a concentration-dependent reduction up to 78%. Finally, Yavuz and coworkers demonstrated a reduced oxidative stress in cases compared to controls in a dose-dependent manner (I.P injection of resveratrol at low dose 1 mg/kg and high dose 10 mg/kg), confirming also reduced lesion size and reduced proliferative scores for the treatment group independent of the dose [42].

Table 2. Studies investigating effects of non-oral intake of phytoestrogens on endometriosis in an animal in vivo model.

Authors	Date	Model	Substance	Cases (n)	Control (n)	Results
Cotroneo et al. [19]	2001	Rats	S.C., genistein: • 50 µg/g (high) • 16.6 µg/g (average) • 5 µg/g (low)	7/8/10	Vehicle (20) or Estrone (7)	Higher and average dose of Genistein and administration of estrone: - increased uterine/body weight ratios - increased uterine PR expression at all doses - supported growth of the implanted tissue in a dose-responsive manner
Laschke et al. [23]	2008	Hamsters	I.P. EGCG 65 mg/kg	7	Vehicle (10)	- inhibited angiogenesis and blood perfusion of endometriotic lesions
Xu et al. [24]	2009	Mice	I.P. EGCG 50 mg/kg	10	Vitamin E (10) Vehicle (10)	- smaller lesions than control animals - down-regulation of VEGFA mRNA expression - down-regulation of MAPK1 and NFKB mRNA expression
Laschke et al. [25]	2010	Hamsters	IP genistein 50/200 mg/kg	Low dose (6) High dose (4)	Vehicle (6)	- blood perfusion and angiogenesis of endometriotic lesions was not affected by Genistein treatment
Xu et al. [29]	2011	Mice	I.P. EGCG 50 mg/kg	10	Vitamin E (10) Vehicle (10)	- decreased lesion size - down-regulation of MMP-9, CXCL3, VEGFC, c-JUN, and IFNγ - suppression of VEGFC mRNA and protein - decreased VEGFC levels in both microvessels and glandular epithelial cells
Ergenoglu et al. [33]	2013	Rats	I.M. resveratrol 10 mg/kg	6	Vehicle (6)	- reduction of implant size - decreased levels of VEGF in peritoneal fluid and plasma - decreased levels of MCP-1 in peritoneal fluid - suppression of VEGF expression in endometriotic tissue
Ricci et al. [35]	2013	Mice	I.P. resveratrol 10–25 mg/kg; EGCG 20–100 mg/kg by esophageal gavage	Resveratrol (29) EGCG (27)	Vehicle (NR)	- both treatments reduced number and volume of lesions - both diminished proliferation and vascular density of endometriotic lesions - both increased apoptosis

Table 2. Cont.

Authors	Date	Model	Substance	Cases (n)	Control (n)	Results
Wang et al. [37]	2013	Mice	I.P. EGCG 50 mg/kg or pro-EGCG 50 mg/kg	EGCG (8) proEGCG (8)	Vitamin E (8) Vehicle (8)	- decreased lesion size - decreased angiogenesis - increased total apoptopic cell numbers
Amaya et al. [38]	2014	Mice	S.C. resveratrol 6/30/60 mg/kg	E2 + 6 mg of Resveratrol (4) E2 + 30 mg of Resveratrol (4) E2 + 60 mg of Resveratrol (4)	E2 (4) E2 + P (4)	- reduction in ESR1 and Ki-67 by the highest dose in eutopic endometrial epithelial cells - reduction in Ki-67 expression by the highest dose in endometrial stroma
Matsuzaki et al. [40]	2014	Mice	I.P. EGCG 50 mg/kg	NR	NR	- lower scores for both Sirius red and Masson trichrome staining
Yavuz et al. [42]	2014	Rats	I.P resveratrol 1/10 mg/kg	Low dose (8) High dose (8)	Vehicle (8)	- lower implants volume in cases independently from dose - reduced oxidative stress in cases compared to controls in a dose-dependent manner - proliferative scores for glandular tissue and stromal tissue were lower in cases
Bayoglu Tekin et al. [43]	2015	Mice	I.M. resveratrol 30 mg/kg S.C. 1 mg/kg single dose LA	Resveratrol (NR) LA and resveratrol (NR)	Vehicle (NR) LA (NR)	- reduced implant volumes, histopathological grade and immuno-reactivity to MMP-2, MMP-9 and VEGF - decreased plasma and peritoneal fluid levels of IL-6, IL-8 and TNF-α
Singh et al. [45]	2015	Mice	I.P. EGCG and doxycycline (NPs) at a dose of 40 mg/kg body weight	50	10	- decreased ROS and LPO, MMP-2 and MMP-9 activity - decreased angiogenesis and microvessel density
Jouhari et al. [52]	2018	Rats	S.C. 100 mg/kg silymarin	8	Vehicle (8) Letrozole (8) Cabergoline (8)	- smaller volume of implants - lower mean score of the histopathological evaluation of the implants

Table 2. Cont.

Authors	Date	Model	Substance	Cases (n)	Control (n)	Results
Wei et al. [58]	2018	Mice	I.P. nobiletin 10, 20 mg/kg	Low dose Nobiletin (3) High dose Nobiletin (3)	3 (endometriosis) 3 (sham)	- reduced lesion size - lower PCNA and VEGF immunostaining - higher E-cadherin staining - decreased levels of IL-6, IL-1β, and MMP-3 - reduced levels of TNF-α and MMP-1 - reduced phosphorylation of IKKα, IκBα and p65 factors
Ding et al. [60]	2019	Mice	I.P. scutellarin • 15 mg/kg • 7.5 mg/kg	Low dose (9) High dose (9)	Vehicle (9)	- reduction of lesion weight, improved hyperalgesia, reduced proliferation, angiogenesis, and fibrogenesis of the lesions - reduced the platelet activation rate in peripheral blood
Ham et al. [61]	2019	Mice	I.P. silibinin 100 μL	15	Vehicle (15)	- reduced average size of lesions - decreased expression of TNF-α, IL-1β, and IL-6 mRNA
Park et al. [68]	2019	Mice	I.P. quercetin 35 mg/kg	15	Vehicle (15)	- decreased lesion volume - decreased Ccnd1 mRNA
Park et al. [69]	2019	Mice	I.P. luteolin 40 mg/kg/day	6	Vehicle (6)	- reduced endometriotic lesions growth - decreased mRNA expression of Ccne1, Cdk2 and Cdk4
Park et al. [76]	2020	Mice	I.P. myricetin 30 mg/kg	10	Vehicle (10)	- decreased lesion size - decreased Ccne1 mRNA expression

Only statistically significant effects ($p < 0.05$) were reported. *Legend*: S.C = subcutaneous; PR = progesterone receptor; I.P = intraperitoneal; EGCG = epigallocatechin-3-gallate; E2 = 17b-estradiol; NR = not reported; VEGF = vascular endothelial growth factor; MAPK1 = mitogen activated protein kinase 1; NFKB = nuclear factor kappa B; MMP = matrix metalloproteinase; CXCL3 = chemokine (C-X-C motif) ligand 3; IFNγ = interferon γ; I.M. = intramuscular; MCP-1 = monocyte chemotactic protein 1; proEGCG = prodrug of green tea epigallocatechin-3-gallate; P = progesterone; ESR1 = estrogen receptor α; LA = leuprolide acetate; IL = interleukin; TNF-α = tumor necrosis factor-α; NPs = synthesized nanoparticles; ROS = reactive oxygen species; LPO = lipid peroxidation; EM = endometriosis; PCNA = proliferating cell nuclear antigen; IKKα = IκB kinase; Ccnd1 = cyclin D1; DMSO = dimethyl sulfoxide; Ccne1 = cyclin e1; Cdk = cyclin-dependent kinase.

Table 3. Studies investigating the effects of phytoestrogen oral intake on endometriosis in an animal in vivo model.

Authors	Date	Model	Substance	Cases (n)	Control (n)	Results
Cotroneo et al. [19]	2001	rats	Genistein 250/1000 mg/kg AIN-76A diet	12 + 11 (lower/higher dietary intake)	Vehicle (17)	- increased uterine PRB by the higher dietary intake
Yavuz et al. [22]	2007	rats	Genistein 500 mg/kg	10	Raloxifene at 10 mg/kg or no vehicle (10 + 13)	- smaller area and lower histological scores of endometriotic lesions
Bruner-Tran et al. [26]	2011	mice	Resveratrol 6 mg	20	Vehicle (16)	- decreased number of endometrial implants per mouse by 60% and the total volume of lesions per mouse by 80%
Chen et al. [27]	2011	rats	Puerarin • High (600 mg/kg) • Medium (200 mg/kg) • Low (60 mg/kg)	45 (15 each)	Danazol at dose of 80 mg/kg or vehicle (15 + 15)	- inhibition of growth of ectopic implants for both Puerarin and Danazol - inhibition of P450 aromatase expression and reduction of estrogen levels in endometriotic tissue using the low dose
Rudzitis-Auth et al. [32]	2012	mice	Xanthohumol 100 mM	8	Vehicle (8)	- decreased lesion growth and volume - suppression of peritoneal and mesenteric endometriotic lesions - reduced proliferation and PI3-J protein
Rudzitis-Auth et al. [36]	2013	mice	Resveratrol 40 mg/kg	10	Vehicle (10)	- lower lesion volume and size - reduced number of PCNA-positive stromal cells - lower Ki-67-positive glandular cells - inhibition of angiogenesis
Ricci et al. [35]	2013	mice	EGCG 20 or 100 mg/kg	18 (9 each)	Vehicle (9)	- reduction of mean number and volume of endometriotic lesions - reduced vascular density - increased apoptosis
Demirel et al. [39]	2014	rats	Extract of Achillea bierbersteinii N-Hexane EtOAc MeOH	18	Vehicle or 6 buserelin acetate 20 mg/weekly sc (12)	- decreased endometriotic volume in EtOAc and buserelin groups - reduced peritoneal TNF-α in EtOAc and reference, VEGF in both and IL-6 in EtOAc

Table 3. *Cont.*

Authors	Date	Model	Substance	Cases (n)	Control (n)	Results
Ozcan Censoy et al. [44]	2015	rats	Resveratrol 60 mg/kg/day	7	Vehicle or leuprolide acetate at 1 mg/kg depot (7 + 8)	- Both resveratrol and leuprolide acetate reduced mean surface areas of endometriotic implants - reduced VEGF score in endometriotic implants - reduced peritoneal and serum VEGF and MCP-1
Di Paola et al. [46]	2016	rats	mPEA\PLD 10 mg/kg	5	Vehicle (5)	- decreased cyst diameter, histological injury score, mast cells number and VEGF, ICAM-1 expression - increased fibrosis score and NGF - less pain behaviors
Ferella et al. [51]	2018	mice	Wogonin 20 mg/kg/day	12	Vehicle (11)	- increased percentage of apoptotic cells
Nahari et al. [54]	2018	rats	Sylimarin (SMN) 50 mg/kg/day	6	Vehicle (6)	- decreased endometriotic-like lesions size and percentage of cell proliferation, angiogenesis, GDNF, grfα and Bcl-6b. - enhanced fibrosis and apoptosis - enhanced ERK1/2 expression.
Melekoglu et al. [53]	2018	rats	Nerolidol 100 mg/kg or Hesperidin 50 mg/kg	16 (8 each)	(8)	- lower volume, more evident in nerolidol group - increased GSH, SOD and GPx
Takaoka et al. [57]	2018	mice	DRIA food at 0.06%	NR	Vehicle (NR)	- decreased number, weight and Ki-67 proliferative activity of endometriotic-like lesions - decreased IL-6, IL-8 and COX-2
Ilhan et al. [62]	2019	rats	Extract of *Urtica dioica* • N-Hexane • EtOAc • MeOH - Fraction A - Fraction B - Fraction C - Fraction D	18 (6 each)	Vehicle or buserelin acetate 20 mg/weekly sc (12)	- decreased adhesion score, endometriotic implant volume, peritoneal TNF-α, VEGF and IL-6 in MeOH, reference and Fraction C

Table 3. Cont.

Authors	Date	Model	Substance	Cases (n)	Control (n)	Results
Ilhan et al. [63]	2019	rats	Extract of *Anthemis austriaca* • N-Hexane • EtOAc • MeOH - Fraction A - Fraction B - Fraction C (Quercetin and Apigenin) - Fraction D	18 (6 each)	Vehicle or buserelin acetate 20 mg/weekly sc (12)	- decreased endometriotic implant volume and adhesion score, peritoneal TNF-α, VEGF and IL-6 in EtOAc, MeOH, and reference - decreased adhesion score and endometriotic implants volume and peritoneal IL-6 and VEGF in Fraction A and in Fraction C - decreased peritoneal TNF-α in Fraction C
Kapoor et al. [64]	2019	rats	Narigenin 50 mg/kg/day: • Only the day of endometriosis induction • Every day for 21 days	12 (6 each)	oral dienogest at dose of 0.3 mg/kg/day for 21 days or nothing (12 endometriosis)(6 sham controls)	Both Narigenin and Dienogest: - suppression of endometriotic lesion growth and reduced lesion weight by inducing apoptosis, cellular ROS and damaging mitochondrial membrane. - inhibition of NO release and restoration of TNFα level - reduced TAK1 levels by 3-fold at dose of 1 μM and 5 μM, reduced VEGF by 2 and 4-fold at dose of 1 μM and 5 μM - mitigation of the expression of Nrf2, its repressor and effector molecule reduced number of cells migrating at 1 μM and 5 μM - reduced expression of MMP-2 and MMP-3
Bina et al. [70]	2020	rats	*Achillea cretica* (A.C.) extract once a day at dose of • 100 mg/kg/day; • 200 mg/kg/day; • 400 mg/kg/day	18 (6 each)	Vehicle or letrozole (12 endometriosis) (6 sham controls)	- reduced size of implanted tissue, mean score of the histopathological evaluation of the implants, thickness of epithelial layer. - decreased serum TNF-α and both serum and tissue IL-6 levels after treatment with A.C. 100, 400 and letrozole. - reduced tissue TNF-α and both serum and tissue VEGF levels after treatment with A.C. 100 and letrozole

Table 3. *Cont.*

Authors	Date	Model	Substance	Cases (n)	Control (n)	Results
Hsu et al. [72]	2020	mice	ISL and estrogens (10 mg/kg/day) • 1 mg/kg (LI) • 5 mg/kg (HI)	12 (6 each)	Vehicle (6)	- smaller volume of lesions - decreased tissue VEGF level in HI - decreased serum IL-1β in HI cand decreased tissue IL-1β in HI e LI. - decreased serum and tissue IL-6 levelincreased Bax, cleaved-caspase-3 and E-Cadherin expression in HI. - decreased bcl-2, ER-β, N-Cadherin, Snail and Slug expression.
Ilhan et al. [73]	2020	rats	Extract of *Melilotus officinalis* (kaempferol, quercetin, and coumarin derivatives) at 100 mg/kg/day • N-Hexane • EtOAc • MeOH - Fraction A - Fraction B - Fraction C - Fraction D	18 (6 each)	Vehicle or buserelin acetate 20 mg/weekly sc (12)	Both MeOH, Fraction C and buserelin acetate: - decreased endometriotic implants volume and peritoneal TNF-α, VEGF and IL-6 levels - decreased endometriotic implant adhesion score, volume and IL-6 in Fraction B

Only statistically significant effects ($p < 0.05$) were reported. *Legend*: PRB, progesterone receptor type B; EcSC = ectopic endometrial stromal cells; EGCG = epigallocatechin gallate; EtOAc = ethyl acetate; MeOH = methanol; TNF alfa = tumor necrosis factor alfa; VEGF = vascular endothelial growth factor; IL = interleukin; MCP-1 = monocyte chemoattractant protein-1; mPEA\PLD = micronized palmitoylethanolamide/polydatin; ICAM-1 = intercellular adhesion molecule-1; NGF = nerve growth factor; GDNF = glial cell line-derived neurotrophic factor; grfα = receptor of GDNF; ERK1/2 = extracellular signal-regulated kinases; GSH = glutathione; SOD = superoxide dismutase; GPx = glutathione peroxidase; DRIA = daidzein-rich isoflavone aglycones; NR = not reported; COX = cyclooxygenase; ROS = reactive oxygen species; NO = nitric oxide; Nrf2 = nuclear factor erythroid 2-related factor; MMP = matrix metalloproteinases; ISL = isoliquiritigenin; HI = high dose of ISL; LI = low dose of ISL; ER = estrogen receptor; H&E = hematoxylin and eosin; PCNA = proliferating cell nuclear antigen.

The potential role for the genistein to sustain endometriosis has been explored by Cotroneo et al. and Laschke et al. [19,25]. Totally in disagreement with the other studies in this context, the subcutaneous and intraperitoneal injections of genistein was shown to sustain the growth of the implanted tissue in a dose-responsive manner [19] and not to sustain the neoangiogenesis and blood perfusion of endometriotic lesions [25]. When measuring uterine receptor expression, the treatment resulted in a significantly uterine decreased expression of ER-α protein and in an increased progesterone receptor (PR) expression at all doses compared to controls [19]. When administered orally, the same group of authors found that genistein determined an increase of uterine PR type B (PRB) at higher dietary dose. By contrast, in his previous research Yavuz et al. demonstrated that administered orally genistein resulted in smaller areas of endometriotic lesions and lower histological scores if compared with control animals [22].

Subcutaneous administration of silymarin [52] and intraperitoneal injection of silibinin, scutellarin, nobiletin, quercetin and myricetin have all been shown to reduce lesion size in mice and rats [58,60,61,68,76]. Ham et al. also found that the expression of TNF-α, IL-1β, and IL-6 mRNA decreased to 80.4%, 73.8%, and 96.5% respectively in the endometriotic lesions upon intraperitoneal silibinin treatment in mice [61]. Since scutellarin is traditionally used as a potent antiplatelet agent, Ding et al. evaluated its potential therapeutic effect showing also improved hyperalgesia in both low-dose and high-dose and changes consistent with reduced proliferation, angiogenesis, and fibrogenesis of the lesions. Moreover, this flavonoid also significantly reduced the platelet activation rate in peripheral blood when administered intraperitoneally in mice [60]. Intraperitoneal-injected nobiletin was shown to be effective on the activation of NF-κB in endometriotic cells, mainly targeting on the activity of IκB kinases (IKKs) and reducing p65 phosphorylation level [58]. A potential anti-proliferative role on endometriosis through cell cycle regulation has been demonstrated by Park et al. upon intraperitoneal administration of myricetin, quercetinin or luteolin in a mouse model [68,69,76].

In a rat model of endometriosis, oral administration of Puerarin inhibited the growth of ectopic implants and reduced estrogens levels in endometriotic tissue even when administered at low dose and without systemic adverse effects [27].

The potential therapeutic action of Xanthohumol, a flavonoid belonging to the same family of resveratrol, has been investigated by Rudzitis [32]. Similarly to resveratrol, oral Xanthohumol was able to reduce lesion growth by decreasing cell proliferation. Similar results were obtained with the oral administration of Sylimarin, Naringenin and Wogonin, plant-derived flavonoids [51,54,64]. Melekoglu et al. have evaluated the effect of hesperidin, a flavanone glycoside found in citrus fruit, on endometriosis development in a rat model observing lower lesion volumes and increased levels of antioxidant parameters when administered orally at dose of 50 mg/kg for 14 days [53].

Oral isoliquiriteginin (ISL), a flavonoid found in liquorice, has been found not only to decrease lesion volume but also to reduce serum and tissue VEGF, IL1β and IL-6 and to increase Bax, Bcl-2 and E-cadherin [72]. Other authors have investigated the effect of a daidzein-rich isoflavone aglycones diet [57] or of extract of different plants known to contain several PE such as *Achileea bierbersteinii* [39], *Urtica dioica* and *Anthemis austriaca* [62,63], *Melilotus officinalis* [73] and *Achillea critica* [70] on endometriosis lesions. All of them have been found to decrease the volume of lesion and adhesion scores. Also, decreased concentration TNF-α were observed both in peritoneal [62,63] and in serum and tissue samples [70]. Moreover, *Urtica dioica*, *Anthemis austriaca*, *Melilotus officinalis* and *Achillea critica* (AC) extract were able to reduce peritoneal VEGF and IL-6 compared to controls. The anti-inflammatory properties of AC were observed in the ability to reduce serum TNF-α, VEGF and IL-6 as well.

3.1.3. Phytoestrogen Dietary Intake and the Risk of Endometriosis in Humans

Table 4 shows the results of the seven studies that have investigated the effects of PE intake on endometriosis in humans. The first study that evaluated the effects of intaking soy products such as genistein and daidzein found an inverse association between the isoflavone intake and the risk of undergoing premenopausal hysterectomy for benign gynecological conditions, including endometriosis [18]. Similar results have been obtained in a case-control study evaluating urinary levels of genistein and daidzein in 138 women. Levels of isoflavones were found to be inversely correlated to stage III-IV of the disease. Frequency of ER-2 gene RsaI polymorphism was also assessed. A significant association was noted between specific genotypes of ER-2 RsaI polymorphism and genistein levels in risk of advanced endometriosis. Since altered estrogen or soy isoflavone signal transduction thanks to ER-2 gene polymorphisms may be directly responsible for susceptibility to severe endometriosis, the authors suggested that isoflavones may play a more effective role among the ER-2 RsaI R/r + R/R genotype than the r/r genotype, although the latter itself is likely to be protective for endometriosis [21]. Three studies have evaluated the effects of resveratrol on endometriosis women [31,49,65].

Table 4. Studies investigating the effect of phytoestrogen oral intake on humans.

Authors	Date	Study Design	Substance and Duration	Age (Years, Mean)	Case (n)	Control (n)	Results
Nagata et al. [18]	2001	prospective cohort study	Genistein, Daidzein in one year	35–54 42.9 ± 4.4	1172	n.a.	- decreased risk of hysterectomy for pain: RR (95% CI) 0.35 (0.13 ± 0.97)
Tsuchiya et al. [21]	2007	case-control study	Urinary levels of Genistein/Daidzein, NR	20–45 Stage I-II: 32.3 ± 3.2 Stage III-IV: 32.6 ± 3.7	79 (stage I–II n = 31; stage III–IV n = 48)	59	- inversely associated with stage III-IV with aOR 0.21 (95% CI = 0.06–0.76) for Genistein and 0.29 (0.08–1.03) for Daidzein levels - ER-2 RsaI R/r + R/R genotype more frequent than the r/r genotype in advanced stages
Maia et al. [31]	2012	retrospective study	Resveratrol 30 mg for 2–6 months	24–40 31 ± 4	OC+ resveratrol (26)	OC (16)	- reduction in pain scores, with 82% of patients reporting complete resolution of dysmenorrhea and pelvic pain after 2 months - lower COX-2 expression in eutopic endometrium at immunohistochemistry - lower aromatase expression in eutopic endometrium at immunohistochemistry
Mendes da Silva et al. [49]	2017	randomized clinical trial	Resveratrol 40 mg for 42 days	20–50 35.4 ± 7.1	22	Placebo (22)	- no difference in pain scores between groups [median difference: 0.75, 95% confidence interval: −1.6 to 2.3]
Signorile et al. [56]	2018	prospective cohort study	Quercetin 200 mg, titrated Turmeric 20 mg, titrated Parthenium 19.5 mg for three months	34 ± NR	Group I (30 patients treated with all the ingredients); Group II (30 patients treated with only linseed oil and 5 MTHF calcium salt)	Group III, placebo (30)	- significant reduction of headache (from 14% to 4%), cystitis (from 12% to 2%), muscles ache (from 4% to 1%), irritable colon (from 15% to 6%), dysmenorrhea (from 62% to 18%) and dyspareunia (from 30% to 15%), CPP (from 62% to 18%) - reduction of serum PGE2 level
Kodarahmian et al. [65]	2019	placebo-controlled, parallel, randomized double-blind exploratory clinical trial	Resveratrol. 400 mg for 12–14 weeks	18–37 30.19 ± 2.4	17	Placebo (17)	- reduced MMP-2 and MMP-9 mRNA and protein levels in eutopic endometrium - reduced level of MMP-2 and MMP-9 in endometrial fluid and serum
Youseflu et al. [77]	2020	case-control study on dietary data	Isoflavones, lignans, coumestrol, in one year	15–45 yo 31.01 ± 6.56	78	78	- reduced risk of endometriosis for Isoflavones [OR 0.38 (0.33–0.83)], Lignan [OR 0.49 (0.46–0.52)], and Coumestrol [OR 0.38 (0.15–0.96)] assumption

Only statistically significant effects ($p < 0.05$) were reported. Legend: n.a = not applicable; RR = rate ratios; CI = confidence interval; aOR = adjusted odds ratio; ER-2 = estrogen receptor-2; LPS = laparoscopy; HYS = hysteroscopy; OC = oral contraceptive; COX-2 = cyclo-oxygenase-2; SD = standard deviation; MTHF = methyltetrahydrofolate; CPP = chronic pelvic pain; PGE2 = prostaglandin E2; MMP = matrix metalloproteinase, NR = not reported. According to Maia and coworkers, the addition of 30 mg of resveratrol to the oral contraceptives (OC) regimen resulted in a further significant reduction in pain scores after 2 months of treatment, with complete resolution of dysmenorrhea and pelvic pain reported in 82% of cases [31]. Additionally, COX-2 and aromatase expression were significantly lower in the eutopic endometrium of patients using the combination of OC with resveratrol compared with those using OC alone [31]. Kodarahmian and colleagues investigated the effects of resveratrol on MMP-2 and MMP-9 levels in endometriosis patients (n = 34) who were randomly divided into treatment (n = 17 patients treated with 400 mg of resveratrol) and control (n = 17 patients treated with placebo) women. Reduced levels of both MMP-2 and MMP-9 mRNA and protein were found in eutopic endometrium as well as lower concentrations in serum and endometrial fluid following the administration of resveratrol for 12–14 weeks [65]. A randomized controlled trial conducted by da Mendes da Silva and colleagues randomized subjects to receive monophasic OC for 42 days in addition to 40 mg of resveratrol or placebo in order to compare them for the reduction of pain scores. In contrast with other studies, pain scores after treatment were not significantly different between groups leading the authors to conclude that daily use of resveratrol combined with continuous use of a OC, was not superior to a OC alone for the treatment of pain in women with endometriosis [49]. The study conducted by Signorile et al., evaluated the effects of quercetin, titrated turmeric and titrated parthenium in a dietary supplement with linoleic acid, alpha linolenic acid, nicotinamide and 5-methyltetrahydrofolate calcium salt in patients affected by endometriosis. The authors found a significant reduction of headache, cystitis, muscles ache, irritable colon, dysmenorrhea, dyspareunia and chronic pelvic pain (CPP) in treated patients compared to patients treated with a composition comprising only of linseed oil and 5-methyltetrahydrofolate calcium salt and to the placebo group. Moreover, they reported reduction of serum dosage of PGE2 in patients treated with the dietary supplements for three months [56]. A case control study collected dietary data from 78 women with a laparoscopically confirmed endometriosis and 78 patients with normal pelvis using a food frequency questionnaire (FFQ) as a validated semi-quantitative questionnaire and analyzing PE type in each dietary item. The logistic regression model observed inverse associations between the consumption of PE, total isoflavones (especially related to formononetin and glycitein) and endometriosis risk. Additionally, high consumption of lignans (secoisolariciresinol, lariciresinol, matairesinol) and coumestrol in the third quartile resulted in a reduced risk of endometriosis. The authors concluded supporting the role of PE consumption in limiting the progression of endometriosis due to its inflammatory nature and the hormonal basis of the disease [77].

4. Discussion

Most of the available therapies for endometriosis are hormonal-based therapies able to establish either a hypo-estrogenic or a hyper-progestogenic milieu [80–82]. Phytoestrogens are a heterogeneous group of naturally occurring compounds in plants structurally similar to estrogens [15]. They are characterized by a phenolic ring, which determines their agonist or antagonist properties, and two hydroxyl groups which are crucial for the binding to ER [15]. Classified into three main classes, PE include flavonoids (i.e., puerarin, genistein, coumestrol, EGCG, naringenin, quercetin), lignans (i.e., eneterolactone), and stilbenes (i.e., resveratrol) [14,83]. Flavonoids are characterized by a typical structure C6–C3–C6 with two rings of benzene A and B linked by a chain of 3 carbons cycled through an atom of oxygen [84]. Based on the connection, the position, the degree of saturation, oxidation, and hydroxylation of the B and C rings, they are commonly divided into isoflavones and coumestans [15,84–86]. Genistein and daidzein (up to 90% of isoflavones) are present in soybeans [87]. Among coumestans, coumestrol is one of the most studied and considered as an endocrine disruptor due to the high affinity in binding ERs [88], with an estrogenic activity greater than that of other isoflavones due to the position of its two hydroxyl groups [89]. It is present in a variety of plants including soybeans, clover, alfalfa sprouts, sunflower seeds, spinach, and legumes. Flavones, a subgroup of flavonoids whose main compound is apigenin, are characterized by a double bond between C2 and C3 that may induce cell cycle arrest and DNA damage in some cell types [90,91]. The skeleton and the position of phenolic group are the main characteristics of another flavonoid subgroup, named flavonols, of which quercetin and kaempferol are the most predominant components in plants [86]. Epicatechin, thought to be responsible for the main health effects of cocoa is another flavonoid compound found in unfermented cocoa beans. Epigallocatechin gallate (EGCG), formed by the ester of epigallocatechin and gallic acid, is present in green tea. Both of them have been associated with antioxidant and chemopreventive effects in several cell types [92,93]. Another flavonoid, narigenin, found in all citric fruits, seems to increase antioxidant defenses by limiting lipid peroxidation and protein carbonylation [85,94]. Lignans are non-flavonoid PE commonly found in grains, nuts, coffee and tea, cocoa, flaxseed, and some fruits [95]. According to some evidence, these PE are capable of mimicking the antioxidant effects of some hormones [96]. Finally, stilbenes are non-flavonoid PE of which the most studied is resveratrol, a compound with two phenolic rings connected by a styrene double bond, found in a wide variety of dietary foods, including grapes, wine, nuts, and berries [97–99]. Several in vitro and in vivo studies reported anti-cancer, antioxidant, anti-aging, anti-inflammatory and anti-pathogen properties of resveratrol [97,100,101].

Based on the results presented herein, these compounds may have some effects on the disease establishment. According to in vitro findings, 19 out of 22 studies reported the ability of PE to induce anti-proliferative, anti-inflammatory and proapoptotic effects on endometriotic cells. Only three studies did not find any positive effect exerted by PE in vitro [20,35,71]. Various mechanisms have been proposed to explain this in vitro action including the alteration of cell cycle proteins, the activation/inactivation of regulatory pathways, modification of ROS levels. Two considerations should be done in relation to the in vitro results obtained: 1. among the 22 published studies, nine were written by the same Chinese group [50,55,61,66–69,75,76]. Therefore, confirmatory findings by independent groups need to be obtained. 2. many studies have used cell lines as a model for endometriotic lesions. A number of immortalized cell lines deriving from endometriosis have been established by either forcing cells to survive through a cell crisis or by the introduction of one or more oncogene(s). However, genetic authentication and biological validation of these lines was disregarded by most authors. For instance, no STR profile was publicly available. Moreover, we have recently demonstrated that some of these endometriotic cell lines express ER-α but are PR-negative [8]. Since signaling initiated by both ER-α and PR is necessary for endometrial physiology, it is of foremost importance that cells are thoroughly characterized prior to each experiment for the maintenance of the proper phenotype and for their receptor status. This concept should be applied also to PE treatment of cells.

In line with in vitro findings, also results derived from animal models of endometriosis generally supported a beneficial effect of the compounds in reducing lesion growth and development. Indeed, a role of PE in limiting ectopic implants has been shown in 36 out of 38 studies independent of the specific drug used. Only two studies did not find any positive effect exerted by PE in in vivo experimental models [19,25] and both studies investigated the possible role of genistein in the treatment of induced models of endometriosis. Mechanisms proposed to explain this effect include decreased angiogenesis and microvessel density, enhanced fibrosis and apoptosis and alteration in MMP activity. Rats and mice offer attractive preclinical models of reproductive disorders because they are easily bred, they can be genetically manipulated, their reproductive system is well understood, and their small size means large quantities of drugs are not required for testing allowing for multiple replicates. In the context of endometriosis, these advantages apply but laboratory rats and mice do not exhibit spontaneous cyclical decidualization and menstruation. Therefore, although uterine tissue has been used to generate endometriosis-like lesions, the lesions are not formed from tissue undergoing active breakdown and remodeling as might be the case in women or menstruating primates. Therefore, similar to cell lines, experimental animal models of endometriosis are not devoid of limits. Due to their divergence from humans in key aspects of reproductive physiology, current experimental systems for the study of endometriosis are a very imperfect model [102]. As a matter of fact, most of the treatment for endometriosis used in experimental models provided satisfactory results while being of poor efficacy in humans [18,21,31,49,56,65,77].

As a matter of fact, the huge amount of in vitro and in vivo animal findings did not correspond to consistent literature in women affected. Randomized trials were only two using resveratrol and outcomes evaluated included pain score and MMP activity [49,65]. Quercitin was also shown to be able to reduce pain in a prospective cohort study [56]. Reasons for a limited reporting of PE effects in endometriosis patients is unclear. We cannot exclude that negative results have not been published. Alternatively, being natural compounds, they are viewed as dietary supplements and regularly prescribed with poor controls on outcomes. Certainly, based on results of experimental models, PE effect deserves to be investigated in more depth in future or ongoing clinical trials.

5. Conclusions

Phytoestrogens are naturally-occurring plant compounds that share a similar chemical structure and function to the estrogens found in the human body. Foods rich in phytoestrogens include soy, fruits, vegetables, spinach, sprouts, beans, cabbages, and grains. The effect of diet on hormonal activity, inflammatory markers, and the immune system means that the food choices women make might play a key role in the development of endometriosis. Furthermore, endometriosis has been shown to be related to prolonged exposure to the hormone estrogen in the absence of progesterone and to a prolonged inflammatory environment in the pelvis. Although there is consistent evidence, deriving from in vitro or in vivo animal model studies, for phytoestrogens' biological properties in endometriosis, only a few studies have been published regarding their use in patients with endometriosis, with inconsistent results. Phytoestrogens have many favorable characteristics, such as anti-proliferative, anti-angiogenic, anti-inflammatory, pro-apoptotic and anti-oxidant properties, which could make them a viable alternative in the future for the control and prevention of endometriosis. More powered and well-designed trials are needed to better investigate PE effects in women affected by endometriosis.

Supplementary Materials: The following are available online at https://www.mdpi.com/article/10.3390/nu13082532/s1, Figure S1: Risk of bias assessment according to the risk of bias tool by Clarity Group [79].

Author Contributions: Conceptualization, L.B., M.S., R.V. and P.V.; Methodology, P.V.; Validation, P.V., M.C. and J.O.; Investigation, L.B., M.S., R.V., C.D. and N.S.; Resources, L.B., M.S., R.V., C.D. and N.S.; Data Curation, L.B., M.S. and R.V.; Writing—Original Draft Preparation, L.B., M.S., R.V., C.D. and N.S.; Writing—Review and Editing, P.V., J.O. and M.C.; Visualization, P.V., J.O. and M.C.; Supervision, P.V., J.O. and M.C.; Project Administration, P.V. All authors have read and agreed to the published version of the manuscript.

Funding: This research received no external funding.

Institutional Review Board Statement: Not applicable.

Informed Consent Statement: Not applicable.

Data Availability Statement: Data sharing is not applicable to this article as no new data were created or analyzed in this study.

Conflicts of Interest: The authors declare no conflict of interest with respect to the research, authorship and/or publication of this article.

References

1. Parazzini, F.; Esposito, G.; Tozzi, L.; Noli, S.; Bianchi, S. Epidemiology of endometriosis and its comorbidities. *Eur. J. Obstet. Gynecol. Reprod. Biol.* **2017**, *209*, 3–7. [CrossRef]
2. Vercellini, P.P.; Vigano, P.; Somigliana, E.; Fedele, L. Endometriosis: Pathogenesis and treatment. *Nat. Rev. Endocrinol.* **2013**, *10*, 261–275. [CrossRef]
3. Vigano, P.; Candiani, M.; Monno, A.; Giacomini, E.; Vercellini, P.P.; Somigliana, E. Time to redefine endometriosis including its pro-fibrotic nature. *Hum. Reprod.* **2018**, *33*, 347–352. [CrossRef]
4. Vigano, P.; Ottolina, J.; Bartiromo, L.; Bonavina, G.; Schimberni, M.; Villanacci, R.; Candiani, M. Cellular components contributing to fibrosis in endometriosis: A literature review. *J. Minim. Invasive Gynecol.* **2020**, *27*, 287–295. [CrossRef]
5. Huhtinen, K.; Stahle, M.; Perheentupa, A.; Poutanen, M. Estrogen biosynthesis and signaling in endometriosis. *Mol. Cell Endocrinol.* **2012**, *358*, 146–154. [CrossRef]
6. Kyama, C.M.; Debrock, S.; Mwenda, J.M.; D'Hooghe, T.M. Potential involvement of the immune system in the development of endometriosis. *Reprod. Biol. Endocrinol.* **2003**, *1*, 123. [CrossRef]
7. Zondervan, K.T.; Becker, C.M.; Koga, K.; Missmer, S.A.; Taylor, R.N.; Viganò, P. Endometriosis. *Nat Rev Dis Primers* **2018**, *19*, 4–9. [CrossRef]
8. Romano, A.; Xanthoulea, S.; Giacomini, E.; Delvoux, B.; Alleva, E.; Vigano, P. Endometriotic cell culture contamination and authenticity: A source of bias in in vitro research? *Hum. Reprod.* **2020**, *35*, 364–376. [CrossRef]
9. Stratton, P.; Berkley, K.J. Chronic pelvic pain and endometriosis: Translational evidence of the relationship and implications. *Hum. Reprod. Update* **2011**, *17*, 327–346. [CrossRef]
10. Goncalves, G.A. p27(kip1) as a key regulator of endometriosis. *Eur. J. Obstet. Gynecol. Reprod. Biol.* **2018**, *221*, 1–4. [CrossRef]
11. Harris, H.R.; Chavarro, J.E.; Malspeis, S.; Willett, W.C.; Missmer, S.A. Dairy-food, calcium, magnesium and vitamin D intake and endometriosis: A prospective cohort study. *Am. J. Epidemiol.* **2013**, *177*, 420–430. [CrossRef] [PubMed]
12. Harris, H.R.; Eke, A.C.; Chavarro, J.E.; Missmer, S.A. Fruit and vegetable consumption and risk of endometriosis. *Hum. Reprod.* **2018**, *33*, 715–727. [CrossRef]
13. Parazzini, F.; Viganò, P.; Candiani, M.; Fedele, L. Diet and endometriosis risk: A literature review. *Reprod. Biomed. Online* **2013**, *26*, 323–336. [CrossRef]
14. Nikolić, I.L.; Savić-Gajić, I.M.; Tačić, A.D.; Savić, I.M. Classification and biological activity of phytoestrogens: A review. *Adv. Technol.* **2017**, *6*, 96–106. [CrossRef]
15. Roca, P.; Sastre-Serra, J.; Nadal-Serrano, M.; Pons, D.G.; Blanquer-Rossello, M.D.; Oliver, J. Phytoestrogens and mitochondrial biogenesis in breast cancer. Influence of estrogen receptors ratio. *Curr. Pharm. Des.* **2014**, *20*, 5594–5618. [CrossRef]
16. Kirichenko, T.V.; Myasoedova, V.A.; Orekhova, V.A.; Ravani, A.L.; Nikitina, N.A.; Grechko, A.V.; Sobenin, I.A.; Orekhov, A.N. Phytoestrogen-rich natural preparation for treatment of climacteric syndrome and atherosclerosis prevention in Perimenopausal women. *Phytother. Res.* **2017**, *31*, 1209–1214. [CrossRef]
17. Shukla, V.; Chandra, V.; Sankhwar, P.; Popli, P.; Kaushal, J.B.; Sirohi, V.K.; Dwivedi, A. Phytoestrogen genistein inhibits EGFR/PI3K/NF-kB activation and induces apoptosis in human endometrial hyperplasial cells. *RSC Adv.* **2015**, *5*, 56075–56085. [CrossRef]
18. Nagata, C.; Takatsuka, N.; Kawakami, N.; Shimizu, H. Soy product intake and premenopausal hysterectomy in a follow-up study of Japanese women. *Eur. J. Clin. Nutr.* **2001**, *55*, 773–777. [CrossRef]
19. Cotroneo, M.S.; Lamartiniere, C.A. Pharmacologic, but not dietary, genistein supports endometriosis in a rat model. *Toxicol. Sci.* **2001**, *61*, 68–75. [CrossRef]
20. Edmunds, K.M.; Holloway, A.C.; Crankshaw, D.J.; Agarwal, S.K.; Foster, W.G. The effects of dietary phytoestrogens on aromatase activity in human endometrial stromal cells. *Reprod. Nutr. Dev.* **2005**, *45*, 709–720. [CrossRef]

21. Tsuchiya, M.; Miura, T.; Hanaoka, T.; Iwasaki, M.; Sasaki, H.; Tanaka, T.; Nakao, H.; Katoh, T.; Ikenoue, T.; Kabuto, M.; et al. Effect of soy isoflavones on endometriosis: Interaction with estrogen receptor 2 gene polymorphism. *Epidemiology* **2007**, *18*, 402–408. [CrossRef]
22. Yavuz, E.; Oktem, M.; Esinler, I.; Toru, S.A.; Zeyneloglu, H.B. Genistein causes regression of endometriotic implants in the rat model. *Fertil. Steril.* **2007**, *88*, 1129–1134. [CrossRef] [PubMed]
23. Laschke, M.W.; Schwender, C.; Scheuer, C.; Vollmar, B.; Menger, M.D. Epigallocatechin-3-gallate inhibits estrogen-induced activation of endometrial cells in vitro and causes regression of endometriotic lesions in vivo. *Hum. Reprod.* **2008**, *23*, 2308–2318. [CrossRef]
24. Xu, H.; Lui, W.T.; Chu, C.Y.; Ng, P.S.; Wang, C.C.; Rogers, M.S. Anti-angiogenic effects of green tea catechin on an experimental endometriosis mouse model. *Hum. Reprod.* **2009**, *24*, 608–618. [CrossRef]
25. Laschke, M.W.; Schwender, C.; Vollmar, B.; Menger, M.D. Genistein does not affect vascularization and blood perfusion of endometriotic lesions and ovarian follicles in dorsal skinfold chambers of Syrian golden hamsters. *Reprod. Sci.* **2010**, *17*, 568–577. [CrossRef] [PubMed]
26. Bruner-Tran, K.L.; Osteen, K.G.; Taylor, H.S.; Sokalska, A.; Haines, K.; Duleba, A.J. Resveratrol inhibits development of experimental endometriosis in vivo and reduces endometrial stromal cell invasiveness in vitro. *Biol. Reprod.* **2011**, *84*, 106–112. [CrossRef]
27. Chen, Y.; Chen, C.; Shi, S.; Han, J.; Wang, J.; Hu, J.; Liu, Y.; Cai, Z.; Yu, C. Endometriotic implants regress in rat models treated with puerarin by decreasing estradiol level. *Reprod. Sci.* **2011**, *18*, 886–891. [CrossRef] [PubMed]
28. Wang, D.; Liu, Y.; Han, J.; Zai, D.; Ji, M.; Cheng, W.; Xu, L.; Yang, L.; He, M.; Ni, J.; et al. Puerarin suppresses invasion and vascularization of endometriosis tissue stimulated by 17β-estradiol. *PLoS ONE* **2011**, *6*, e25011. [CrossRef]
29. Xu, H.; Becker, C.M.; Lui, W.T.; Chu, C.Y.; Davis, T.N.; Kung, A.L.; Birsner, A.E.; D'Amato, R.J.; Wai Man, G.C.; Wang, C.C. Green tea epigallocatechin-3-gallate inhibits angiogenesis and suppresses vascular endothelial growth factor C/vascular endothelial growth factor receptor 2 expression and signaling in experimental endometriosis in vivo. *Fertil. Steril.* **2011**, *96*, 1021–1028. [CrossRef]
30. Cheng, W.; Chen, L.; Yang, S.; Han, J.; Zhai, D.; Ni, J.; Yu, C.; Cai, Z. Puerarin suppresses proliferation of endometriotic stromal cells partly via the MAPK signaling pathway induced by 17ß-estradiol-BSA. *PLoS ONE* **2012**, *7*, e45529. [CrossRef]
31. Maia, H.; Haddad, C.; Pinheiro, N.; Casoy, J. Advantages of the association of resveratrol with oral contraceptives for management of endometriosis-related pain. *Int. J. Womens Health* **2012**, *4*, 543–549. [CrossRef] [PubMed]
32. Rudzitis-Auth, J.; Körbel, C.; Scheuer, C.; Menger, M.D.; Laschke, M.W. Xanthohumol inhibits growth and vascularization of developing endometriotic lesions. *Hum. Reprod.* **2012**, *27*, 1735–1744. [CrossRef]
33. Ergenoglu, A.M.; Yeniel, A.O.; Erbas, O.; Aktug, H.; Yildirim, N.; Ulukus, M.; Taskiran, D. Regression of endometrial implants by resveratrol in an experimentally induced endometriosis model in rats. *Reprod. Sci.* **2013**, *20*, 1230–1236. [CrossRef]
34. Ji, M.; Liu, Y.; Yang, S.; Zhai, D.; Zhang, D.; Bai, L.; Wang, Z.; Yu, J.; Yu, C.; Cai, Z. Puerarin suppresses proliferation of endometriotic stromal cells in part via differential recruitment of nuclear receptor coregulators to estrogen receptor-α. *J. Steroid Biochem. Mol. Biol.* **2013**, *138*, 421–426. [CrossRef] [PubMed]
35. Ricci, A.G.; Olivares, C.N.; Bilotas, M.A.; Bastón, J.I.; Singla, J.J.; Meresman, G.F.; Barañao, R.I. Natural therapies assessment for the treatment of endometriosis. *Hum. Reprod.* **2013**, *28*, 178–188. [CrossRef] [PubMed]
36. Rudzitis-Auth, J.; Menger, M.D.; Laschke, M.W. Resveratrol is a potent inhibitor of vascularization and cell proliferation in experimental endometriosis. *Hum. Reprod.* **2013**, *28*, 1339–1347. [CrossRef] [PubMed]
37. Wang, C.C.; Xu, H.; Man, G.C.; Zhang, T.; Chu, K.O.; Chu, C.Y.; Cheng, J.T.; Li, G.; He, Y.X.; Qin, L.; et al. Prodrug of green tea epigallocatechin-3-gallate (Pro-EGCG) as a potent anti-angiogenesis agent for endometriosis in mice. *Angiogenesis* **2013**, *16*, 59–69. [CrossRef] [PubMed]
38. Amaya, S.C.; Savaris, R.F.; Filipovic, C.J.; Wise, J.D.; Hestermann, E.; Young, S.L.; Lessey, B.A. Resveratrol and endometrium: A closer look at an active ingredient of red wine using in vivo and in vitro models. *Reprod. Sci.* **2014**, *21*, 1362–1369. [CrossRef]
39. Demirel, M.A.; Suntar, I.; Ilhan, M.; Keles, H.; Kupeli Akkol, E. Experimental endometriosis remission in rats treated with Achillea biebersteinii Afan: Histopathological evaluation and determination of cytokine levels. *Eur. J. Obstet. Gynecol. Reprod. Biol.* **2014**, *175*, 172–177. [CrossRef]
40. Matsuzaki, S.; Darcha, C. Antifibrotic properties of epigallocatechin-3-gallate in endometriosis. *Hum. Reprod.* **2014**, *29*, 1677–1687. [CrossRef]
41. Taguchi, A.; Wada-Hiraike, O.; Kawana, K.; Koga, K.; Yamashita, A.; Shirane, A.; Urata, Y.; Kozuma, S.; Osuga, Y.; Fujii, T. Resveratrol suppresses inflammatory responses in endometrial stromal cells derived from endometriosis: A possible role of the sirtuin 1 pathway. *J. Obstet. Gynaecol. Res.* **2014**, *40*, 770–778. [CrossRef]
42. Yavuz, S.; Aydin, N.E.; Celik, O.; Yilmaz, E.; Ozerol, E.; Tanbek, K. Resveratrol successfully treats experimental endometriosis through modulation of oxidative stress and lipid peroxidation. *J. Cancer Res. Ther.* **2014**, *10*, 324–329. [CrossRef]
43. Bayoglu Tekin, Y.; Guven, S.; Kirbas, A.; Kalkan, Y.; Tumkaya, L.; Guvendag Guven, E.S. Is resveratrol a potential substitute for leuprolide acetate in experimental endometriosis? *Eur. J. Obstet. Gynecol. Reprod. Biol.* **2015**, *184*, 1–6. [CrossRef]
44. Cenksoy, O.P.; Oktem, M.; Erdem, O.; Karakaya, C.; Cenksoy, C.; Erdem, A.; Guner, H.; Karabacak, O. A potential novel treatment strategy: Inhibition of angiogenesis and inflammation by resveratrol for regression of endometriosis in an experimental rat model. *Gynecol. Endocrinol.* **2015**, *31*, 219–224. [CrossRef]

45. Singh, A.K.; Chakravarty, B.; Chaudhury, K. Nanoparticle-assisted combinatorial therapy for effective treatment of endometriosis. *J. Biomed. Nanotechnol.* **2015**, *11*, 789–804. [CrossRef]
46. Di Paola, R.; Fusco, R.; Gugliandolo, E.; Crupi, R.; Evangelista, M.; Granese, R.; Cuzzocrea, S. Co-micronized palmitoylethanolamide/polydatin treatment causes endometriotic lesion regression in a rodent model of surgically induced endometriosis. *Front. Pharmacol.* **2016**, *7*, 382. [CrossRef] [PubMed]
47. Taguchi, A.; Koga, K.; Kawana, K.; Makabe, T.; Sue, F.; Miyashita, M.; Yoshida, M.; Urata, Y.; Izumi, G.; Tkamura, M.; et al. Resveratrol enhances apoptosis in endometriotic stromal cells. *Am. J. Reprod. Immunol.* **2016**, *75*, 486–492. [CrossRef] [PubMed]
48. Kim, J.H.; Woo, J.H.; Kim, H.M.; Oh, M.S.; Jang, D.S.; Choi, J.H. Anti-endometriotic effects of pueraria flower extract in human endometriotic cells and mice. *Nutrients* **2017**, *9*, 212. [CrossRef]
49. Mendes da Silva, D.; Gross, L.A.; Neto, E.P.G.; Lessey, B.A.; Savaris, R.F. The use of resveratrol as an adjuvant treatment of pain in endometriosis: A randomized clinical trial. *J. Endocr. Soc.* **2017**, *1*, 359–369. [CrossRef]
50. Park, S.; Lim, W.; Bazer, F.W.; Song, G. Naringenin induces mitochondria-mediated apoptosis and endoplasmic reticulum stress by regulating MAPK and AKT signal transduction pathways in endometriosis cells. *Mol. Hum. Reprod.* **2017**, *23*, 842–854. [CrossRef] [PubMed]
51. Ferella, L.; Bastón, J.I.; Bilotas, M.A.; Singla, J.J.; González, A.M.; Olivares, C.N.; Meresman, G.F. Active compounds present in Rosmarinus officinalis leaves and Scutellaria baicalensis root evaluated as new therapeutic agents for endometriosis. *Reprod. Biomed. Online* **2018**, *37*, 769–782. [CrossRef]
52. Jouhari, S.; Mohammadzadeh, A.; Soltanghoraee, H.; Mohammadi, Z.; Khazali, S.; Mirzadegan, E.; Lakpour, N.; Fatemi, F.; Zafardoust, S.; Mohazzab, A.; et al. Effects of silymarin, cabergoline and letrozole on rat model of endometriosis. *Taiwan J. Obstet. Gynecol.* **2018**, *57*, 830–835. [CrossRef] [PubMed]
53. Melekoglu, R.; Ciftci, O.; Eraslan, S.; Cetin, A.; Basak, N. The beneficial effects of nerolidol and hesperidin on surgically induced endometriosis in a rat model. *Gynecol. Endocrinol.* **2018**, *34*, 975–980. [CrossRef] [PubMed]
54. Nahari, E.; Razi, M. Silymarin amplifies apoptosis in ectopic endometrial tissue in rats with endometriosis; implication on growth factor GDNF, ERK1/2 and Bcl-6b expression. *Acta Histochem.* **2018**, *120*, 757–767. [CrossRef]
55. Park, S.; Lim, W.; Bazer, F.W.; Song, G. Apigenin induces ROS-dependent apoptosis and ER stress in human endometriosis cells. *J. Cell Physiol.* **2018**, *233*, 3055–3065. [CrossRef]
56. Signorile, P.G.; Viceconte, R.; Baldi, A. Novel dietary supplement association reduces symptoms in endometriosis patients. *J. Cell Physiol.* **2018**, *233*, 5920–5925. [CrossRef]
57. Takaoka, O.; Mori, T.; Ito, F.; Okimura, H.; Kataoka, H.; Tanaka, Y.; Koshiba, A.; Kusuki, I.; Shigehiro, S.; Amami, T.; et al. Daidzein-rich isoflavone aglycones inhibit cell growth and inflammation in endometriosis. *J. Steroid. Biochem. Mol. Biol.* **2018**, *181*, 125–132. [CrossRef]
58. Wei, Y.; Shao, X. Nobiletin alleviates endometriosis via down-regulating NF-κB activity in endometriosis mouse model. *Biosci. Rep.* **2018**, *38*, BSR20180470. [CrossRef]
59. Arablou, T.; Delbandi, A.A.; Khodaverdi, S.; Arefi, S.; Kolahdouz-Mohammadi, R.; Heidari, S.; Mohammadi, T.; Aryaeian, N. Resveratrol reduces the expression of insulin-like growth factor-1 and hepatocyte growth factor in stromal cells of women with endometriosis compared with nonendometriotic women. *Phytother. Res.* **2019**, *33*, 1044–1054. [CrossRef]
60. Ding, D.; Cai, X.; Zheng, H.; Guo, S.W.; Liu, X. Scutellarin suppresses platelet aggregation and stalls lesional progression in mouse with induced endometriosis. *Reprod. Sci.* **2019**, *26*, 1417–1428. [CrossRef] [PubMed]
61. Ham, J.; Kim, J.; Bazer, F.W.; Lim, W.; Song, G. Silibinin-induced endoplasmic reticulum stress and mitochondrial dysfunction suppress growth of endometriotic lesions. *J. Cell Physiol.* **2019**, *234*, 4327–4341. [CrossRef]
62. Ilhan, M.; Ali, Z.; Khan, I.A.; Taştan, H.; Küpeli Akkol, E. Bioactivity-guided isolation of flavonoids from Urtica dioica L. and their effect on endometriosis rat model. *J. Ethnopharmacol.* **2019**, *243*, 112100. [CrossRef]
63. Ilhan, M.; Ali, Z.; Khan, I.A.; Tastan, H.; Kupeli Akkol, E. Promising activity of Anthemis austriaca Jacq. on the endometriosis rat model and isolation of its active constituents. *Saudi Pharm. J.* **2019**, *27*, 889–899. [CrossRef]
64. Kapoor, R.; Sirohi, V.K.; Gupta, K.; Dwivedi, A. Naringenin ameliorates progression of endometriosis by modulating Nrf2/Keap1/HO1 axis and inducing apoptosis in rats. *J. Nutr. Biochem.* **2019**, *70*, 215–226. [CrossRef] [PubMed]
65. Kodarahmian, M.; Amidi, F.; Moini, A.; Kashani, L.; Shabani Nashtaei, M.; Pazhohan, A.; Bahramrezai, M.; Berenjian, S.; Sobhani, A. The modulating effects of Resveratrol on the expression of MMP-2 and MMP-9 in endometriosis women: A randomized exploratory trial. *Gynecol. Endocrinol.* **2019**, *35*, 719–726. [CrossRef]
66. Ryu, S.; Bazer, F.W.; Lim, W.; Song, G. Chrysin leads to cell death in endometriosis by regulation of endoplasmic reticulum stress and cytosolic calcium level. *J. Cell Physiol.* **2019**, *234*, 2480–2490. [CrossRef] [PubMed]
67. Park, S.; Lim, W.; Song, G. Delphinidin induces antiproliferation and apoptosis of endometrial cells by regulating cytosolic calcium levels and mitochondrial membrane potential depolarization. *J. Cell Biochem.* **2019**, *120*, 5072–5084. [CrossRef]
68. Park, S.; Lim, W.; Bazer, F.W.; Whang, K.Y.; Song, G. Quercetin inhibits proliferation of endometriosis regulating cyclin D1 and its target microRNAs in vitro and in vivo. *J. Nutr. Biochem.* **2019**, *63*, 87–100. [CrossRef]
69. Park, S.; Lim, W.; You, S.; Song, G. Ameliorative effects of luteolin against endometriosis progression in vitro and in vivo. *J. Nutr. Biochem.* **2019**, *67*, 161–172. [CrossRef] [PubMed]
70. Bina, F.; Daglia, M.; Santarcangelo, C.; Baeeri, M.; Abdollahi, M.; Nabavi, S.M.; Tabarrai, M.; Rahimi, R. Phytochemical profiling and ameliorative effects of Achillea cretica L. on rat model of endometriosis. *J. Ethnopharmacol.* **2020**, *254*, 112747. [CrossRef]

71. Hernandes, C.; de Oliveira, R.N.; de Souza Santos, A.H.; Malvezzi, H.; de Azevedo, B.C.; Gueuvoghlanian-Silva, B.Y.; Pereira, A.M.S.; Podgaec, S. The Effect of rutin and extracts of uncaria guianensis (Aubl.) J. F. gmeland on primary endometriotic cells: A 2D and 3D study. *Molecules* **2020**, *13*, 1325. [CrossRef]
72. Hsu, Y.W.; Chen, H.Y.; Chiang, Y.F.; Chang, L.C.; Lin, P.H.; Hsia, S.M. The effects of isoliquiritigenin on endometriosis in vivo and in vitro study. *Phytomedicine* **2020**, *77*, 153214. [CrossRef]
73. Ilhan, M.; Ali, Z.; Khan, I.A.; Taştan, H.; Küpeli Akkol, E. The regression of endometriosis with glycosylated flavonoids isolated from Melilotus officinalis (L.) Pall. in an endometriosis rat model. *Taiwan J Obstet. Gynecol.* **2020**, *59*, 211–219. [CrossRef] [PubMed]
74. Khazaei, M.R.; Rashidi, Z.; Chobsaz, F.; Niromand, E.; Khazaei, M. Inhibitory effect of resveratrol on the growth and angiogenesis of human endometrial tissue in an In Vitro three-dimensional model of endometriosis. *Reprod. Biol.* **2020**, *20*, 484–490. [CrossRef] [PubMed]
75. Park, W.; Park, M.Y.; Song, G.; Lim, W. 5,7-Dimethoxyflavone induces apoptotic cell death in human endometriosis cell lines by activating the endoplasmic reticulum stress pathway. *Phytother. Res.* **2020**, *34*, 2275–2286. [CrossRef] [PubMed]
76. Park, S.; Song, G.; Lim, W. Myricetin inhibits endometriosis growth through cyclin E1 down-regulation in vitro and in vivo. *J. Nutr. Biochem.* **2020**, *78*, 108328. [CrossRef]
77. Youseflu, S.; Jahanian Sadatmahalleh, S.H.; Mottaghi, A.; Kazemnejad, A. Dietary phytoestrogen intake and the risk of endometriosis in iranian women: A case-control study. *Int. J. Fertil. Steril.* **2020**, *13*, 296–300.
78. Page, M.J.; McKenzie, J.E.; Bossuyt, P.M.; Boutron, I.; Hoffmann, T.C.; Mulrow, C.D.; Shamseer, L.; Tetzlaff, J.M.; Akl, E.A.; Brennan, S.E.; et al. The PRISMA 2020 statement: An updated guideline for reporting systematic reviews. *BMJ* **2021**, *29*, 372.
79. EFSA Scientific Committee; Benford, D.; Halldorsson, T.; Jeger, M.J.; Knutsen, H.K.; More, S.; Naegeli, H.; Noteborn, H.; Ockleford, C.; Ricci, A.; et al. The principles and methods behind EFSA's guidance on uncertainty analysis in scientific assessment. *EFSA J.* **2018**, *16*, 5122.
80. Agarwal, S.K.; Daniels, A.; Drosman, S.R.; Udoff, L.; Foster, W.G.; Pike, M.C.; Spicer, D.V.; Daniels, J.R. Treatment of endometriosis with the GnRHa deslorelin and add-back estradiol and supplementary testosterone. *Biomed. Res. Int.* **2015**, *2015*, 934164. [CrossRef] [PubMed]
81. Abu Hashim, H. Potential role of aromatase inhibitors in the treatment of endometriosis. *Int. J. Womens Health* **2014**, *6*, 671–680. [CrossRef]
82. Nawathe, A.; Patwardhan, S.; Yates, D.; Harrison, G.R.; Khan, K.S. Systematic review of the effects of aromatase inhibitors on pain associated with endometriosis. *BJOG* **2008**, *115*, 818–822. [PubMed]
83. Cos, P.; De Bruyne, T.; Apers, S.; Berghe, D.V.; Pieters, L.; Vlietinck, A.J. Phytoestrogens: Recent developments. *Planta Med.* **2003**, *69*, 589–599.
84. Wang, T.-Y.; Li, Q.; Bi, K. Bioactive flavonoids in medicinal plants: Structure, activity and biological fate. *Asian J. Pharm. Sci.* **2018**, *13*, 12–23. [CrossRef] [PubMed]
85. Panche, A.N.; Diwan, A.D.; Chandra, S.R. Flavonoids: An overview. *J. Nutr. Sci.* **2016**, *5*, e47. [CrossRef]
86. Graf, B.A.; Milbury, P.E.; Blumberg, J.B. Flavonols, flavones, flavanones and humanhealth: Epidemiological evidence. *J. Med. Food* **2005**, *8*, 281–290. [CrossRef]
87. Chan, K.K.L.; Siu, M.K.Y.; Jiang, Y.-X.; Wang, J.-J.; Leung, T.H.Y.; Ngan, H.Y.S. Estrogen receptor modulators genistein, daidzein and ERB-041 inhibit cell migration, invasion, proliferation and sphere formation via modulation of FAK and PI3K/AKT signaling in ovarian cancer. *Cancer Cell Int.* **2018**, *18*, 65. [CrossRef]
88. Kuiper, G.G.J.M.; Carlsson, B.; Grandien, K.; Enmark, E.; Häggblad, J.; Nilsson, S.; Gustafsson, J.-A. Comparison of the ligand binding specificity and transcript tissue distribution of estrogen receptors and β. *Endocrinology* **1997**, *138*, 863–870. [CrossRef] [PubMed]
89. Konar, N. Non-isoflavone phytoestrogenic compound contents of various legumes. *Eur. Food Res. Technol.* **2013**, *236*, 523–530. [CrossRef]
90. Onzalez-Mejia, M.E.; Voss, O.H.; Murnan, E.J.; Dose, A.I. Apigenin-induced apoptosis of leukemia cells is mediated by a bimodal and differentially regulated residue-specific phosphorylation of heat-shock protein–27. *Cell Death Dis.* **2010**, *1*, e64. [CrossRef]
91. Cos, P.; Ying, L.; Calomme, M.; Hu, J.P.; Cimanga, K.; Van Poel, B.; Pieters, L.; Vlietinck, A.A.J.; Berghe, D.V. Structure–activity relationship and classification of flavonoids as inhibitors of xanthine oxidase and superoxide scavengers. *J. Nat. Prod.* **1998**, *61*, 71–76. [CrossRef] [PubMed]
92. Shay, J.; Elbaz, H.A.; Lee, I.; Zielske, S.P.; Malek, M.H.; Hüttemann, M. Molecular mechanisms and therapeutic effects of (-)-epicatechin and other polyphenols in cancer, inflammation, diabetes and neurodegeneration. *Oxidative Med. Cell. Longev.* **2015**, *181260*, 1–13. [CrossRef] [PubMed]
93. Yang, C.S.; Wang, H. Cancer preventive activities of tea catechins. *Molecules* **2016**, *21*, 1679. [CrossRef]
94. Salehi, B.; Fokou, P.V.T.; Sharifi-Rad, M.; Zucca, P.; Pezzani, R.; Martins, N.; Sharifi-Rad, J. The Therapeutic potential of naringenin: A Review of clinical trials. *Pharmaceuticals* **2019**, *12*, 11. [CrossRef]
95. Durazzo, A.; Lucarini, M.; Camilli, E.; Marconi, S.; Gabrielli, P.; Lisciani, S.; Gambelli, L.; Aguzzi, A.; Novellino, E.; Santini, A.; et al. Dietary lignans: Definition, description and research trends in databases development. *Molecules* **2018**, *23*, 3251. [CrossRef]
96. Cotterchio, M.; Boucher, B.; Kreiger, N.; Mills, C.A.; Thompson, L.U. Dietary phytoestrogen intake—Lignans and isoflavones—And breast cancer risk (Canada). *Cancer Causes Control* **2007**, *19*, 259–272. [CrossRef]

97. Xiao, Q.; Zhu, W.; Feng, W.; Lee, S.S.; Leung, A.W.; Shen, J.; Gao, L.; Xu, C. A review of resveratrol as a potent chemoprotective and synergistic agent in cancer chemotherapy. *Front. Pharmacol.* **2019**, *9*, 1534. [CrossRef]
98. Sirerol, J.A.; Rodríguez, M.L.; Mena, S.; Asensi, M.A.; Estrela, J.M.; Ortega, A.L. Role of natural stilbenes in the prevention of cancer. *Oxidative Med. Cell. Longev.* **2015**, *2016*, 1–15. [CrossRef] [PubMed]
99. Berman, A.Y.; Motechin, R.A.; Wiesenfeld, M.Y.; Holz, M.K. The therapeutic potential of resveratrol: A review of clinical trials. *NPJ Precis. Oncol.* **2017**, *1*, 1–9. [CrossRef]
100. Nawaz, W.; Zhou, Z.; Deng, S.; Ma, X.; Ma, X.; Li, C.; Shu, X. Therapeutic versatility of resveratrol derivatives. *Nutrients* **2017**, *9*, 1188. [CrossRef]
101. Ko, J.-H.; Sethi, G.; Um, J.-Y.; Shanmugam, M.K.; Arfuso, F.; Kumar, A.P.; Bishayee, A.; Ahn, K.S. The role of resveratrol in cancer therapy. *Int. J. Mol. Sci.* **2017**, *18*, 2589. [CrossRef] [PubMed]
102. Dinsdale, N.; Nepomnaschy, P.; Crespi, B. The evolutionary biology of endometriosis. *Evol. Med. Public Health* **2021**, *9*, 174–191. [CrossRef] [PubMed]

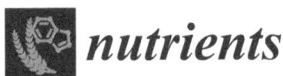

Article

Altered Umbilical Cord Blood Nutrient Levels, Placental Cell Turnover and Transporter Expression in Human Term Pregnancies Conceived by Intracytoplasmic Sperm Injection (ICSI)

Enrrico Bloise [1,2,*,†], Jair R. S. Braga [2,3,†], Cherley B. V. Andrade [2], Guinever E. Imperio [2,4,5], Lilian M. Martinelli [1], Roberto A. Antunes [2,3,6], Karina R. Silva [7], Cristiana B. Nunes [8], Luigi Cobellis [9], Flavia F. Bloise [2], Stephen G. Matthews [4,5,10,11], Kristin L. Connor [12] and Tania M. Ortiga-Carvalho [2]

1. Departamento de Morfologia, Universidade Federal de Minas Gerais, Belo Horizonte, MG 31270-910, Brazil; lilianmassara@gmail.com
2. Laboratório de Endocrinologia Translacional, Instituto de Biofísica Carlos Chagas Filho, Universidade Federal do Rio de Janeiro, Rio de Janeiro, RJ 21941-902, Brazil; jairbraga@me.ufrj.br (J.R.S.B.); cherley@biof.ufrj.br (C.B.V.A.); guinever.imperio@mail.utoronto.ca (G.E.I.); robertoantunes@fertipraxis.com.br (R.A.A.); flaviabloise@biof.ufrj.br (F.F.B.); taniaort@biof.ufrj.br (T.M.O.-C.)
3. Maternidade Escola, Universidade Federal do Rio de Janeiro, Rio de Janeiro, RJ 22240-000, Brazil
4. Department of Physiology, Temerty Faculty of Medicine, University of Toronto, Toronto, ON M5S 1A8, Canada; Stephen.Matthews@utoronto.ca
5. Lunenfeld-Tanenbaum Research Institute, Sinai Health System, Toronto, ON M5G 1X5, Canada
6. Fertipraxis-Centro de Reprodução Humana, Rio de Janeiro, RJ 22640-902, Brazil
7. Laboratório de Endocrinologia Molecular, Instituto de Biofísica Carlos Chagas Filho, Universidade Federal do Rio de Janeiro, Rio de Janeiro, RJ 21941-902, Brazil; ribeiro.ks@gmail.com
8. Departamento de Anatomia Patológica e Medicina Legal, Universidade Federal de Minas Gerais, Belo Horizonte, MG 30130-100, Brazil; cristianabnunes@gmail.com
9. Dipartimento della Donna, del Bambino e di Chirurgia Generale e Specialistica, Università degli Studi della Campania "Luigi Vanvitelli", 80138 Napoli, Italy; luigi.cobellis@unicampania.it
10. Department of Obstetrics and Gynaecology, Temerty Faculty of Medicine, University of Toronto, Toronto, ON M5S 1A8, Canada
11. Department of Medicine, Temerty Faculty of Medicine, University of Toronto, Toronto, ON M5S 3H2, Canada
12. Health Sciences, Carleton University, Ottawa, ON K1S 5B6, Canada; kristin.connor@carleton.ca
* Correspondence: ebloise@icb.ufmg.br; Tel.: +55-31-3409-2783
† These authors contributed equally to this work.

Abstract: Assisted reproductive technologies (ART) may increase risk for abnormal placental development, preterm delivery and low birthweight. We investigated placental morphology, transporter expression and paired maternal/umbilical fasting blood nutrient levels in human term pregnancies conceived naturally ($n = 10$) or by intracytoplasmic sperm injection (ICSI; $n = 11$). Maternal and umbilical vein blood from singleton term (>37 weeks) C-section pregnancies were assessed for levels of free amino acids, glucose, free fatty acids (FFA), cholesterol, high density lipoprotein (HDL), low density lipoprotein (LDL), very low-density lipoprotein (VLDL) and triglycerides. We quantified placental expression of GLUT1 (glucose), SNAT2 (amino acids), P-glycoprotein (P-gp) and breast cancer resistance protein (BCRP) (drug) transporters, and placental morphology and pathology. Following ICSI, placental SNAT2 protein expression was downregulated and umbilical cord blood levels of citrulline were increased, while FFA levels were decreased at term ($p < 0.05$). Placental proliferation and apoptotic rates were increased in ICSI placentae ($p < 0.05$). No changes in maternal blood nutrient levels, placental GLUT1, P-gp and BCRP expression, or placental histopathology were observed. In term pregnancies, ICSI impairs placental SNAT2 transporter expression and cell turnover, and alters umbilical vein levels of specific nutrients without changing placental morphology. These may represent mechanisms through which ICSI impacts pregnancy outcomes and programs disease risk trajectories in offspring across the life course.

Keywords: assisted reproductive technology (ART); intracytoplasmic sperm injection (ICSI); amino acids; citrulline; glucose; lipids; free fatty acids (FFA); placenta; proliferation; apoptosis; GLUT1; SNAT2; P-gp and BCRP

1. Introduction

The advance of assisted reproductive technology (ART) allows the birth of thousands of children every year for individuals otherwise unable to conceive naturally [1,2]. However, several reports indicate that ART pregnancies may potentially be at higher risk for preterm birth, placenta praevia, placenta accreta, retained placenta, villous edema, abnormal placental growth, altered placental weight and having babies with low birthweight [3,4]. The mechanisms by which ART affect pregnancy outcomes may originate from maternal ovarian stimulation procedures; gamete/embryo manipulation and in vitro culture conditions, such as culture medium composition, culture substrate stiffness/rigidity, oxygen tension, pH, embryo culture duration; and embryo transfer methodologies, among others. In response to these stressors the embryo may adapt its growth kinetics, leading to altered fetoplacental growth and subsequent phenotypes [2].

Ultrastructural assessment of the human placenta following conception with ART revealed a thicker placental barrier and fewer microvilli at the apical membrane of syncytiotrophoblasts [5], suggesting compromised placental transport function. Placental transport efficiency may indirectly be assessed by calculating the fetal:placental (F:P) weight ratio [6]. Reduced F:P weight ratio has been observed in animal models and human population-based studies with in vitro fertilization (IVF) or intracytoplasmic sperm injection (ICSI) techniques [2,7–10]. An altered F:P ratio may be a marker of a suboptimal intrauterine environment, which is known to increase risk for cardiovascular and metabolic diseases in offspring during adult life [11].

The placenta supplies nutrients to the fetus by simple diffusion, facilitated or active transporter-mediated processes and by endocytosis/exocytosis [12,13]. Transplacental glucose transport is predominantly mediated by GLUT1 and GLUT3 transporters [14–16], whereas neutral amino acids are transported into the fetal circulation via the sodium-dependent neutral amino acid transporters (SNATs), isoforms I, II and IV [16,17]. Glucose and amino acid transport efficiency depend upon placental size and F:P weight ratio [7,18]. Term newborns from mouse pregnancies conceived by IVF have lower birthweight but exhibit higher placental weight and reduced F:P weight ratio. Additionally, mouse placentae following IVF are less efficient in transporting amino acids [7], and exhibit decreased mRNA expression of *Glut* and *Snat* transporters [7,10]. Further, impaired nutrient delivery to the fetus may contribute to the low birthweight commonly reported in ART newborns [2], and is likely to program postnatal developmental trajectories and life-long disease risk. However, less is known about the effects of specific ARTs, such as ICSI, on placental development and nutrient transport efficiency in human pregnancy, including whether changes in placental development and function influence fetal nutrient levels.

Placental efflux transport has also been shown to vary according to placental size. Activity of the transporter P-glycoprotein (P-gp) was inversely correlated with placental size in mouse pregnancy, since larger placentae within a litter were more efficient in effluxing P-gp substrates compared to smaller placentae [19]. P-gp belongs to the ATP-binding cassette (ABC) superfamily of efflux transporters and, with the efflux transporter breast cancer resistance protein (BCRP), comprise the best investigated of the ABC transporters in the placenta, namely the multidrug resistance (MDR) transporters. MDR transporters are localized to the apical membrane of the syncytiotrophoblast and prevent the entry of a number of drugs and toxicants from the maternal circulation into the fetal compartment, therefore functioning as major placental efflux gatekeepers against fetal exposure to potentially teratogenic compounds [20]. Despite their key roles in fetal protection, placental P-gp and BCRP have not been previously investigated in the context of ICSI. In this context, since placental size may vary after ART [2,4,9], it is possible that placental expression of P-gp and BCRP in ICSI pregnancies may be impacted.

Given the evidence from animal models and human studies showing differences in placental size and F:P weight ratio in pregnancies conceived by ART [9], and the importance of both nutrient and efflux transporters in supporting optimal fetal development and protection during pregnancy, we hypothesized that ICSI placentae would have reduced nutrient transport efficiency, and that ICSI may result in increased risk of fetal exposure to drugs and toxins in utero via altered placental MDR transport.

2. Materials and Methods

2.1. Patients

Two groups of healthy patients (control naturally conceived (CON)) and ICSI) were recruited by the medical staff of the "Maternidade Escola" from the Universidade Federal do Rio de Janeiro—Hospital system, in Rio de Janeiro city, Brazil. The study was approved by the Research Ethics Board from "Maternidade Escola"—Universidade Federal do Rio de Janeiro (project number CAAE: 30214214.0.0000.5275). In Brazil, the ICSI procedure prevails over IVF regardless of the male infertility factor, therefore we recruited ICSI rather than IVF conceived pregnancies in our study. Inclusion criteria comprised singleton pregnancies naturally conceived (>37 weeks' gestation; CON, $n = 10$) or conceived by ICSI with fresh embryo transfer (>37 weeks' gestation; ICSI, $n = 11$; $n = 9$ primary infertility and $n = 2$ tubal factor infertility), delivered by elective C-section without signs of labor, recruited from June 2015 until December 2017. Informed written consent was obtained from each patient prior to inclusion in the study. Clinical data were collected during patient enrollment and interviews. Exclusion criteria comprised vaginal delivery, spontaneous onset of term labor, smoking, congenital uterine anomalies, cervical incompetence, uterine malformations, polyhydramnios, multiple gestations and fetal–maternal complications (infectious diseases, thyroid disease, asthma, cardiovascular diseases, diabetes, hypertension, preeclampsia, abruption placentae, and fetal malformation). There were no other complications or comorbidities documented in the cohort at the time of recruitment.

2.2. Blood Sampling and Placental Tissue Collection

Paired maternal/umbilical fasting blood (8 h prior to C-section) and placental tissues were collected from women undergoing elective C-sections (with no labor). Maternal blood was collected from a peripheral vein immediately before the C-section procedure. Umbilical cord venous blood sampling was performed by an experienced OB-GYN, under sterile conditions, in a single clamped segment on the neonatal side of the umbilical cord immediately after birth, following neonatal separation from the cord and prior to placental delivery. Blood samples were harvested in heparinized sterile vacuum blood collection tubes and centrifuged at 3000 rpm for 15 min at 4 °C. The harvested plasma was then aliquoted and stored at −80 °C until analysis.

Placental villous tissue collection was performed as previously described [21]. In brief, placental core sampling was performed using cuts made to a core depth to avoid the maternal decidua, the chorionic plate or any area of thrombosis, infarcts or other abnormalities. Therefore, only placental villous tissue from term placentae was selected. Placental fragments were washed in 0.9% sterile saline, quickly dried and immediately placed in RNALater (Thermo Fischer Scientific, São Paulo, Brazil) for downstream mRNA expression analysis, or fixed overnight in buffered 4% paraformaldehyde (Sigma-Aldrich, São Paulo, Brazil), for histopathological, TUNEL and immunohistochemistry analyses.

2.3. Analysis of Maternal and Umbilical Venous Blood Nutrient Contents

Assessment of nutrient concentrations in the umbilical venous blood and matched maternal blood was performed according to routine protocols by a commercial laboratory specialized in conducting genetic, biochemical, and metabolic analyses of neonates, (DLE® Genética Humana e Doenças Raras, located in Rio de Janeiro, Brazil).

Free amino acid levels of aspartic acid, glutamic acid, alanine, arginine, phenylalanine, glycine, methionine, ornithine, serine, tyrosine, threonine, tryptophan, valine, asparagine, isoleucine, leucine, lysine, taurine, citrulline and histidine, were measured by Liquid Chromatography/Tandem Mass Spectrometry (LC-MS/MS) method. Serum glucose, cholesterol, HDL, LDL, VLDL and triglyceride levels were measured by the enzymatic colorimetric method. Free fatty acids (FFA) were quantified by the kinetic spectrophotometry method, according to the DLE laboratory specifications for each test.

2.4. Quantitative Real-Time PCR (qPCR)

qPCR was performed as described previously [21–23]. Total RNA was isolated from placental villous tissue (~30 mg) using TRIzol Reagent (TRIzol Reagent; Life Technologies, USA). RNA concentration and purity were assessed with Implen NanoPhotometer (Implen GmbH, Munich, DE, Germany). Only samples with a 260 nm/280 nm absorbance ratio higher than 1.8 were included in the study. For cDNA synthesis, 1000 ng of total RNA were reverse-transcribed into cDNA using a High Capacity cDNA Reverse Transcription Kit (Applied Biosystems, San Francisco, CA, USA). mRNA levels of genes of interest were assessed with intron-spanning primers (Table 1) by qPCR using HOT FIREPol Evagreen qPCR Supermix (Solis, Denmark) and the Master Cycler Realplex system (Eppendorf, Germany). The following cycling conditions were performed: combined initial denaturation at 50 °C (2 min) and 95 °C (10 min), followed by 40 cycles of denaturation at 95 °C (15 s), annealing at 60 °C (30 s) and extension at 72 °C (45 s). Assay efficiency ranged from 95–105%. Genomic DNA contamination was ruled out using reverse transcriptase-negative samples and melting curve analysis extracted from each reaction. Gene expression was normalized to the geometric mean of three stably expressed reference genes: peptidyl-propyl isomerase B (PPIB), 14-3-3 protein zeta/delta (YWHAZ) and TATA-binding protein (TBP) (Table 1). Relative gene expression was calculated according to LinReg method, qPCR efficiency was $100 \pm 10\%$.

Table 1. List of Primer sequences used in this study.

Gene	Primer Sequences	Reference
SLC38A1 (SNAT1)	F: 5'-GTGTATGCTTTACCCACCATTGC-3' R: 5'-GCACGTTGTCATAGAATGTCAAGT-3"	[24]
SLC38A2 (SNAT2)	F: 5'-AGATCAGAATTGGCACAGCATA-3' R: 5'-ACGAAACAATAAACACCACCTTAA-3'	[24]
SLC38A4 (SNAT4)	F: 5'-GAGGACAATGGGCACAGTTAGT-3' R: 5'-TTGCCGCCCTCTTTGGTTAC-3'	[24]
SLC2A1 (GLUT1)	F: 5'-ATCAACCGCAACGAGGAGAAC-3' R: 5'-CACCACAAACAGCGACACGAC-3'	[25]
SLC2A3 (GLUT3)	F: 5'-TCAGGCTCCACCCTTTGCGGA-3' R: 5'-TGGGGTGACCTTCTGTGTCCCC-3'	[26]
ABCB1 (P-gp)	F: 5'-AGCAGAGGCCGCTGTTCGTT-3' R: 5'-CCATTCCGACCTCGCGCTCC-3'	[27]
ABCG2 (BCRP)	F: 5'-TGGAATCCAGAACAGAGCTGGGGT-3' R: 5'-AGAGTTCCACGGCTGAAACACTGC-3'	[27]
PPIB	F: 5' GAGACTTCACCAGGGG -3' R: 5'- CTGTCTGTCTTGGTGCTCTCC-3'	[28]
YWHAZ	F: 5'-ACTTTTGGTACATTGTGGCTTCAA-3' R: 5'-CCGCCAGGACAAACCAGTAT-3'	[28]
TBP	F: 5'-TGCACAGGAGCCAAGAGTGAA-3' R: 5'-CACATCACAGCTCCCCACCA-3'	[28]

2.5. Histopathological, Immunohistochemistry and TUNEL Assessment of CON and ICSI Placentae

Paraffin-embedded placental tissue was cut into 5-µm stepped serial cross-sections, and every sixth section was stained with either hematoxylin and eosin (H&E) for histopathological analysis or subjected to immunohistochemical or TUNEL analysis.

Morphometric analysis consisted of evaluating the volumetric proportions of the cellular components of the placentae as well as the presence of trophoblast pathologies that could be attributed to the method of conception. The volumetric proportion analysis in CON and ICSI placentae was undertaken by two separate examiners blinded to groups estimating the following histological components: syncytiotrophoblasts, syncytial knots, cytotrophoblasts, connective tissue, and blood vessel. Captured images were superimposed with a grid of equidistant points (25 µm). 1000 points were counted per placenta; equivalent to an area of, on average, 655,288.7 µm^2. The volumetric ratio (VR) of each component was calculated as VR = NP × 100/1000, where NP = number of equivalent points for each histological component [22,23]. Analysis and image acquisition were performed in a Zeiss Axiolab 1 photomicroscope (Carl Zeiss, White Plains, NY, EUA), coupled to a CCD camera (Leica DFC345FX). Morphometric analysis was performed using the Fiji ImageJ 1.0 (ImageJ, Madison, WI, USA) program.

Histopathological analysis was undertaken by a single experienced pathologist blinded to groups, in three random placental sections per patient. Placental pathological features investigated were: villous edema, microcalcification, chronic villitis (presence of inflammatory cells infiltrating the villous stroma), ischemic or infarction changes (defined by the presence of localized dead or devitalized chorionic villi and noticeable villous agglutination or early infarction), avascular villi, increased peri-villous fibrin (accumulation of fibrin or fibrinoid material in the intervillous space), and intervillous thrombi (laminated clots within the intervillous space) [29–31]. These pathological features were deemed either present or absent in CON and ICSI placentae [30].

For immunohistochemistry, following deparaffinization in three xylene immersions and rehydration in descending gradients of ethanol, endogenous peroxidase activity was blocked with 3% H_2O_2 in methanol for 10 min and washed in PBS. Antigen retrieval was performed by preheating sections in 10 mmol/L sodium citrate (pH 6.0). Sections were again washed in PBS before blocking in 3% PBS/BSA for 1 h. Sections were incubated overnight at 40 °C, with the following primary antibodies: anti-Ki67 antibody (Spring Bioscience, Pleasanton, CA, USA), anti-GLUT1 (1: 100—ab652, Abcam, SP, Brasil), anti-SNAT 2 (1: 200—LS-C179270, LSBio, Seattle, WA, EUA), anti-P-gp (1:500—Mdr1[sc-55510]; Santa Cruz Biotechnology, Dallas, TX, USA) and anti-Bcrp (1:100—Bcrp [MAB4146]; Merck Millipore, Burlington, MA, USA). Followed by slide washing and incubation with biotin-conjugated secondary antibody (SPD-060-Spring Bioscience, Pleasanton, CA, USA) for 1 h. Sections were then re-washed in PBS (3× for 10 min each time), incubated with streptavidin-HRP (30 min; SPD-060-Spring Bioscience, Pleasanton, CA, USA) and submitted to chromogenic detection of horseradish peroxidase (HRP) activity by 3,3′-diaminobenzidine (DAB) reagent (DAB peroxidase substrate kit, SPD-060-Spring Bioscience, Pleasanton, CA, USA). The immune reaction was also performed in the absence of the primary antibody (negative control) to monitor nonspecific binding of the secondary antibody.

The terminal deoxynucleotidyl transferase dUTP nick end labeling (TUNEL) analysis was undertaken to assess apoptotic nuclei ratio, using the ApopTag® In Situ Peroxidase Detection Kit (S7100—Merck Millipore, Danvers, MA, USA), according to the manufacturer's instructions. TUNEL reaction was also performed omitting TdT as negative control. Slides were counterstained with hematoxylin, dehydrated in ascending grades of ethanol, clarified in three xylene immersions and cover-slipped. Slides were visualized with a high-resolution Olympus DP72 (Olympus Corporation, Tokyo, Japan) camera coupled to the Olympus BX53 light microscope (Olympus Corporation, Tokyo, Japan). Scoring of immunosignals was performed as previously described with adaptations [32–34], using STEPanizer software [35]. A total of 30 digital images were captured per placental fragment of each patient. In each image, Ki-67 and TUNEL nuclei immunostaining were quantified and the resulting value was divided by the area of the total image, which yielded an estimate for the number of proliferative or apoptotic nuclei present in the whole tissue (number of nuclei/area of tissue). Quantification of GLUT 1, SNAT2, P-gp and BCRP immunostaining was performed using the Image Pro Plus 5.0 software (Media Cybernetics, Maryland, Rockville, MD, USA) mask tool, where immunostaining of the percentage area of viable tissue was quantified (with negative/empty spaces excluded) [32–34].

2.6. Statistical Analysis

Outliers were identified using the ROUT method (GraphPad Prism 7.0 software). Differences between conception groups for clinical data, immunohistochemistry, qPCR and morphological comparisons were determined by normality test using D'Agostino-Pearson normality test followed by unpaired t-test or non-parametric Mann-Whitney test. Data are presented as means ± standard deviation (SD) or median and interquartile range (IQR). Nutrient outcome measures in maternal and cord blood were tested for normality and unequal variances (Levene test, JMP v14.3). Data that were non-normal were transformed to achieve normality, where possible. Differences between conception groups for outcome measures were determined by t-test, or Welch ANOVA, or Wilcoxon test for non-parametric data ($p < 0.05$, JMP v14.3). Nutrient data are presented as means ± SD or median and IQR. Data transformed for analyses are presented as untransformed values. There were no sex differences in any nutrients investigated in the cord blood (data not shown), thus analyses between CON and ICSI groups are inclusive of newborn sex. There was a total of 10 CON and 11 ICSI participants who had nutrient levels measured in maternal blood and umbilical vein blood. Some participants did not have a measured value for a nutrient, and/or statistical outliers were removed, resulting in lower final n-numbers for specific nutrient measures (which are reported for each nutrient in the tables). Fisher's exact test was performed to evaluate placental histopathological findings between groups (GraphPad Prism 7.0 software). Correlations between maternal pre-pregnancy BMI and levels of nutrients in maternal circulation, or between levels of nutrients in maternal circulation and umbilical vein circulation, were determined by Pearson or Spearman correlation analyses. Data are presented as Pearson's correlation coefficient or Spearman's rho. Statistical differences were set at $p < 0.05$.

3. Results

3.1. Clinical Data

There were no differences in maternal age, initial (first trimester) and final (term) body mass index (BMI), maternal weight gain across pregnancy, gestational age at delivery, birth weight, placental weight or F:P weight ratio between conception groups (Table 2).

Table 2. Clinical and biometric profile of the pregnancies enrolled in the study.

Parameter	CON (n = 10)	ICSI (n = 11)	p-Value
Maternal age (years)	32.50 ± 7.71	35.36 ± 6.61	NS
Gestational age at delivery (days)	271.6 ± 2.37	272.0 ± 3.79	NS
Weight gain (kg; 12 weeks-birth)	10.31 ± 4.44	14.30 ± 5.90	NS
Initial maternal BMI (kg/m^2)	25.62 ± (19.0–29.4)	23.58 ± (21.7–28.3)	NS
Final maternal BMI (kg/m^2)	29.57 ± 3.17	28.59 ± 2.53	NS
Newborn sex	M (4); F (6)	M (6); F (5)	
Birthweight (g)	3365 ± 318	3199 ± 194	NS
Placental weight (g)	592.6 ± (359–689)	547.8 ± 22.21 (438–655)	NS
Newborn head circumference (cm)	35.00 ± 0.97	34.41 ± 1.36	NS
Newborn length (cm)	48.20 ± 1.69	48.77 ± 1.65	NS
Fetal/Placental Weight ratio	5.81 ± 0.98	5.94 ± 0.91	NS
Apgar 1'/Apgar 5'	9/10	9/10	NS

Data are mean ± SD or median (IQR). Groups were analyzed using Unpaired t-test or Mann-Whitney Test. newborn. CON = naturally conceived, ICSI = intracytoplasmic sperm injection. NS = not significant.

3.2. ICSI Impairs Placental SNAT 2 Immunostaining

We determined the placental mRNA expression of major transporter systems. We did not detect statistical differences in the mRNA expression levels of the neutral amino acid transporters, *SLC38A1* (encoding SNAT1), *SLC38A2* (SNAT2) and *SLC38A4* (SNAT 4); in the glucose transporters, *SLC2A1* (GLUT1) and *SLC2A3* (GLUT3); and in the MDR transporters *ABCB1* (P-gp) and *ABCG2* (BCRP) (Supplementary Figure S1). GLUT1 and SNAT2 are two major placental glucose and amino acid transporters, and their immunostaining was detected in the membrane and cytoplasm of syncytiotrophoblasts, in endothelial cells of fetal blood vessels and in the cytoplasm of placental connective tissue (to a lesser extent). SNAT2 immunostaining was decreased in ICSI placentae ($p < 0.05$) and there were no changes in the semiquantitative expression levels of placental GLUT1 transporter (Figure 1A–H). P-gp and BCRP were immunolocalized in the apical membrane and cytoplasm of syncytiotrophoblasts, whereas BCRP was also localized in endothelial cells of fetal blood vessels and in placental connective tissue. There were no changes in immunostaining of P-gp and BCRP between groups (Figure 1I–P).

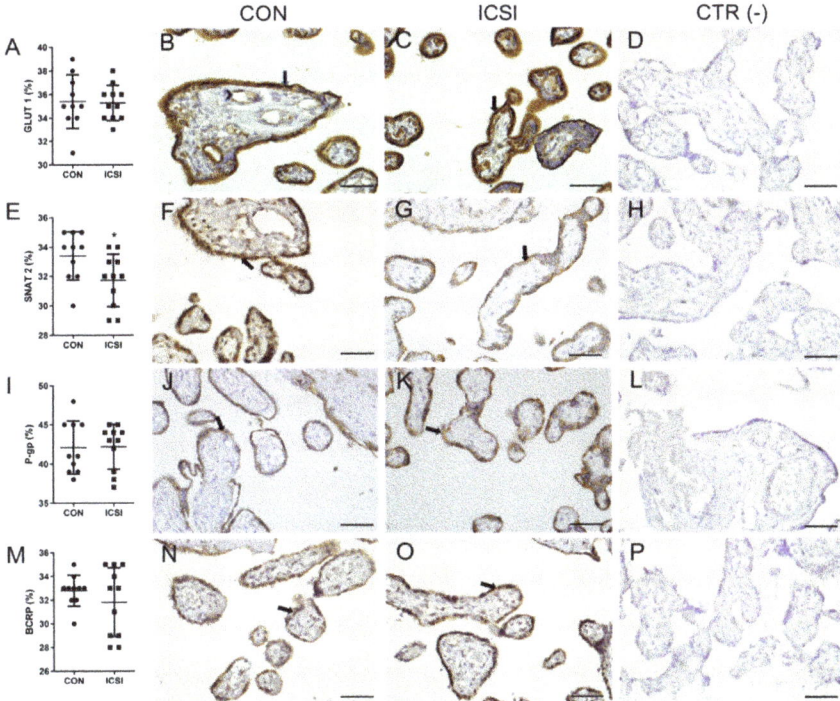

Figure 1. The amino acid transporter SNAT2 is downregulated in the human ICSI placenta. Semiquantitative staining scores (**A,E,I,M**) and corresponding representative immunostaining photomicrographies of placental GLUT1 (**B,C**), SNAT2 (**F,G**), P-gp (**J,K**) and BCRP (**N,O**) in control naturally conceived (CON; $n = 10$/group) and ICSI ($n = 11$/group) term placentae. All transporters were predominantly localized to the membrane and cytoplasm of syncytiotrophoblasts. Staining of GLUT1, SNAT2 and BCRP were also detected, to a lesser extent, in endothelial cells of fetal blood vessels and in the cytoplasm of placental connective tissue. (**D,H,L,P**) negative controls. Data are presented as media ± SD. (**A,E,I,M**) statistical differences were analyzed using Unpaired *t*-test. * $p < 0.05$. Arrows indicate the syncytium; arrow heads indicate fetal blood cells. Scale bar = 50 µm.

3.3. Venous umbilical Cord Blood from ICSI Term Pregnancies Exhibit Specific Changes in Nutrient Levels

We next evaluated maternal and umbilical cord blood levels of free amino acids in CON and ICSI pregnancies to identify possible changes that could be attributed to the method of conception. Levels of aspartic acid, glutamic acid, alanine, arginine, phenylalanine, glycine, methionine, ornithine, serine, tyrosine, threonine, tryptophan and valine were consistently detected in the maternal and venous umbilical cord blood in CON and ICSI pregnancies, whereas citrulline and histidine were not detected in some participants (Figure 2).

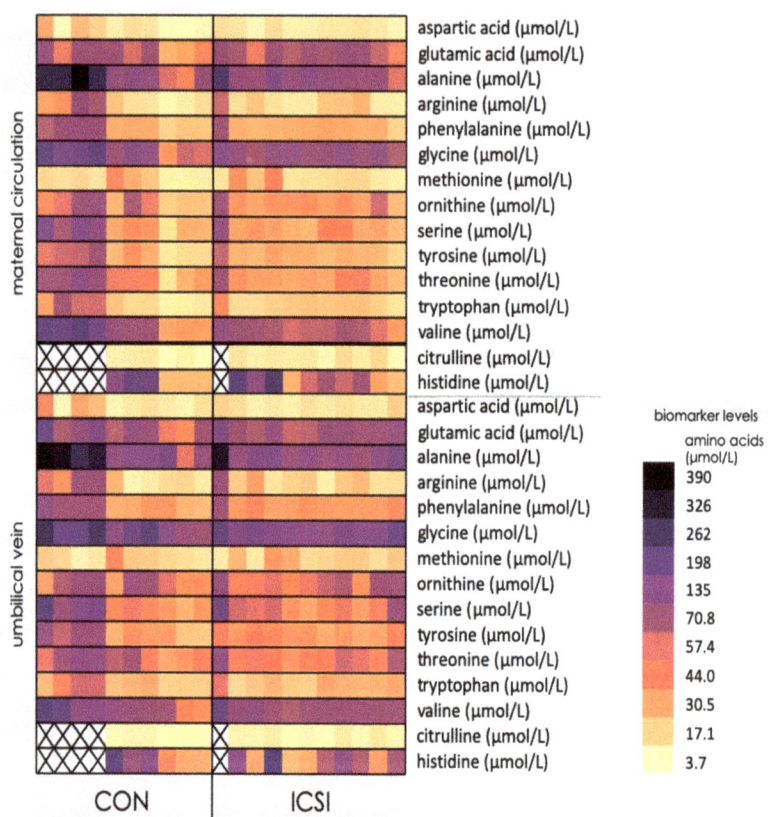

Figure 2. Heatmap of free amino acid levels in maternal circulation and umbilical vein in control, naturally conceived (CON; n = 10) and ICSI (n = 11) term pregnancies. Each column represents the nutrient profile of an individual pregnancy (maternal and umbilical vein). Darker colors indicate higher biomarker concentrations whereas lighter colors indicate lower biomarker concentrations. X = no value measured. Refer to Supplementary Tables S1 and S2 for values.

Levels of asparagine, isoleucine, leucine, lysine and taurine, were not detected in most participants and were therefore not analyzed for statistical differences (Supplementary Tables S1 and S2). Overall, there were more CON mothers with blood levels of free amino acids within the reference ranges than ICSI mothers, despite that the majority of the subjects had amino acid levels below the reference ranges (Supplementary Figure S2). There were no differences in the levels of free amino acids in maternal circulation between CON and ICSI (Table 3 and Supplementary Table S1), however, citrulline concentration was increased in venous cord blood of ICSI-conceived newborns compared to newborns conceived naturally ($p < 0.05$, Table 3). Umbilical cord levels of the other amino acids measured (aspartic acid, glutamic acid, alanine, arginine, phenylalanine, glycine, methionine, ornithine, serine, tyrosine, threonine, tryptophan, valine and histidine) did not differ between CON and ICSI (Supplementary Table S2).

Table 3. Citruline and free fatty acid concentrations in maternal and umbilical vein circulations with natural conception and ICSI.

Nutrient	CON	ICSI	p-Value
	Maternal circulation		
Citrulline (μmol/L)	8.2 ± 3.0 (6)	10.7 ± 3.1 (10)	NS
Free fatty acids (mmol/L)	0.89 ± 0.19 (9)	0.75 ± 0.28 (10)	NS
	Umbilical Vein Circulation		
Citrulline (μmol/L)	6.5 ± 1.6 (6)	8.5 ± 1.9 (10)	0.0385
Free fatty acids (mmol/L)	0.24 ± 0.05 (10)	0.14 ± 0.08 (10)	0.0057

Data are mean ± SD. n for each variable indicated in parentheses. NS = not significant. CON = naturally conceived; ICSI = intracytoplasmic sperm injection.

We observed higher maternal blood levels of FFA, lipids and lipoproteins in the maternal circulation compared to umbilical cord blood in CON and ICSI pregnancies (Figure 3). Overall, both CON and ICSI mothers demonstrated normal blood levels of HDL cholesterol, but both groups overall exhibited high levels of all other lipids/lipoproteins (Supplementary Figure S3). There were no differences in the levels of FFA (Table 3), glucose, lipids or lipoproteins in maternal blood between CON and ICSI groups (Supplementary Table S1). However, FFA levels were lower in cord blood of ICSI-conceived newborns compared to newborns conceived naturally ($p < 0.01$, Table 3), whereas levels of other lipids/lipoproteins and glucose did not differ between groups (Supplementary Table S2).

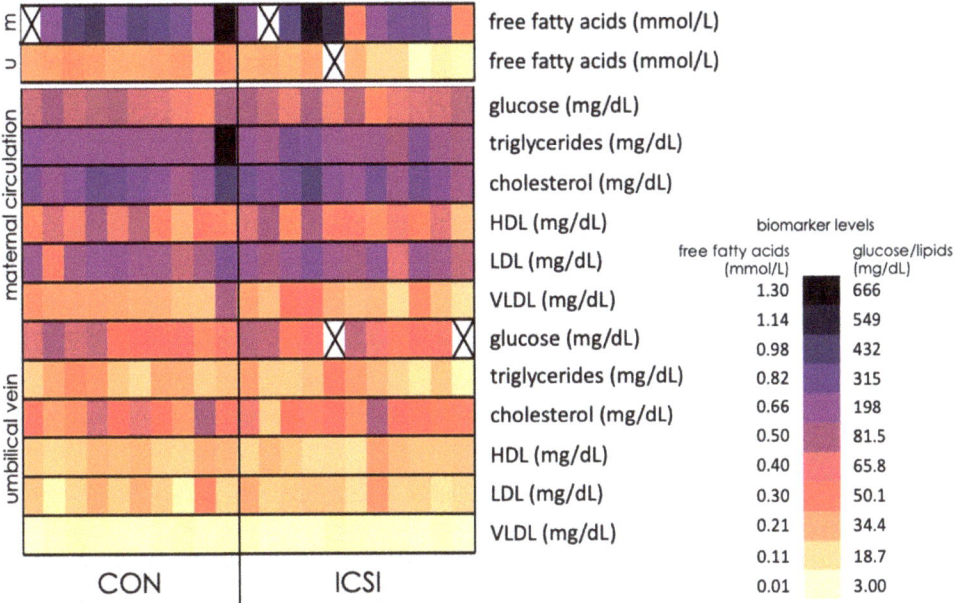

Figure 3. Heatmap of free fatty acids, glucose and lipid biomarker levels in maternal circulation and umbilical vein in control naturally conceived (CON; $n = 10$) and ICSI ($n = 11$). Each column represents the nutrient profile of an individual pregnancy (maternal and umbilical vein). Darker colors indicate higher biomarker concentrations and lighter colors indicate lower biomarker concentrations. X = no value measured. Refer to supplementary Tables S1 and S2 for values. m = maternal circulation. u = umbilical vein.

Next, we explored relationships between key clinical variables and outcome measures in our cohort. Maternal pre-pregnancy BMI was not correlated with circulating maternal nutrient levels, except a slight negative correlation between pre-pregnancy BMI and glutamic acid levels (r = −0.439, p = 0.046). Second, we observed significant positive correlations between all circulating nutrient levels in mothers with their levels in the umbilical vein, with the exception of triglycerides, HDL, VLDL and methionine (Table 4).

Table 4. Correlations between maternal circulating nutrient levels and the same nutrient level in umbilical vein from CON and ICSI pregnancies.

Nutrient	Spearman's Rho	p-Value
Free fatty acids (mmol/L)	0.6757	0.002
Glucose (mg/dL)	0.5271	0.02
Triglycerides (mg/dL)	0.2182	NS
Cholesterol (mg/dL)	0.4717	0.03
HDL (mg/dL)	0.0095	NS
LDL (mg/dL)	0.5436	0.01
VLDL (mg/dL)	−0.0250	NS
Aspartic acid (µmol/L)	0.6824	0.0007
Glutamic acid (µmol/L)	0.5143	0.02
Alanine (µmol/L)	0.5896	0.005
Arginine (µmol/L)	0.6998	0.0004
Phenylalanine (µmol/L)	0.5055	0.02
Glycine (µmol/L)	0.7351	0.0001
Methionine (µmol/L)	0.4297	NS
Ornithine (µmol/L)	0.6701	0.0009
Serine (µmol/L)	0.7165	0.0003
Tyrosine (µmol/L)	0.7545	<0.0001
Threonine (µmol/L)	0.8078	<0.0001
Tryptophan (µmol/L)	0.6359	0.002
Valine (µmol/L)	0.9299	<0.0001
Citrulline (µmol/L)	0.7900	0.0003
Histidine (µmol/L)	0.6461	0.007

NS = not significant. $p < 0.05$ (Spearman's rho (ρ)).

We also explored potential relationships between umbilical vein FFA and citrulline levels. We did not find any relationship between levels of these nutrients (r = −0.362, p = 0.18) for the whole cohort, or when exploring relationships within each of the CON (p = −0.529, p = 0.28) and ICSI groups (p = 0.185, p = 0.63).

3.4. Placental Proliferation and Apoptosis Are Increased in the Human ICSI Placenta

Since altered proliferation and apoptosis have been previously described in the mouse IVF placenta [7,36], we investigated whether the human ICSI placenta would exhibit differences in parameters related to cellular proliferation (placental staining of the Ki67 proliferation marker) and apoptosis (TUNEL staining). Increased Ki67 staining ($p < 0.0001$) was detected in the nuclei of cytotrophoblasts and connective tissue (to a lesser extent), whereas increased apoptotic immunosignals ($p < 0.0001$) were visible in the nuclei of syncytiotrophoblasts, cytotrophoblasts and connective tissue of ICSI placentae (Figure 4). Next, to evaluate whether these changes would be associated with any specific placental pathologies, we undertook histopathological analyses. We did not detect any placental pathologies that could be specifically attributed to the method of conception (Supplementary Table S3). Further, we also investigated the impact of ICSI in the number of placental histological components by performing a volumetric proportion analyses. No changes in the number of syncytiotrophoblasts, cytotrophoblasts, connective tissue, blood vessels or syncytial knots were observed between groups (Figure 5).

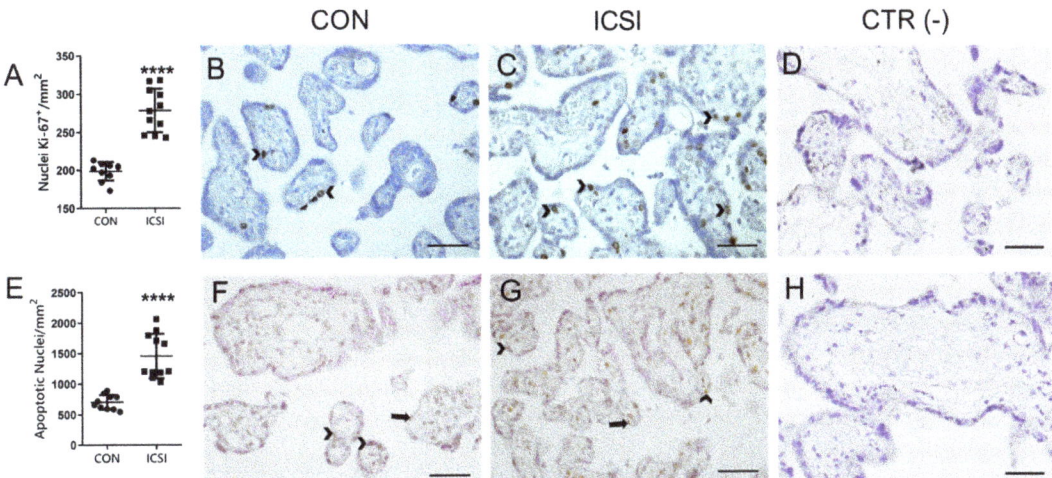

Figure 4. Placental proliferation and apoptosis are increased in the human ICSI placenta. Semiquantitative staining scores (**A,E**) and corresponding representative immunostaining photomicrographies of Ki67 (**B,C**) and TUNEL (**F,G**) obtained from term human naturally (CON; $n = 10$) conceived and ICSI ($n = 11$) placentae. (**D,H**) negative controls. (**A,E**) data are presented as mean ± SD. Statistical differences were analyzed using Unpaired t-test. **** $p < 0.0001$. Arrows indicate syncytium nuclear staining; arrowheads indicate cytotrophoblastic nuclear staining. Scale bar = 50 µm.

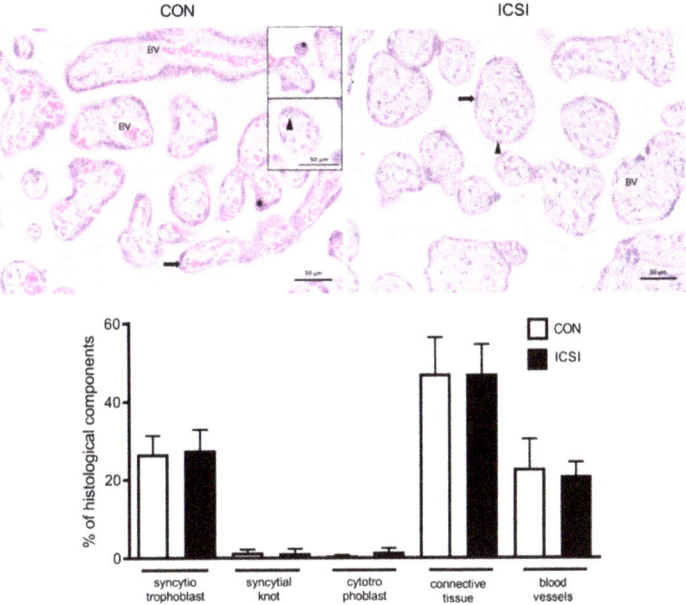

Figure 5. ICSI does not alter placental volumetric proportion. Representative histological photomicrographies of control naturally conceived (CON; $n = 10$) and ICSI ($n = 11$) placentae and correspondent volumetric proportion analyses of the number of syncytiotrophoblasts, cytotrophoblasts, connective tissue, blood vessels, and syncytial knots. Data presented as mean ± SD. $p < 0.05$ Arrows indicate the syncytium, arrow heads indicate cytotrophoblasts, indicate the syncytium knots and BV= blood vessels (fetal). Scale bar = 50 µm.

4. Discussion

This is the first study to comprehensively quantify placental nutrient and MDR transporters and maternal and umbilical nutrient levels, in ICSI compared to naturally conceived pregnancies, to better understand the mechanisms that may explain poor pregnancy outcomes in pregnancies conceived with ICSI. Using a cohort from Brazil, we found that ICSI pregnancies had placentae with decreased SNAT2 protein expression, had significant increase in venous umbilical cord citrulline and decreased FFA levels at term. We also observed increased markers of proliferation and apoptosis in ICSI placentae. These alterations may potentially disrupt placental development and transport potential.

In our study, contrary to our hypothesis, there were no changes in placental or birth weights or F:P weight ratio, suggesting that alterations in these parameters may not be common findings in pregnancies conceived by ICSI (vs. other forms of ART), or, alternatively, that other comorbidities often associated with sub- and infertility, but controlled for or absent in our study (e.g., maternal complications, elevated maternal BMI), explain more of the differences seen in fetoplacental weights following ART procedures [2,37]. This is consistent with the lack of differences between ICSI and CON participants in our study for maternal age, weight gain and BMI, amongst other clinical data. Further, although greater placental weight and lower F:P ratio were reported in pregnancies conceived by ART (ICSI and IVF) in a large Scandinavian based-population study [9], these differences in findings may also be attributed to sample size and/or to population ethnicity and other demographics (Scandinavian vs. Brazilian). Our findings are also in contrast with those described in mice conceived by IVF, which exhibited lower fetal weight, higher placental weight and lower F:P ratio [7,10]. It is important to note that there have been reports showing species-specific placental and fetal phenotypic adaptations in response to ART [2].

We detected lower protein expression levels of the neutral amino acid transporter SNAT2 in ICSI placentae, whereas GLUT1 (glucose) and P-gp/BCRP (drug) immunostaining remained unchanged. mRNA levels of *SLC38A2* (encoding SNAT2) and other transporter systems were not different between ICSI and CON groups, suggesting that ICSI alters placental protein levels of SNAT2 without changing its corresponding mRNA levels, at least in term no labor C-section placentae. Placental SNAT2 has been reported to be highly regulated by a variety of environmental factors including in vitro culture conditions [7], hormones (glucocorticoid exposure) [24,38,39], pH, oxygen tension [40], high fat diet [41], maternal protein restriction [42] and in obstetric conditions such as intrauterine growth restriction (IUGR) [43,44]. SNAT2 transports neutral amino acids such as alanine, asparagine, cysteine, glutamine, glycine, histidine, methionine, proline and serine and its activity is upregulated when cell growth and increased protein synthesis is required [17]. This is consistent with our finding of increased rates of cell proliferation and apoptosis in ICSI placentae, which may explain, at least in part, the altered placental SNAT2 expression levels observed.

Despite altered SNAT2 protein levels, there were no changes in SNAT2 amino acid substrates in the venous umbilical cord blood of ICSI pregnancies. However, we did find higher cord blood citrulline levels with ICSI. Citrulline was detected in 6 out of 10 CON pregnancies and 9 out of 11 ICSI pregnancies. This is the first report to show alterations in citrulline levels that could be attributed to ICSI procedures. Citrulline can originate from ornithine by actions of the ornithine carbamyl/carbamoyl transferase (OTC) or be released as by-product resulted from enzymatic nitric oxide synthesis from arginine by endothelial nitric oxide synthase (eNOS), inflammatory (iNOS) or neuronal NOS (nNOS) [45–47]. Of interest, placental citrulline synthesis and transport is not well understood, but may occur via distinct transporter systems as reported in other cell types [44,46]. Enterocytes may uptake citrulline using B (0,+), L, and b (0,+) amino acid transport systems [48], whereas in human umbilical vein cells (HUVECs), citrulline, along with arginine, is transported via the cationic amino acid transporter system y+/CATs [49]. Citrulline transmembrane transport occurring via Na+-dependent systems in rat small intestine and proximal tubular kidney cells have also been documented [47,50,51]. Of importance, citrulline levels in fetal plasma were increased in nutrient restricted (70% of control diet) pregnant baboons at mid-pregnancy, with no alterations in fetal and placental weight, i.e., prior to the onset of IUGR [45]. Importantly, nitric oxide (NO) derived from (eNOS) activity controls placental vascular tone and an imbalance of endothelial eNOS/arginase activity may contribute to vascular dysfunction in IUGR umbilical and placental vessels [52]. In our study, we excluded pregnancies with complications such as IUGR and pre-eclampsia, but given that ART-conceived pregnancies have higher IUGR and pre-eclampsia risk [4], further studies should investigate the maternal and fetal citrulline levels in ICSI pregnancies complicated by these conditions.

We observed a decrease in serum FFA levels in venous cord blood of ICSI newborns. Placental transport of FFA occurs via several transport mechanisms [16,53] and when visually comparing the heatmaps of the maternal versus the umbilical vein lipids and lipoproteins, it is possible to identify lower levels of these lipid biomarkers in the umbilical vein, showing that lipid transfer into the fetal circulation is largely controlled by the placenta. Future studies are necessary to investigate placental lipid metabolism and transfer in ICSI pregnancies to understand the mechanisms leading to lower FFA levels in ICSI newborns, and the impact this may have on fetal development. Although there were no differences in maternal levels of lipids and lipoproteins between ICSI and CON, overall, both groups of mothers had levels of FFA, cholesterol, triglycerides and lipoproteins above the recommended reference ranges. This may suggest that the placenta is adapting to lipid excess in order to regulate supply to the fetus. Further, taken with our finding that most mothers had lower circulating levels of free amino acids than recommended reference ranges for adults, our data suggests that participants in our study had a suboptimal nutritional profile. Future studies could cross-validate blood biomarker findings with validated food frequency questionnaires to better understand participant nutritional profiles and whether these, or the ART procedure itself, contribute to the outcomes observed, including lower FFA levels in cord blood from ICSI pregnancies. Since maternal malnutrition alters materno–fetal FFA transfer in pregnancy [54], disrupts placental expression of fatty acid transporters in mice [53] and in ewes [55] and significant lower cholesterol levels in the ICSI mouse placenta have been reported [56], it is conceivable that placental fatty acid transport is altered following ICSI in human pregnancies. This clearly requires further investigation.

Correlation analyses identified that, apart from triglycerides, HDL, VLDL and methionine, umbilical vein nutrient levels were positively associated with maternal levels of these nutrients. This demonstrates that even though the syncytium trophoblast barrier controls fetal nutrient transfer through the action of diverse mechanisms [13,16], the umbilical cord nutrient profile is directly dependent upon the maternal nutritional status. In our cohort, maternal pre-pregnancy BMI had limited influence on maternal blood nutrient levels. Further, the lack of correlation between umbilical cord citrulline and FFA levels in ICSI pregnancies suggests that ICSI impacts levels of these nutrients in the umbilical cord, possibly through independent, currently unknown mechanisms.

The placenta has high energetic demands throughout pregnancy, which increase exponentially at term [57]. Placentomegaly has been detected at term ICSI mouse [58] and human (IVF and ICSI-conceived) placentae [9], accompanied by significantly lower birthweights compared to spontaneously conceived pregnancies [9]. With this in mind, and the altered placental turnover we observed by increased rates of proliferation and apoptosis in ICSI placentae, it is possible that ICSI placentae are reallocating energetic and metabolic resources to a greater degree than CON, such that these metabolic substrates are used by the placenta to guarantee proper placental size (or its overgrowth)—a hypothesis that clearly requires further investigation. This, however, could have detrimental effects for the fetus, such as decreased transfer of key nutrients, consistent with our finding of lower umbilical cord serum FFA levels in ICSI newborns.

A consequence of decreased levels of specific nutrients in the fetal blood is reprogramming of fetal metabolism which may, in the short-term, ensure proper fetal growth, (here reflected by normal birthweight found in the ICSI group), but in the long-term, this adaptation may predispose offspring to cardiometabolic diseases in adult life, as demonstrated extensively in the developmental origins of health and disease (DOHaD) field [59]. Further, it is possible that changes in nutrient levels in the umbilical cord of ICSI newborns is one of the mechanisms through which excessive gamete and embryo manipulation inherent to ART procedures may program ART conception to altered developmental trajectories and life-long disease risk.

Increased placental apoptosis may be indicative of intrauterine stress, as commonly associated with excessive manipulation of gametes and embryos in ART reproductive cycles [2]. Importantly, given the increase in placental Ki67 staining, we can infer that ICSI placentae are capable of circumventing increased apoptotic rates and maintain cellular allostasis by increasing levels of cell proliferation. The increased proliferation/cell division rates herein observed were not associated with changes in the volumetric ratio of the various placental cell types or specific placental-related pathologies, and thus, allowed adequate placental and fetal growth, at least in later stages in pregnancy.

As to the other transporter systems investigated in this study, we did not observe differences in placental expression levels of GLUT1, P-gp and BCRP transporters in the CON and ICSI groups. Dong et al. [60] found increased levels of GLUT1 in placentae from ART pregnancies, which contrasts with our findings. Such differences may result from patient inclusion criteria in both studies, since the ART group in Dong's study consisted of pregnancies conceived by IVF and ICSI, delivered both by vaginal and C-section modes [60], whereas in this report, we only recruited ICSI pregnancies which delivered by C-section with no labor. Accordingly, we did not find differences in glucose levels in the maternal and venous umbilical cord blood, which matches our findings in placental GLUT1 expression. Further, the lack of differences in placental P-gp and BCRP expression between groups, suggests a preserved protective function of these efflux transporters in ICSI pregnancies, at least in later stages of pregnancy.

Strengths of our study include our comprehensive quantification of the maternal and umbilical cord blood nutrient milieux in ICSI and naturally conceived pregnancies, which allowed us to better capture potential differences in nutrient availability and transfer to the fetus than inferring these based on placental transporter expression alone. Further, our study is one of the few to examine ICSI exposures or placental outcomes in pregnant populations from the Global South, filling a large gap in our understanding of the mechanisms driving fetoplacental development and the programming of later health trajectories in underrepresented populations. As our groups were similar for clinical characteristics, particularly variables associated with subfertility and adverse pregnancy outcomes, all differences described are likely to be attributed to the ICSI method of conception and/or to the intrinsic risk factors inherent to the various causes of the couples' infertility that were not measured here. One potential limitation of our study is the relatively small number of patients enrolled in each group, warranting caution when considering the implications or translatability of our findings to other contexts. Nevertheless, our findings provide preliminary data for larger observational trials. For example, our groups were well-matched for key potential covariates including mode of delivery (all were C-section with no labor), initial and final maternal BMI and newborn fetal sex rates, and we did not include pregnancies with fetal–maternal, endocrine or metabolic complications or other comorbidities. Thus, we were able to study the effects of ICSI more accurately. In addition, due to our limited sample size, we were not able to robustly investigate the effects of sex on placental outcomes. Future studies should be powered to look at sex differences in the placenta from naturally conceived and ICSI conceived pregnancies. Another potential limitation of our study is the semiquantitative nature of the protein measurements. Nevertheless, such analyses enabled us to identify transporter protein expression not only in the syncytiotrophoblast layer of the placenta, but also in endothelial cells of fetal blood vessels and in the connective tissue.

5. Conclusions

We provide some of the first evidence for altered cord blood citrulline and FFA levels in human term pregnancies conceived by ICSI, associated with increased placental cellular turnover (increased rates of placental cell proliferation and apoptosis) and reduced SNAT2 protein abundance. Our data suggest that ICSI may have subtle, but important, effects on placental function without gross alterations in placental size, histology or pathology. Newborns conceived through ICSI may thus be potentially exposed to stressors in utero, which can result in metabolic adaptations, at least in late pregnancy, highlighting the need for follow-up studies to understand postnatal endocrine and metabolic phenotypes and how ICSI and altered placental function may explain these. The present study improves our understanding of the mechanisms that may contribute to poor pregnancy and postnatal outcomes in ICSI pregnancies and offspring, and adds to the dearth of evidence on placental development and function in pregnancies from the Global South.

Supplementary Materials: The following are available online at https://www.mdpi.com/article/10.3390/nu13082587/s1. Table S1: Nutrient concentrations in maternal circulation with natural conception and ICSI; Table S2: Nutrient concentrations in umbilical vein circulation with natural conception and ICSI; Table S3: Histopathology in placentae from naturally conceived and ICSI conceived pregnancies; Figure S1: ICSI does not alter mRNA expression levels of major placental transporter systems; Figure S2: Free amino acids in circulation of mothers who conceived naturally (CON) or with ICSI; Figure S3: Free fatty acid and lipids in circulation of mothers who conceived naturally (CON) or with ICSI.

Author Contributions: Conceptualization, E.B., L.M.M., R.A.A., C.B.N., L.C., K.L.C. and T.M.O.-C.; Data curation, E.B., J.R.S.B., C.B.V.A., F.F.B. and K.L.C.; Formal analysis, E.B., J.R.S.B., C.B.V.A., G.E.I., L.M.M., C.B.N., F.F.B. and K.L.C.; Funding acquisition, E.B., S.G.M. and T.M.O.-C.; Investigation, E.B., J.R.S.B., C.B.V.A., K.L.C. and T.M.O.-C.; Methodology, J.R.S.B., C.B.V.A., G.E.I., L.M.M., K.R.S., C.B.N., F.F.B. and K.L.C.; Project administration, E.B. and T.M.O.-C.; Resources, E.B., T.M.O.-C.; Software, K.L.C.; Supervision, E.B., C.B.V.A., L.C. and T.M.O.-C.; Visualization, E.B. and C.B.V.A.; Writing—original draft, E.B., J.R.S.B., C.B.V.A. and K.L.C.; Writing—review & editing, E.B., G.E.I., R.A.A., K.R.S., L.C., F.F.B., S.G.M., K.L.C. and T.M.O.-C. All authors have read and agreed to the published version of the manuscript.

Funding: This study was also supported by the Conselho Nacional de Desenvolvimento Científico e Tecnológico (CNPq, grant numbers: 402343/2012-3; 401605/2013-2; 422441/2016-3, 306525/2019-4, 310578/2020-5), Fundação de Amparo à Pesquisa do Estado do Rio de Janeiro (FAPERJ, CNE, CNE /E26/292798/2018) and Coordenação de Aperfeiçoamento Pessoal de Nível Superior (CAPES, finance Code 001; CAPES-Print fellowship to E.B.).

Institutional Review Board Statement: This study was conducted according to the guidelines of the Declaration of Helsinki, and approved by the Research Ethics Board from "Maternidade Escola" —Universidade Federal do Rio de Janeiro (project number CAAE: 30214214.0.0000.5275).

Informed Consent Statement: Informed consent was obtained from all subjects involved in the study.

Data Availability Statement: The data that support the findings of this study are available from the corresponding author upon reasonable request.

Acknowledgments: The authors thank the donors for the human specimens used in this study. We thank Nathalia L. Silva for technical assistance. Graphical abstract was created with BioRender.com.

Conflicts of Interest: The authors declare no conflict of interest.

References

1. Dyer, S.; Chambers, G.M.; de Mouzon, J.; Nygren, K.G.; Zegers-Hochschild, F.; Mansour, R.; Ishihara, O.; Banker, M.; Adamson, G.D. International Committee for Monitoring Assisted Reproductive Technologies world report: Assisted Reproductive Technology 2008, 2009 and 2010. *Hum. Reprod.* **2016**, *31*, 1588–1609. [CrossRef]
2. Bloise, E.; Feuer, S.K.; Rinaudo, P.F. Comparative intrauterine development and placental function of ART concepti: Implications for human reproductive medicine and animal breeding. *Hum. Reprod. Update* **2014**, *20*, 822–839. [CrossRef]

3. Vannuccini, S.; Ferrata, C.; Perelli, F.; Pinzauti, S.; Severi, F.M.; Reis, F.M.; Petraglia, F.; Di Tommaso, M. Peripartum and postpartum outcomes in uncomplicated term pregnancy following ART: A retrospective cohort study from two Italian obstetric units. *Hum. Reprod. Open* **2018**, *2018*, hoy012. [CrossRef]
4. Feuer, S.K.; Camarano, L.; Rinaudo, P.F. ART and health: Clinical outcomes and insights on molecular mechanisms from rodent studies. *Mol. Hum. Reprod.* **2013**, *19*, 189–204. [CrossRef]
5. Zhang, Y.; Zhao, W.; Jiang, Y.; Zhang, R.; Wang, J.; Li, C.; Zhao, H.; Gao, L.; Cui, Y.; Zhou, Z.; et al. Ultrastructural Study on Human Placentae from Women Subjected to Assisted Reproductive Technology Treatments. *Biol. Reprod.* **2011**, *85*, 635–642. [CrossRef] [PubMed]
6. Desforges, M.; Sibley, C.P. Placental nutrient supply and fetal growth. *Int. J. Dev. Biol.* **2010**, *54*, 377–390. [CrossRef] [PubMed]
7. Bloise, E.; Lin, W.; Liu, X.; Simbulan, R.; Kolahi, K.S.; Petraglia, F.; Maltepe, E.; Donjacour, A.; Rinaudo, P. Impaired Placental Nutrient Transport in Mice Generated by in Vitro Fertilization. *Endocrinology* **2012**, *153*, 3457–3467. [CrossRef] [PubMed]
8. Delle Piane, L.; Lin, W.; Liu, X.; Donjacour, A.; Minasi, P.; Revelli, A.; Maltepe, E.; Rinaudo, P.F. Effect of the method of conception and embryo transfer procedure on mid-gestation placenta and fetal development in an IVF mouse model. *Hum. Reprod.* **2010**, *25*, 2039–2046. [CrossRef]
9. Haavaldsen, C.; Tanbo, T.; Eskild, A. Placental weight in singleton pregnancies with and without assisted reproductive technology: A population study of 536 567 pregnancies. *Hum. Reprod.* **2012**, *27*, 576–582. [CrossRef]
10. Chen, S.; Sun, F.; Huang, X.; Wang, X.; Tang, N.; Zhu, B.; Li, B. Assisted reproduction causes placental maldevelopment and dysfunction linked to reduced fetal weight in mice. *Sci. Rep.* **2015**, *5*, 10596. [CrossRef]
11. Risnes, K.R.; Romundstad, P.R.; Nilsen, T.I.L.; Eskild, A.; Vatten, L.J. Placental Weight Relative to Birth Weight and Long-term Cardiovascular Mortality: Findings From a Cohort of 31,307 Men and Women. *Am. J. Epidemiol.* **2009**, *170*, 622–631. [CrossRef]
12. Sibley, C.P.; Turner, M.A.; Cetin, I.; Ayuk, P.; Boyd, C.A.R.; D'Souza, S.W.; Glazier, J.D.; Greenwood, S.L.; Jansson, T.; Powell, T. Placental Phenotypes of Intrauterine Growth. *Pediatr. Res.* **2005**, *58*, 827–832. [CrossRef] [PubMed]
13. Burton, G.J.; Fowden, A.L.; Thornburg, K.L. Placental Origins of Chronic Disease. *Physiol. Rev.* **2016**, *96*, 1509–1565. [CrossRef]
14. Schmon, B.; Hartmann, M.; Jones, C.J.; Desoye, G. Insulin and Glucose Do not Affect the Glycogen Content in Isolated and Cultured Trophoblast Cells of Human Term Placenta. *J. Clin. Endocrinol. Metab.* **1991**, *73*, 888–893. [CrossRef] [PubMed]
15. Desoye, G.; Shafrir, E. Placental metabolism and its regulation in health and diabetes. *Mol. Aspects Med.* **1994**, *15*, 505–682. [CrossRef]
16. Lager, S.; Powell, T.L. Regulation of Nutrient Transport across the Placenta. *J. Pregnancy* **2012**, *2012*, 179827. [CrossRef] [PubMed]
17. Bröer, S. SLC38 Family of Transporters for Neutral Amino Acids. In *Handbook of Neurochemistry and Molecular Neurobiology*; Lajtha, A., Reith, M.E.A., Eds.; Springer: Boston, MA, USA, 2007; pp. 327–338. ISBN 978-0-387-30347-5. [CrossRef]
18. Coan, P.M.; Angiolini, E.; Sandovici, I.; Burton, G.J.; Constância, M.; Fowden, A.L. Adaptations in placental nutrient transfer capacity to meet fetal growth demands depend on placental size in mice: Adaptations in placental nutrient transfer capacity. *J. Physiol.* **2008**, *586*, 4567–4576. [CrossRef]
19. Bloise, E.; Bhuiyan, M.; Audette, M.C.; Petropoulos, S.; Javam, M.; Gibb, W.; Matthews, S.G. Prenatal Endotoxemia and Placental Drug Transport in The Mouse: Placental Size-Specific Effects. *PLoS ONE* **2013**, *8*, e65728. [CrossRef]
20. Bloise, E.; Ortiga-Carvalho, T.M.; Reis, F.M.; Lye, S.J.; Gibb, W.; Matthews, S.G. ATP-binding cassette transporters in reproduction: A new frontier. *Hum. Reprod. Update* **2016**, *22*, 164–181. [CrossRef] [PubMed]
21. Imperio, G.E.; Javam, M.; Lye, P.; Constantinof, A.; Dunk, C.E.; Reis, F.M.; Lye, S.J.; Gibb, W.; Matthews, S.G.; Ortiga-Carvalho, T.M.; et al. Gestational age-dependent gene expression profiling of ATP-binding cassette transporters in the healthy human placenta. *J. Cell. Mol. Med.* **2019**, *23*, 610–618. [CrossRef] [PubMed]
22. Martinelli, L.M.; Fontes, K.N.; Reginatto, M.W.; Andrade, C.B.V.; Monteiro, V.R.S.; Gomes, H.R.; Silva-Filho, J.L.; Pinheiro, A.A.S.; Vago, A.R.; Almeida, F.R.C.L.; et al. Malaria in pregnancy regulates P-glycoprotein (P-gp/Abcb1a) and ABCA1 efflux transporters in the Mouse Visceral Yolk Sac. *J. Cell. Mol. Med.* **2020**, *24*, 10636–10647. [CrossRef]
23. Martinelli, L.M.; Reginatto, M.W.; Fontes, K.N.; Andrade, C.B.V.; Monteiro, V.R.S.; Gomes, H.R.; Almeida, F.R.C.L.; Bloise, F.F.; Matthews, S.G.; Ortiga-Carvalho, T.M.; et al. Breast cancer resistance protein (Bcrp/Abcg2) is selectively modulated by lipopolysaccharide (LPS) in the mouse yolk sac. *Reprod. Toxicol.* **2020**, *98*, 82–91. [CrossRef]
24. Audette, M.C.; Greenwood, S.L.; Sibley, C.P.; Jones, C.J.P.; Challis, J.R.G.; Matthews, S.G.; Jones, R.L. Dexamethasone stimulates placental system A transport and trophoblast differentiation in term villous explants. *Placenta* **2010**, *31*, 97–105. [CrossRef] [PubMed]
25. Gao, L.; Lv, C.; Xu, C.; Li, Y.; Cui, X.; Gu, H.; Ni, X. Differential Regulation of Glucose Transporters Mediated by CRH Receptor Type 1 and Type 2 in Human Placental Trophoblasts. *Endocrinology* **2012**, *153*, 1464–1471. [CrossRef] [PubMed]
26. Oliveira, P.F.; Alves, M.G.; Rato, L.; Laurentino, S.; Silva, J.; Sá, R.; Barros, A.; Sousa, M.; Carvalho, R.A.; Cavaco, J.E.; et al. Effect of insulin deprivation on metabolism and metabolism-associated gene transcript levels of in vitro cultured human Sertoli cells. *Biochim. Biophys. Acta BBA-Gen. Subj.* **2012**, *1820*, 84–89. [CrossRef] [PubMed]
27. Lye, P.; Bloise, E.; Javam, M.; Gibb, W.; Lye, S.J.; Matthews, S.G. Impact of bacterial and viral challenge on multidrug resistance in first- and third-trimester human placenta. *Am. J. Pathol.* **2015**, *185*, 1666–1675. [CrossRef] [PubMed]
28. Drewlo, S.; Levytska, K.; Kingdom, J. Revisiting the housekeeping genes of human placental development and insufficiency syndromes. *Placenta* **2012**, *33*, 952–954. [CrossRef] [PubMed]

29. Benirschke, K.; Spinosa, J.C.; McGinniss, M.J.; Marchevsky, A.; Sanchez, J. Partial molar transformation of the placenta of presumably monozygotic twins. *Pediatr. Dev. Pathol. Off. J. Soc. Pediatr. Pathol. Paediatr. Pathol. Soc.* **2000**, *3*, 95–100. [CrossRef]
30. Perni, S.C.; Predanik, M.; Cho, J.E.; Baergen, R.N. Placental pathology and pregnancy outcomes in donor and non-donor oocyte in vitro fertilization pregnancies. *J. Perinat. Med.* **2005**, *33*. [CrossRef] [PubMed]
31. Joy, J.; Gannon, C.; McClure, N.; Cooke, I. Is Assisted Reproduction Associated with Abnormal Placentation? *Pediatr. Dev. Pathol.* **2012**, *15*, 306–314. [CrossRef]
32. Fontes, K.N.; Reginatto, M.W.; Silva, N.L.; Andrade, C.B.V.; Bloise, F.F.; Monteiro, V.R.S.; Silva-Filho, J.L.; Imperio, G.E.; Pimentel-Coelho, P.M.; Pinheiro, A.A.S.; et al. Dysregulation of placental ABC transporters in a murine model of malaria-induced preterm labor. *Sci. Rep.* **2019**, *9*, 11488. [CrossRef]
33. Reginatto, M.; Fontes, K.; Monteiro, V.; Silva, N.; Andrade, C.; Gomes, H.; Imperio, G.; Bloise, F.; Kluck, G.; Atella, G.; et al. Effect of sublethal prenatal endotoxaemia on murine placental transport systems and lipid homeostasis. *Physiology* **2020**. [CrossRef]
34. Andrade, C.B.V.; de Monteiro, V.R.S.; Coelho, S.V.A.; Gomes, H.R.; Sousa, R.P.C.; de Nascimento, V.M.O.; Bloise, F.F.; Matthews, S.G.; Bloise, E.; Arruda, L.B.; et al. ZIKV Disrupts Placental Ultrastructure and Drug Transporter Expression in Mice. *Front. Immunol.* **2021**, *12*, 680246. [CrossRef]
35. Tschanz, S.A.; Burri, P.H.; Weibel, E.R. A simple tool for stereological assessment of digital images: The STEPanizer: TOOL FOR STEREOLOGICAL ASSESSMENT. *J. Microsc.* **2011**, *243*, 47–59. [CrossRef] [PubMed]
36. Raunig, J.M.; Yamauchi, Y.; Ward, M.A.; Collier, A.C. Placental inflammation and oxidative stress in the mouse model of assisted reproduction. *Placenta* **2011**, *32*, 852–858. [CrossRef] [PubMed]
37. Vannuccini, S.; Clifton, V.L.; Fraser, I.S.; Taylor, H.S.; Critchley, H.; Giudice, L.C.; Petraglia, F. Infertility and reproductive disorders: Impact of hormonal and inflammatory mechanisms on pregnancy outcome. *Hum. Reprod. Update* **2016**, *22*, 104–115. [CrossRef] [PubMed]
38. Audette, M.C.; Challis, J.R.G.; Jones, R.L.; Sibley, C.P.; Matthews, S.G. Antenatal Dexamethasone Treatment in Midgestation Reduces System A-Mediated Transport in the Late-Gestation Murine Placenta. *Endocrinology* **2011**, *152*, 3561–3570. [CrossRef] [PubMed]
39. Jones, H.N.; Ashworth, C.J.; Page, K.R.; McArdle, H.J. Cortisol stimulates system A amino acid transport and SNAT2 expression in a human placental cell line (BeWo). *Am. J. Physiol.-Endocrinol. Metab.* **2006**, *291*, E596–E603. [CrossRef]
40. Nelson, D.M.; Smith, S.D.; Furesz, T.C.; Sadovsky, Y.; Ganapathy, V.; Parvin, C.A.; Smith, C.H. Hypoxia reduces expression and function of system A amino acid transporters in cultured term human trophoblasts. *Am. J. Physiol. Cell Physiol.* **2003**, *284*, C310–C315. [CrossRef]
41. Jones, H.N.; Woollett, L.A.; Barbour, N.; Prasad, P.D.; Powell, T.L.; Jansson, T. High-fat diet before and during pregnancy causes marked up-regulation of placental nutrient transport and fetal overgrowth in C57/BL6 mice. *FASEB J.* **2009**, *23*, 271–278. [CrossRef]
42. Rosario, F.J.; Jansson, N.; Kanai, Y.; Prasad, P.D.; Powell, T.L.; Jansson, T. Maternal Protein Restriction in the Rat Inhibits Placental Insulin, mTOR, and STAT3 Signaling and Down-Regulates Placental Amino Acid Transporters. *Endocrinology* **2011**, *152*, 1119–1129. [CrossRef] [PubMed]
43. Jansson, T.; Ylvén, K.; Wennergren, M.; Powell, T.L. Glucose Transport and System A Activity in Syncytiotrophoblast Microvillous and Basal Plasma Membranes in Intrauterine Growth Restriction. *Placenta* **2002**, *23*, 392–399. [CrossRef] [PubMed]
44. Mandò, C.; Tabano, S.; Pileri, P.; Colapietro, P.; Marino, M.A.; Avagliano, L.; Doi, P.; Bulfamante, G.; Miozzo, M.; Cetin, I. SNAT2 expression and regulation in human growth-restricted placentas. *Pediatr. Res.* **2013**, *74*, 104–110. [CrossRef]
45. Pantham, P.; Rosario, F.J.; Weintraub, S.T.; Nathanielsz, P.W.; Powell, T.L.; Li, C.; Jansson, T. Down-Regulation of Placental Transport of Amino Acids Precedes the Development of Intrauterine Growth Restriction in Maternal Nutrient Restricted Baboons. *Biol. Reprod.* **2016**, *95*, 98. [CrossRef] [PubMed]
46. Wijnands, K.; Castermans, T.; Hommen, M.; Meesters, D.; Poeze, M. Arginine and Citrulline and the Immune Response in Sepsis. *Nutrients* **2015**, *7*, 1426–1463. [CrossRef]
47. Ginguay, A.; De Bandt, J.-P. Citrulline production and protein homeostasis. *Curr. Opin. Clin. Nutr. Metab. Care* **2019**, *22*, 371–376. [CrossRef]
48. Bahri, S.; Curis, E.; El Wafi, F.-Z.; Aussel, C.; Chaumeil, J.-C.; Cynober, L.; Zerrouk, N. Mechanisms and kinetics of citrulline uptake in a model of human intestinal epithelial cells. *Clin. Nutr.* **2008**, *27*, 872–880. [CrossRef]
49. Casanello, P.; Sobrevia, L. Intrauterine Growth Retardation Is Associated With Reduced Activity and Expression of the Cationic Amino Acid Transport Systems y+/hCAT-1 and y+/hCAT-2B and Lower Activity of Nitric Oxide Synthase in Human Umbilical Vein Endothelial Cells. *Circ. Res.* **2002**, *91*, 127–134. [CrossRef] [PubMed]
50. Vadgama, J.V.; Evered, D.F. Characteristics of L-Citrulline Transport across Rat Small Intestine In Vitro. *Pediatr. Res.* **1992**, *32*, 472–478. [CrossRef]
51. Mitsuoka, K.; Shirasaka, Y.; Fukushi, A.; Sato, M.; Nakamura, T.; Nakanishi, T.; Tamai, I. Transport characteristics of L-citrulline in renal apical membrane of proximal tubular cells. *Biopharm. Drug Dispos.* **2009**, *30*, 126–137. [CrossRef]
52. Krause, B.J.; Carrasco-Wong, I.; Caniuguir, A.; Carvajal, J.; Faras, M.; Casanello, P. Endothelial eNOS/arginase imbalance contributes to vascular dysfunction in IUGR umbilical and placental vessels. *Placenta* **2013**, *34*, 20–28. [CrossRef]

53. Connor, K.L.; Kibschull, M.; Matysiak-Zablocki, E.; Nguyen, T.T.-T.N.; Matthews, S.G.; Lye, S.J.; Bloise, E. Maternal malnutrition impacts placental morphology and transporter expression: An origin for poor offspring growth. *J. Nutr. Biochem.* **2020**, *78*, 108329. [CrossRef]
54. Hirschmugl, B.; Perazzolo, S.; Sengers, B.G.; Lewis, R.M.; Gruber, M.; Desoye, G.; Wadsack, C. Placental mobilization of free fatty acids contributes to altered materno-fetal transfer in obesity. *Int. J. Obes.* **2021**, *45*, 1114–1123. [CrossRef] [PubMed]
55. Cetin, I.; Parisi, F.; Berti, C.; Mandò, C.; Desoye, G. Placental fatty acid transport in maternal obesity. *J. Dev. Orig. Health Dis.* **2012**, *3*, 409–414. [CrossRef]
56. Raunig, J.M.; Yamauchi, Y.; Ward, M.A.; Collier, A.C. Assisted reproduction technologies alter steroid delivery to the mouse fetus during pregnancy. *J. Steroid Biochem. Mol. Biol.* **2011**, *126*, 26–34. [CrossRef] [PubMed]
57. Vaughan, O.; Fowden, A. Placental metabolism: Substrate requirements and the response to stress. *Reprod. Domest. Anim.* **2016**, *51*, 25–35. [CrossRef] [PubMed]
58. Collier, A.C.; Miyagi, S.J.; Yamauchi, Y.; Ward, M.A. Assisted reproduction technologies impair placental steroid metabolism. *J. Steroid Biochem. Mol. Biol.* **2009**, *116*, 21–28. [CrossRef] [PubMed]
59. Rinaudo, P.; Wang, E. Fetal Programming and Metabolic Syndrome. *Annu. Rev. Physiol.* **2012**, *74*, 107–130. [CrossRef] [PubMed]
60. Dong, J.; Wen, L.; Guo, X.; Xiao, X.; Jiang, F.; Li, B.; Jin, N.; Wang, J.; Wang, X.; Chen, S.; et al. The increased expression of glucose transporters in human full-term placentas from assisted reproductive technology without changes of mTOR signaling. *Placenta* **2019**, *86*, 4–10. [CrossRef]

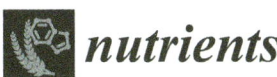

Review

Has Menstruation Disappeared? Functional Hypothalamic Amenorrhea—What Is This Story about?

Karina Ryterska [1,*], Agnieszka Kordek [2] and Patrycja Załęska [1]

[1] Department of Human Nutrition and Metabolomics, Pomeranian Medical University in Szczecin, 70-204 Szczecin, Poland; patrycjaazaleska288@gmail.com
[2] Neonatal Clinic, Pomeranian Medical University in Szczecin, 70-204 Szczecin, Poland; agkordek@pum.edu.pl
* Correspondence: ryterska@pum.edu.pl

Abstract: Functional hypothalamic amenorrhea (FHA) is a very common condition affecting women of procreative age. There are many reasons for this disorder, including a low availability of energy in the diet, low micro- and macronutrient intake, overly intensive physical activity, disturbed regeneration processes, sleep disorders, stress, and psychological disorders. The main determinant is long-term stress and an inability to handle the effects of that stress. FHA is a very complex disorder and often goes undiagnosed. Moreover, therapeutic interventions do not address all the causes of the disorder, which could have implications for women's health. As shown by scientific reports, this condition can be reversed by modifying its causes. This review of the literature aims to update the current knowledge of functional hypothalamic amenorrhea and underscores the complexity of the disorder, with particular emphasis on the nutritional aspects and potential interventions for restoring balance.

Keywords: gynecologic disease; amenorrhea; nutrition; ovary; uterus; stress; low energy; physical activity

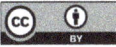

1. Introduction

Functional hypothalamic amenorrhea (FHA) is one of the most common menstruation disorders among women of childbearing age. The diagnosis of FHA is based on the exclusion of other causes of non-menstruation, including organic and anatomical factors [1–4]. This status should be reversible upon the modification of the basic causes.

The main determinant of the disorder is a combination of psychosocial and metabolic stress. Predisposing factors include low energy availability [1], nutrient deficiencies [1,5], excessive physical activity [1,2], a lack of endometrium regeneration [1,2], abnormal sleep [1,2], emotional tension [1,2], unmanageable chronic or severe stress [1,2], and dysfunctional behavior [1,2,5]. A common occurrence in FHA is the co-existence of many components. Previous reports suggested the crucial importance of body weight in the pathogenesis of the disorder. However, it is now clear that functional menstruation disorders are diagnosed in people with wide range of body weight and body fat. Neuroendocrine aberrations may also occur despite a normal body weight [4–6].

In response to the above mentioned factors, the pulsatory secretion of gonadotropin releasing hormone (GnRH) in the hypothalamus is blocked, which results in the abnormal secretion of tropic hormones by the pituitary gland, including follicotropins (FSH) and lutropin (LH) [1,3,7,8]. As a consequence, estrogen production is reduced, and no ovulation occurs. Progesterone is also absent since ovulation is completely blocked. Progesterone is produced by the luteinization of granulosa cells of the ovulating follicle. The entire monthly cycle is deregulated and, over time, becomes completely absent [1,3,7,8].

Although the onomastics suggest a disorder associated with reproductive functions, FHA is closely correlated with the regulation of the entire endocrine system and the neurotransmitter system. The following metabolic and psychological consequences have been described (Figure 1) [7]: The hypothalamus–pituitary–ovary axis ceases to function, and the hypothalamus and pituitary and thyroid glands are affected. These consequences manifest as a reduction in relevant activities. The TSH level decreases or lies at the lower limit of the standard range, as does the T4 level. The T3 concentration is also reduced, and the conversion of T4 to the active metabolite T3 is impaired. T4 is converted into a non-active reverse-T3 that blocks T3 receptors [1,3]. In response to chronic stress, the HPA axis is enhanced at each step of regulation, which results in chronically elevated cortisol levels and subtly regulated rhythms over about 24 h. A reduced concentration of leptin plays a significant role in this process. The characteristic results include reduced glucose, insulin, insulin-like growth factor (IGF-1), and kisspeptin along with elevated ghrelin, growth hormone (GH), Y neuropeptide Y, peptide YY, and beta-endorphin [3,5–9]. Kisspeptin, encoded by the Kiss-1 gene, is a hormone produced in the hypothalamus that plays a key role in the direct stimulation and release of GnRH [1]. Moreover, some studies have suggested a positive correlation between kisspeptin and LH secretory pulses [10]. Kisspeptin may also influence the negative and positive feedback of estrogen [11]. Many reports have emphasized the sensitivity of kisspeptin to the metabolic state of the body and to stress, both acute and chronic [10,11]. It was reported that the higher the cortisol level is, the lower the plasma level of kisspeptin will be [10]. Intriguing observations were described in one study, which observed that the subcutaneous injection of kisspeptin in women with FHA caused the secretion of gonadotropins and an increase in estradiol concentrations [10].

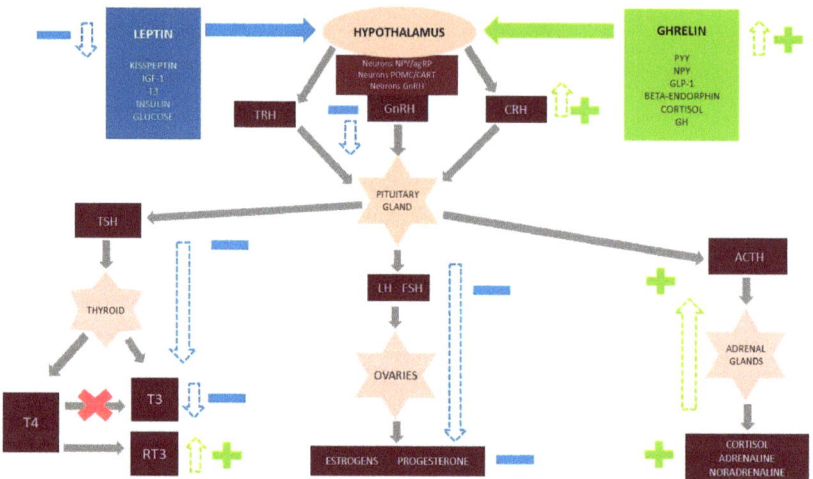

Figure 1. Functional hypothalamic amenorrhea (FHA) and influence on the endocrine system. Figure 1 shows the major hormone axis dysfunction caused by FHA, including the additional important neurohormonal factors that decrease (leptin, kisspeptin, IGF-1, FT3, insulin, and glucose) and increase (ghrelin and peptide YY (PYY), neuropeptide Y (NPY), growth hormone (GH), glucagon-like peptide 1 (GLP-1), beta-endorphins, and cortisol) in FHA. The hypothalamus secretes gonadotropin releasing hormone (GnRH), corticotropin-releasing hormone (CRH), and thyrotropin-releasing hormone (TRH), which then affect the pituitary gland and stimulate it to secrete tropic hormones: lutropin (LH), follicotropins (FSH), adrenocorticotropic hormone (ACTH), and thyroid-stimulating hormone (TSH). These hormones then affect the target organs. In turn, the ovaries, adrenal glands, and thyroid glands secrete hormones specific to them. Under physiological conditions, all hormonal axes are regulated by positive and negative feedback. A decreased concentration of hormones occurs in each of the secretory stages for the hypothalamus–pituitary–ovary (HPO) and hypothalamus–pituitary–thyroid (HPT) axes. Moreover, in the case of the thyroid gland, the conversion of T4 to the metabolically active form of T3 is disturbed. Instead, the inactive form reverse-T3 is produced in excess and blocks the receptors for T3.

As a result of metabolic adaptation, for protective purposes, the low levels of gonadal and thyroid hormones in FHA do not stimulate positive feedback. The HPA axis is also overstimulated at each stage of regulation. As a consequence, there is an increased level of cortisol, which may not have an inhibitory effect with negative feedback at the higher centers of axis regulation.

Notably, changes in menstruation are the latter signs of the disorder. Symptoms such as a lack of ovulation and abridged luteal phase are of primary concern [1,12]. These symptoms occur despite normal monthly bleeding. Without the use of specialized tests, these problems often go unnoticed. Other, more pronounced signals include irregular menstruation, elongated cycles, and spotting, referred to as "oligo-polymenorrhea". The last step is the complete lack of menses. For women who regularly menstruate, menstrual atrophy can occur more than 3 months. On the other hand, in the case of irregular cycles, menstrual atrophy can occur over 6 months [1,7,12].

In light of past scientific reports, it can be concluded that multidirectional operations are needed. Based primarily on a combination of work with the patient's psyche and primary improvement in nutritional status. Consistent activities should include a modification of eating habits and training [13–15].

2. Pathogenicity

2.1. Psychology

In the literature, the psychological profile of women with functional menstruation disorders is quite well characterized. This profile includes perfectionism [16,17], high demands for oneself and others [14], low self-esteem [16], introversion [16], a fear of judgment [16], a strong need for social acceptance [16], problems with communication and social networking [16], a fear of maturity and sexuality, an inability to deal with daily stress and problems [1,16–18], and an inability to define one's emotions [1,16]. In addition, high levels of anxiety [14], depressed mood [14,16], depression [14,16], and sleep disorders have been noted [1,14–18].

Abnormal nutrition and physical activity, an increased focus on diet, and a fear of gaining weight are also common [6,18,19]. These symptoms have been observed despite the elimination of women with clinical nutrition disorders from the sample groups [13,17,20]. Some reports, moreover, suggest that FHA is a milder form of ED (eating disorders) [16], with a much lesser degree of mental disorders and cognitive impairment but even more easily altered thinking and conduct [4]. However, it is important to remain vigilant, as eating disorders can often assume different forms that are not always simple to identify. The first step should always be to consult a doctor and a therapist [13,16,21,22]. The characteristics and attitudes mentioned above can have a very strong influence on the patient's disturbed perception of reality and increased sensitivity to stressors [14,16,17,23,24]. In addition, the inability to modify cognitive patterns, engage in appropriate activities, and reduce stress can increase tension and anxiety. It was also underscored that individual susceptibility to stress is important [14,23], and FHA is most likely to increase through natural means. Some studies suggest that this sensitivity may be genetic [16]. It would be interesting to determine if there is a phenotype forming a system of neurotransmitters that lead to FHA [13,14,16].

In addition, scientific reports show that women's exposure to stress during the prenatal period significantly affects the unborn child and results in increased sensitivity to the HPA axis. Early childhood experiences have similar effects [14,16]. In combination with education, predisposition can significantly contribute to shaping irregular attitudes and problems in life. In addition to cognitive dysfunctions, the stress related to everyday life and an inability to deal with that stress, abnormal sleep patterns, excessive physical activity, and a scarcity of energy from nutrients combine to form a "snowball" mechanism and enhanced reactivity [14,17,18,23,25,26].

Thus, on the one hand, the above characteristics are common in FHA. On the other hand, an imbalance of neurotransmitters, the overstimulation of the HPA axis, elevated cortisol levels, thyroid suppression, and reduced estrogen levels result in an increased occurrence of depressive states and strengthen the characteristics of the disorder [9,25,26].

A similar mechanism affects sleep. Excessive excitation of the sympathetic nervous system, chronic stress, anxiety, and tension are all conducive to sleeping disorders. Moreover, the lack of optimal quantitative and qualitative regeneration at night according to circadian rhythms has numerous health implications, both physical and mental. These implications have a strong negative impact on the whole endocrine economy, especially cortisol and leptin. In addition, a lack of adequate regeneration increases the risk of depression and contributes to greater irritability, deterioration, and decreases in cognitive function and efficient responses. A lack of adequate regeneration also weakens resilience to stress and available psycho-energy resources, thereby making a smaller stimulus produce a much greater effect [27,28].

2.2. Nutrition

In a situation of energy scarcity, the body minimizes its energy expenditures by curtailing less-important functions that are not essential for survival, such as menstruation. Survival becomes the overriding goal in increasing the activation of the sympathetic nervous system during a crisis. The menstrual cycle is an energy-intensive process. After pregnancy, lactation increases the expenditures even more. Caring for two organisms simultaneously then becomes impossible due to a lack of energy, components, and resources for the mother herself. The brain interprets energy scarcity and stress as adverse environmental conditions for the birth of the offspring. All these factors impede reproductive functions and offer protection for the body of the woman and her child. In the literature, this state is described as a reproductive compromise [6–8,18,29,30].

A well-known important determinant for FHA development is low energy availability. This issue is due to a lack of adaptation to the needs of food consumption and/or increased energy expenditures linked to physical activity. Both components frequently occur together. Regardless of the substrate, this condition generates a deficit of energy that translates into metabolic stress on the body. Nutrient deficiencies can be an additional aggravating factor (including of basic macronutrients, minerals, and vitamins) [5,15,20,31–33].

Energy is defined as the energy pool that remains for the body to use to maintain homeostasis, proper functioning, and optimal health. Energy availability (EA) is calculated based on the quantity of calories supplied with the diet after deducting the energy expenditures associated with the training divided by the non-fatty mass of the body [6,8,19,30].

Formula: EA = energy supplied from diet (kcal) − energy expenditure during training (kcal)/non-fat body weight (kg). (1)

This is the most widely cited pattern in the FHA literature alongside low energy availability. Because of its simplicity, this pattern is practical to enumerate [6,30,34]. Unlike classic energy balance, where the measurement is estimated for the total weight of the body, for the EA model in this template, the value of energy is determined in relation to the non-fat body weight. This type of body mass is significantly more active and generates a higher energy cost [35]. In addition, lean body mass (LBM) is generally higher in active individuals, suggesting that this parameter is more accurate. However, this parameter cannot be regarded as universally precise, reliable, or adequate. The estimated demand requires confirming other patterns and assessing the practical applications for each patient. Regardless of the formula used, the calculation of energy consumption expenditures and daily activity alongside controlling food intake under standard conditions may be a mistake and cause a great deal of difficulties [5,36]. Such measures must be taken with a high degree of caution in planning and monitoring [30,32,33].

A 2003 study suggested a threshold of 30 kcal/kg to initiate the disorder [37]. However, in subsequent studies, irregularities were observed in broad ranges, even above the threshold of 30 kcal/kg LBM. Some scientists also observed functional disturbances even when the declared EA was at an optimum level. However, changes in macronutrient consumption and other variables that could contribute to latent low energy availability (LEA) were also recognized [20,38]. However, it was not certain that the patient's reported measurements were correct. Ultimately, with an increase in the deficit, the severity of health consequences also increases [12,30]. Undoubtedly, low energy availability is associated with a serious threat to the organism, which is significant for reproduction functions (Figures 2 and 3) [7,8,19,32].

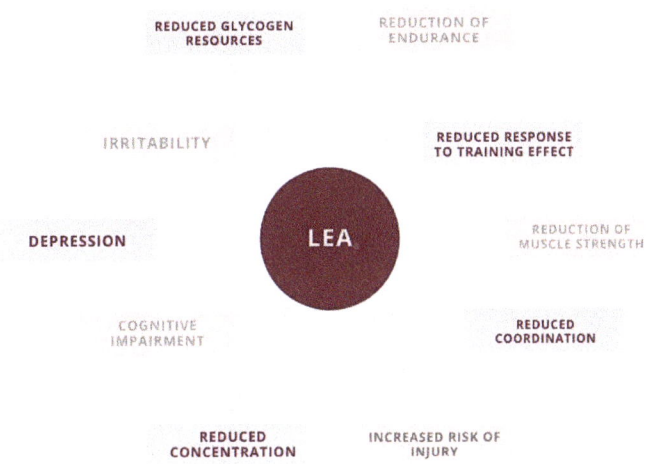

Figure 2. Psychological and physiological implications of low energy availability (LEA).

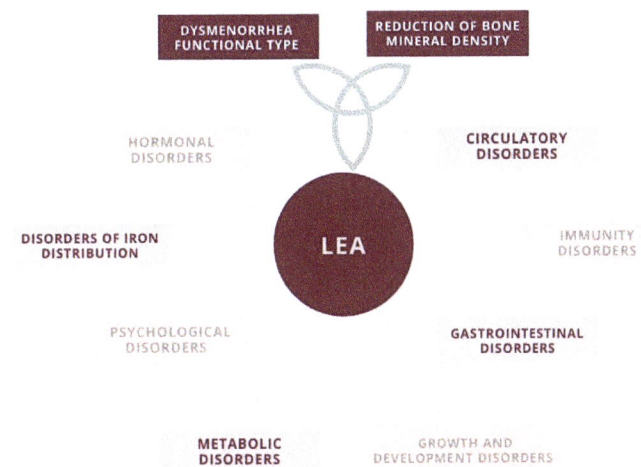

Figure 3. Low energy availability (LEA) and implications in a female athlete triad, including the functional type of dysmenorrhea and a reduction in bone mineral density.

It is presently difficult to estimate the exact energy limits that could contribute to menstrual disorders. This is likely due to a number of factors contributing to energy expenditure and consumption. Each patient's individual sensitivity, which has been consistently emphasized by researchers, also plays a key role [14,18,29,30].

However, there are certain thresholds in the literature that can be used as indicators for measurements. Low EA is determined as $\leq$ 30 kcal (125 kJ)/1 kg Fat Free Mass (FFM) per day. This value is similar to the basal metabolic rate [6,30]. The reduced energy availability risk shall be expressed in the range of 30–45 kcal (125–188 kJ)/1 kg FFM per day. This range is considered to entail a risk of reduced energy availability and is thus recommended only for a short time to reduce body fat. The correct EA is defined as $\geq$ 45 kcal (188 kJ)/1 kg FFM per day. Previous studies noted that this formula provides a ceiling close to "zero" for the energy balance [30,32]. In the event of pre-existing disorders, this value is likely to be necessary to restore lost menstruation and ovulation. The amount of energy spent on scheduled physical activity should also be added to this scheme [6,8].

LEA plays a significant role in the food consumption of FHA women and seems to impact not only the amount of energy delivered but also the distribution of individual macronutrients [5,32]. A lower intake of fat and carbohydrates was recognized in studies monitoring food intake among the sample group [20,39]. Easily digestible carbohydrates are easily accessible, and the supply of dietary fiber and low energy density products is generally high [20]. While the amount of protein supplied is debatable, the protein quantity usually falls within the upper limit of the standard or is even above [20,31–33]. These conclusions indicate the specific and interesting features of eating habits. On the one hand, these habits may result from modern trends in nutrition that do not necessarily coincide with the principles of proper nutrition. On the other hand, some diets correlate with eating disorders or abnormal attitudes. It is also possible to lack sufficient knowledge and mistakenly believe that the consumption of a diet with more fiber, protein, and food with low energy density is beneficial to the health of a physically active person. Each macronutrient has an individualized role in the body, which is also crucial in the context of menstrual function and energy availability. Some studies suggest that an increased participation of dietary fiber and dietary protein could contribute to a widening energy deficit despite the delivery of an optimal amount of energy [20]. Considering the characteristics of both components, fiber and protein, the influence between the two may be multidirectional. It is important for one to ensure an optimal supply of fat and carbohydrates in the diet to support the endocrine system.

Studies increasingly highlight the importance of the continuous availability of readily oxidized fuels [6,21,30,38]. The justification for such fuels is, above all, the sensitivity of LH pulsation to glycogen resources. A previous study noted that short-term deficits in women potentially not at risk affected the luteal phase, which is one of the first symptoms of menstrual abnormalities [12]. Another important nutritional factor is ensuring an appropriate amount of carbohydrates in the diet, as carbohydrates are the primary and fastest energy source for an organism and thus an indicator of energy balance [20]. A low supply of carbohydrates is correlated with the depletion of glycogen, leading to glycogen depletion [38].

Fat, which is a basic feedstock for steroid hormone synthesis, tends to be an insignificant component in the diets of women with menstrual disorders. At the same time, fat intake appears to be essential to ensure that omega-family fatty acids are present in the appropriate concentrations to reduce inflammation in the body [18,22]. For women with FHA, it is worth highlighting the role of omega-3 fatty acids in reducing inflammation associated with a spectrum of interactions [18,22,40]. There are indications that these fatty acids may improve menstrual-cycle-related ailments, as well as fertility [41,42]. Omega-3 fatty acids have also been shown to reduce perceived stress and anxiety in PMS and menopause, which are both states in which the amount of sex hormones is low, as in FHA [41]. Previous research also suggested that omega-3 fatty acids can support the prevention of depression and exert beneficial effects on the cardiovascular system and lipid regulation [40,43,44]—All of which could be affected to a large extent in the women in the sample group [1,9,45].

Studies have also suggested that not only the total amount of calories delivered but also the caloric distribution throughout the day is important for normal hormone pulsation [6], in order to avoid periods of deficiency, which can be translated into hourly deficits in energy availability. These values were correlated with higher cortisol levels and lower levels of T3 and sex hormones [38,46], particularly during the training period, which could significantly increase the exhaustion of resources [6]. The regular distribution of meals during the day and the avoidance of periods of hunger are basic tasks in diet planning.

Apart from the supply of energy and macronutrients, dietary micronutrients and vitamins play an important role in FHA. Vitamin D3 is a significantly deficient component in the general population and is difficult to supplement with one's daily diet [47]. This disorder is exacerbated among the group of women at risk of FHA [9,45,47]. Vitamin D3 has many functions in the body and is one of the key factors involved in the body's skeletal economy. Bone mineral density is extremely sensitive to functional endocrine disruptors [1,9,22]. In addition, there is evidence that bone mineral density can have a positive impact on mood and cognitive function, countering depression, which may provide considerable support for the target group of women [48]. Vitamin D3 may reduce inflammation and hepcidin levels, thereby increasing the absorption of iron [49]. Some studies have suggested that vitamin D deficiency may be associated with impaired fertility, but more evidence is needed. In addition, a correlation was observed between the loss of this component, lengthening of the follicular phase, and reduction of the luteal phase [50].

Calcium has many important functions in the body and is one of the key players in the context of bone mineral density [1,51]. Bone-related disorders are significantly more prevalent in this population of women [9,45,49].

Magnesium has been well-studied in the context of stress, anxiety disorders, and depression [47,51], which are often observed in women with FHA. In the case of magnesium, a vicious cycle was observed [52]. There is evidence that, in response to acute and chronic stress, magnesium resources are depleted, and the urinary output of magnesium is increased. Stressors may have a variety of backgrounds, both psychological and environmental. Sleep deprivation and intense physical exertion are also important [51,52], as is a lack of energy. Lack of energy is the main reason for increases in nutrient deficits. However, a scarcity of magnesium can amplify the symptoms of and susceptibility to both stress and depression [52]. In addition, magnesium performs many important functions in the body and is a co-factor in over 300 enzymatic reactions [52]. There are also reports that magnesium can improve the metabolism of vitamin D3 [53].

Monthly bleeding is not present, or is very rare and mild, in the studied group of women. Thus, such women do not experience increased monthly losses of iron resources. Nevertheless, deficits of iron [22,54] can be observed as the first factor, possibly due to insufficient consumption of iron in the diet and/or the presence of ingredients that limit the absorption of this element, such as excess fiber and phytic acid [17.56]. The second most important factor is increased physical activity, particularly in endurance tests [49]. The third factor is an inflammatory state that contributes to the production of hepcidin, a hormone that blocks the absorption of iron from the gastrointestinal tract. In addition, a deficiency of this element can significantly increase apathy and mood swings and decrease lactation [49].

Folate appears to be an essential component in the normal development and preparation of pregnancy. However, regardless of whether fertilization is a desirable outcome, this nutrient should be adequately supplied in the diet. There are some indications that folates can have a beneficial effect on menstrual cycle regulation and ovulation [41,55,56]. It was suggested that this phenomenon may be related to homocysteine [41,55]. Folate deficiency can contribute to the hypomethylation of DNA and oxidative stress [55]. Previous studies suggested that, in the case of mutations in the MTHR C677T gene and T-allele carriers associated with lower enzyme activity, a lower sensitivity of oocytes to the FSH hormone, reduced oocytes, and reduced estradiol production by granular cells compared to the case with vectors of the wild-type gene can occur [41,56,57]. In addition, folates can support vascular endothelial functions. Women with FHA commonly present folate dysfunctions [1,6,9,19,56].

It was long thought that the most critical factor in FHA development was insufficient body weight. However, the most important diagnostic parameter appears, instead, to be the composition of the body, specifically, fatty tissue content [5,15,31,58]. In athletes, it is recognized that, as a result of the development of greater-than-average muscle mass, the weight of the body can oscillate beyond the normal ranges. However, the athlete's fat levels may be below the recommended minimum. The determination of clear standards is highly debatable and depends on individual factors [15]. However, if the above parameters and BMI are below the recommended standard, they must necessarily be restored to normal values [7,15,22,59]. It is commonly acknowledged that functional disorders can occur in those with broad ranges of both body weight and fat content, even when these parameters are correct and do not change over the years [1,4–6,29,32]. In addition, markers indicating low energy availability are also recognized in these women. Elevated levels of cortisol and ghrelin have been observed alongside reduced levels of sex hormones, T3, glucose, insulin, and leptin [5]. In many cases, the resting metabolic rate is also reduced. As a result of metabolic adaptation, the organism must minimize its expenditures and adapt [19,30,32,60]. Additional factors include psychosocial stress and physical activity, which can exacerbate stress on the body and impede reproduction [4,10,15].

2.3. Physical Activity

The greatest threat to FHA comes from forms of physical exercise in which aesthetics and the weight of the body play an important role, e.g., bodybuilding, dance, and gymnastics [6,15,19,22]. FHA is also common among amateurs [33,61–63], and women are becoming increasingly involved in physical activities. Unfortunately, without proper preparation, adaptation, and knowledge and the supervision of a specialist, there may be many risks.

In recent years, in the pathogenesis of functional menstruation disorders, sport has been primarily considered for inducing significant energy expenditures and compensating for energy consumption—sometimes due to ignorance and errors in the estimation of the exact components of the activity and sometimes due to an intentional, incorrectly designed, and prolonged fat-reduction program. Such issues may also be caused by the deliberate maintenance of a significant energy deficit, exacerbated by the stress of eating disorders or dysfunctional attitudes in these areas. An open and intriguing question is whether physical effort alone can result in hormonal deregulation. Most research discusses the generation of deficits. However, the fact that training itself is a stressor for the organism's body should not be overlooked [2,59]. A systematic review considering the impacts of activity on ovulation noted that high-intensity activity affects the functioning of the reproductive system, particularly when one's BMI is below the norm but also when the BMI is within a suitable range. Many mechanisms could be involved in this relationship [59]. Another study noted the inhibitory effect of exercise on sexual hormone concentrations. Interestingly, this effect was not dependent on energy availability. Attention has also been paid to the need to modify training volume [30].

Physical activity is often considered an excellent way to relieve tension and improve one's mood. Unfortunately, for women with FHA, exercise could worsen their condition. Previous studies noted that, in response to a stress challenge, there is a significant increase in cortisol and a decrease in blood glucose compared to in healthy women [14,17,23,29]. This may indicate the significant depletion of energy resources and a mechanism to promote the organism's mobilization to obtain such resources. This is an intriguing area of study, highlighting the need to consider the sensitivity of FHA women in relation to sporting activities.

Compulsive and physical dependence may also be problematic. These factors may lead to a situation where a person's brain chemistry demands an increase in training load and frequency [13], despite that load being greater than what the individual can handle and/or inappropriate for particular circumstances [2,34,64–66]. This may lead to the phenomenon of over-training and related aberrations, and addiction and compulsion may lead to self-destruction in the mental, physical, and social fields. The characteristics and attitudes of FHA women were found to significantly increase dysfunction [8,34].

It should be noted that training alone is a stressor for an individual. Training stimulates the sympathetic nervous system and increases metabolic stress [2,29,37,58,59,67,68]. Training is often desirable for the development of an athlete. Regular physical activity is essential for staying healthy. The optimal dose and individual adjustment of the training parameters are crucial (they should be appropriate for the situation of the person undergoing training).

Stress and physical effort, in many cases, exacerbate the scarcity of resources and lead to an increase in demand. For amateurs, physical activity is only a supplementary part of life. Such individuals are burdened with many stressors resulting from everyday life, work, and school. Consequently, all components should co-exist, including a training plan, regeneration, and sleep; a diet that takes into account the consumption of not only a sufficient number of calories and macronutrients but also vitamins and minerals; and proper hydration.

3. Actionable Steps for Restoring Balance

Functional menstruation disorders can be characterized as psychosomatic diseases. Considering all the components, in many cases, it is necessary to simultaneously include multidirectional activities for each aspect so that changes can be smoothly implemented and to avoid prolonging the pathological state of the body [17]. Previous studies indicate that the longer the body's decline persists, the longer the time needed to recover, and the more severe the consequences. Hence, time plays a significant role [22,54].

The first step should always be to consult an endocrine gynecologist and obtain a thorough diagnosis to exclude other diseases and control the current state of the body [1,2,69].

A detailed review of the patient's diet, physical activity, feelings of stress, sleep, attitudes towards nutrition, and psychological profile is also crucial. Attention should be paid to whether the patient presents typical features of FHA and if an eating disorder is present. Sufficient data can help to locate the main cause of the problem, and primary causes the most destructive should be addressed first [1,23,24]. Endocrinological guidelines strongly recommend focusing on solving the behavioral issues that contributed to the problem. However, pharmacology is not recommended for first-line treatment because it only masks the return of natural menstruation due to ongoing or worsening undernourishment and exposure to stress [68]. In addition, hormone replacement therapy (HRT) does not affect the functioning of other hormones or improve bone mineral density if the dysfunctional condition is maintained [1,3,15,22].

Firstly, the nutritional status and eating habits of the individual should be assessed. In the vast majority of cases, an increase in energy consumption to the recommended value of 45 kcal/1 kg LBM supplies the amount of energy spent on training activities. The continuous observation of the patient's response, however, remains important. The relevant calculations only provide an estimate, so they are not always entirely accurate [6,8,30,32]. In a study using a 360-kcal energy preparation without changes in sports activity for a period of six months, menstruation with ovulation was observed [39,70]. This study also observed a minimal increase 1.6 kg of body weight, which was adequate given the calories of the products used [39,70]. Another study used a 3-month intervention to increase energy supply and improve eating habits. As a result, 234 kcal of energy was generated, accompanied by an increase in the supply of macronutrients, vitamins, and minerals. Regular menstruation did not resume. However, increase of LH level and increase FSH to LH ratio level was observed and positively correlated with EA [61]. These parameters provide a promising indication of a gradual recovery in the balance and correct functions of the organism. The authors in [54] described cases of two different women who were physically active and had appropriate body weight and body-fat content. In response to an increase in energy availability, improvements in nutritional status markers (increases in T3 and leptin and a decrease in ghrelin) and the resumption of menstruation were noted. In both cases, however, the observed menstruation featured anovulatory cycles with the luteal phase. In addition, a re-stop was observed in the event of a drop in energy availability. Importantly, no target energy level was reached throughout the intervention. Consequently, the imposition of other factors and the lack of consistency could have contributed to the continuation of the problems of FHA [54].

Studies suggest that more attention should also be paid to the redistribution of energy over 24 h to avoid a latent deficit [38,46]. Dietary programming during the training period is particularly important. The regularity of one's meals and a regular distribution according to one's needs also appear to be beneficial. Too large of a gap between meals leads to significant drops in glucose; thus, fasting or intermittent fasting is not advisable. Based on studies analyzing the dietary habits of FHA women and their impact on the physiology and biochemistry of the organism, a key activity seems to be to ensure the balanced participation of macro components according to the recommended standards individually adapted to the patient's situation [22].

Minerals and vitamins also play an important role. Special attention in the literature is given to vitamin D3 and calcium [1,22]. Studies also suggest the possibility of shortages of magnesium, zinc, iron, and folic acid; vitamins A, E, K, and C; and certain B vitamins [1,20,31,33]. The best solution is to address this shortage through one's diet. It is, therefore, important to use high-nutrient-potential foods [22].

In the event of significant deficits or difficulties in meeting one's dietary needs, targeted supplementation needs to be considered. In the study group, deficits in vitamins and minerals were a serious problem. On the one hand, excess stress, physical activity, and associated inflammation lead to increased expenditures of, and demands for, nutrients [51]. Moreover, low energy availability can impair basic metabolism, which in itself can exacerbate deficits [22]. In addition, an excess supply of dietary fiber can make it difficult to absorb certain nutrients [20], and an insufficiency of nutrient resources exerts metabolic stress on the organism and may hinder basic life processes [22,47,51]. Additionally, stress may negatively affect digestive enzymes and gut microbiota, which may result in the abnormal uptake of nutrients from the intake of food and/or their endogenous production [51].

Vitamin D3 is essential for the proper functioning of an organism but is difficult to acquire through food. It is thus recommended to include vitamin D3 supplements in one's diet [48]. The dose should be selected following a previous examination of the blood concentration and tailored to each person's individual needs. Another source of vitamin D3 is exposure to sunlight [48]. The concentration of calcium in the blood must be continuously monitored, and densitometry should also be performed in clinical settings [1]. The calcium availability in a patient's diet should not be a problem, especially if the patient consumes dairy products. In addition, vitamin D3 supplementation should be considered to allow for a more efficient use of this element by the skeletal system [49]. Magnesium should also be easy to acquire through one's diet. However, in the event of a magnesium deficit, it is worth considering supplementation. In particular, magnesium supplementation appears to be beneficial for women with menstrual disorders, not only those with functional disorders [71]. An adequate supply of magnesium can have a positive effect on a person's mood, facilitate adaptation to stressful conditions, and reduce irritability. In addition, magnesium can benefit the initiation and quality of sleep [52]. In a previous study, exposure to severe mental and physical stressors, acute chronic stress, and physical effort were correlated with lower levels of zinc in the serum and plasma; zinc was also observed to have positive effects on the efficacy of antidepressants and lower cortisol levels [51]. Another intriguing observation was a reduction in inflammation and oxidative stress [72]. Iron supplementation can have a number of negative effects on one's health. For example, excess iron can lower the concentration of leptin. The best solution seems to be an extended diagnosis and to address the shortage through one's diet as far as possible. Supplementation should be used as a last resort and only under the ongoing supervision of a doctor. The best solution for securing a supply of folic acid appears to be its consumption within one's diet because the folic acid in food products occurs in a methylated form. In the case of mutations such as those of the MTHFR C677T gene, synthetic folic acid supplementation is not effective. In this case, it is worth considering folic acid's methylated form. Other factors involved in methylation should also be considered, such as vitamins B2, B6, and B12 and zinc [41,55]. Any decision should be made after consultation with a specialist and introduced on a case-by-case basis. The omega-3 fatty acids mentioned in the previous section play an important role in the functions of the body and have beneficial effects [40]. Determining the appropriate supply for one's daily diet and the optimal balance between omega-3 and omega-6 fatty acids could, however, pose a significant challenge. The concentrations of individual omega-3 acids are also a key factor [40,43].

Only a few vitamins and minerals have been mentioned in this article. It is important to stress that each of the aforementioned nutrients is needed for the proper functioning of an organism, especially in the case of significant loads. B vitamins, especially folic acid, and antioxidants should not be neglected. To a large extent, the demand for nutrients allows a well-balanced diet to be achieved. It would also be beneficial to include recreational food in the diets of women with FHA (i.e., foods that are slightly more processed and have a higher energy density). Firstly, these foods will increase the quantity of calories delivered in a relatively simple way. Secondly, they could positively influence the psyches and satisfy the needs of FHA women. These measures would contribute to easing tension and preventing the use of drugs. The removal of such nutritional restrictions would help to improve nutritional relationships, encourage good eating habits, and facilitate healthy functioning [20].

A major factor to consider is the reduction of stressors. Physical activity, despite its many advantages, is one of these stressors. For women with FHA and malnutrition, its effect is compounded [14,23,29,58]. The issue of functional menstruation disorders is, moreover, common among athletes. Hence, a number of studies have focused on the above group. These researchers focused on using non-volatile training parameters. However, the modifications of those parameters were subject to energy consumption, and interventions produced varying results (also positive). This has led to the belief that physical activity can remain at a similar level over the long term. However, it is not appropriate to compare professionally trained trainers to amateurs with fewer training pressures, which could introduce further modifications. It is certainly not appropriate to generalize measures for applications requiring training units and the development of peak sport performance. Moreover, recreational athletes do not always have a professional training plan adapted to their current capabilities that reasonably accounts for the necessary regeneration periods. Studies suggest that excessive physical activity can occur among FHA women, which may be caused by eating disorders or other dysfunctions [13,34].

The complete avoidance of planned activities without the agreement of the patient does not appear to be an optimal solution. The avoidance of such activities may be stressful and generate anxiety when the sport is a daily routine, especially when it is related to eating disorders, compulsion, and/or addiction. In the above situation, it is important not to drive and support destructive behavior. On the other hand, it is worth considering modifications based on a compromise with the patient and coming to an agreement with solutions that are safe for that particular context. To minimize health risks, it should also be ensured that regeneration and nutritional status are maximized. Research further suggests the need to alter the training variables, such as by a reduction in the volume and intensity of the training [30,59]. It would also be beneficial to reduce the training frequency and introduce longer regeneration times, e.g., every other day. The types of training could also be altered. For example, yoga and related outdoor activities have a high potential to improve mental and physical health and do not generate increased excitability of the sympathetic nervous system; instead, they may have the opposite effect. However, resistance may be caused by patients' anxiety in response to changing their exercise patterns, increasing their energy, and reducing their training parameters [6]. It is very important that experts make the patient aware of these issues. Patients should also work with a psychotherapist to reduce the relevant barriers and improve their psychological states [1,13,17,22]. Interventional studies on the use of psychotherapy in the treatment of FHA are already sufficient. The studies to date suggest including both cognitive and behavioral therapy due to promising results indicating the resumption of menstrual function with ovulation, increased leptin and T3 concentrations, and a decrease in ghrelin and cortisol levels [18,23,24]. Body weight also did not change, which is an additional positive aspect [18,23,24]. More research needs to be conducted in this area. However, given the low risk of undesirable activities, the pathogenesis of the problem, the characteristics of the group, and the benefits already examined, therapy appears to be an important element of recovery. This measure is not only likely to contribute to the correction of dysfunctional attitudes and thoughts but can also enable stress to be properly handled and diminished. In addition, nutrition and physical activity can be extremely beneficial. Ultimately, the benefits of psychotherapy seem to be significant in both psychosocial and physical terms [14,16–18,23,24].

4. Conclusions

Considering the overall pathogenesis of FHA, the most sensible approach is to combine improved nutritional status with physical activity and psychotherapy and work on daily stress. A broad range of relaxation techniques can complement these measures [14]. In addition, it is important to ensure that a patient obtains a good quality and quantity of sleep [27]. It is always important to bear in mind the individual sensitivity of the patient and maintain observations.

It is important to continuously and consistently maintain the initiated changes. The present study demonstrates that, the longer the time of decay, the more the time needed to regulate that decay. Changes, such as body weight reductions, are not recommended for 6 to 12 months after standardization. In addition, latent irregularities, such as a lack of ovulation and an abridged luteal phase, should also be prevented. This study indicates that the stressors occurring during the first phase of the cycle influence the delay of ovulation, leading to luteal dysfunction [30]. It is also important to ensure the continuous observation of the patient and a sensible approach both during and outside the recovery and maintenance period. Moreover, the individualization of interventions is crucial, and an interdisciplinary approach seems to be the best solution for promoting a promising prognosis.

Author Contributions: K.R., P.Z. and A.K. wrote the manuscript. All authors have read and agreed to the published version of the manuscript.

Funding: This research received no external funding.

Institutional Review Board Statement: Not applicable.

Informed Consent Statement: Not applicable.

Data Availability Statement: Not applicable.

Conflicts of Interest: The authors declare no conflict of interest.

References

1. Gordon, C.M.; Ackerman, K.E.; Berga, S.L.; Kaplan, J.R.; Mastorakos, G.; Misra, M.; Murad, M.H.; Santoro, N.F.; Warren, M.P. Functional Hypothalamic Amenorrhea: An Endocrine Society Clinical Practice Guideline. *J. Clin. Endocrinol. Metab.* **2017**, *102*, 1413–1439. [CrossRef]
2. Lania, A.; Gianotti, L.; Gagliardi, I.; Bondanelli, M.; Vena, W.; Ambrosio, M.R. Functional Hypothalamic and Drug-Induced Amenorrhea: An Overview. *J. Endocrinol. Investig.* **2019**, *42*, 1001–1010. [CrossRef]

3. Sowińska-Przepiera, E.; Andrysiak-Mamos, E.; Jarząbek-Bielecka, G.; Walkowiak, A.; Osowicz-Korolonek, L.; Syrenicz, M.; Kędzia, W.; Syrenicz, A. Functional Hypothalamic Amenorrhoea–Diagnostic Challenges, Monitoring, and Treatment. *Endokrynol. Pol.* **2015**, *66*, 252–268. [CrossRef] [PubMed]
4. Sophie Gibson, M.E.; Fleming, N.; Zuijdwijk, C.; Dumont, T. Where Have the Periods Gone? The Evaluation and Management of Functional Hypothalamic Amenorrhea. *J. Clin. Res. Pediatr. Endocrinol.* **2020**, *12*, 18–27. [CrossRef]
5. Kyriakidis, M.; Caetano, L.; Anastasiadou, N.; Karasu, T.; Lashen, H. Functional Hypothalamic Amenorrhoea: Leptin Treatment, Dietary Intervention and Counselling as Alternatives to Traditional Practice-Systematic Review. *Eur. J. Obstet. Gynecol. Reprod. Biol.* **2016**, *198*, 131–137. [CrossRef] [PubMed]
6. De Souza, M.J.; Koltun, K.J.; Etter, C.V.; Southmayd, E.A. Current Status of the Female Athlete Triad: Update and Future Directions. *Curr. Osteoporos. Rep.* **2017**, *15*, 577–587. [CrossRef] [PubMed]
7. The Physiology of Functional Hypothalamic Amenorrhea Associated with Energy Deficiency in Exercising Women and in Women with Anorexia Nervosa. -PubMed-NCBI. Available online: https://www.ncbi.nlm.nih.gov/pubmed/26953710 (accessed on 11 May 2019).
8. Elliott-Sale, K.J.; Tenforde, A.S.; Parziale, A.L.; Holtzman, B.; Ackerman, K.E. Endocrine Effects of Relative Energy Deficiency in Sport. *Int. J. Sport Nutr. Exerc. Metab.* **2018**, *28*, 335–349. [CrossRef] [PubMed]
9. Meczekalski, B.; Katulski, K.; Czyzyk, A.; Podfigurna-Stopa, A.; Maciejewska-Jeske, M. Functional Hypothalamic Amenorrhea and Its Influence on Women's Health. *J. Endocrinol. Investig.* **2014**, *37*, 1049–1056. [CrossRef] [PubMed]
10. Podfigurna, A.; Maciejewska-Jeske, M.; Meczekalski, B.; Genazzani, A.D. Kisspeptin and LH pulsatility in patients with functional hypothalamic amenorrhea. *Endocrine* **2020**, *70*, 635–643. [CrossRef]
11. Iwasa, T.; Matsuzaki, T.; Yano, K.; Mayila, Y.; Irahara, M. The roles of kisspeptin and gonadotropin inhibitory hormone in stress-induced reproductive disorders. *Endocr. J.* **2018**, *65*, 133–140. [CrossRef]
12. Williams, N.I.; Leidy, H.J.; Hill, B.R.; Lieberman, J.L.; Legro, R.S.; De Souza, M.J. Magnitude of Daily Energy Deficit Predicts Frequency but Not Severity of Menstrual Disturbances Associated with Exercise and Caloric Restriction. *Am. J. Physiol. Endocrinol. Metab.* **2015**, *308*, E29–E39. [CrossRef] [PubMed]
13. Tranoulis, A.; Soldatou, A.; Georgiou, D.; Mavrogianni, D.; Loutradis, D.; Michala, L. Adolescents and Young Women with Functional Hypothalamic Amenorrhoea: Is It Time to Move beyond the Hormonal Profile? *Arch. Gynecol. Obstet.* **2020**, *301*, 1095–1101. [CrossRef] [PubMed]
14. Pauli, S.A.; Berga, S.L. Athletic Amenorrhea: Energy Deficit or Psychogenic Challenge? *Ann. N. Y. Acad. Sci.* **2010**, *1205*, 33–38. [CrossRef]
15. Roberts, R.E.; Farahani, L.; Webber, L.; Jayasena, C. Current Understanding of Hypothalamic Amenorrhoea. *Ther. Adv. Endocrinol.* **2020**, *11*. [CrossRef] [PubMed]
16. Bomba, M.; Corbetta, F.; Bonini, L.; Gambera, A.; Tremolizzo, L.; Neri, F.; Nacinovich, R. Psychopathological Traits of Adolescents with Functional Hypothalamic Amenorrhea: A Comparison with Anorexia Nervosa. *Eat. Weight. Disord.* **2014**, *19*, 41–48. [CrossRef] [PubMed]
17. Berga, S.L.; Marcus, M.D.; Loucks, T.L.; Hlastala, S.; Ringham, R.; Krohn, M.A. Recovery of Ovarian Activity in Women with Functional Hypothalamic Amenorrhea Who Were Treated with Cognitive Behavior Therapy. *Fertil. Steril.* **2003**, *80*, 976–981. [CrossRef]
18. Neuroprotection via Reduction in Stress: Altered Menstrual Patterns as a Marker for Stress and Implications for Long-Term Neurologic Health in Women. Available online: https://www.ncbi.nlm.nih.gov/pmc/articles/PMC5187947/ (accessed on 31 January 2020).
19. Mountjoy, M.; Sundgot-Borgen, J.K.; Burke, L.M.; Ackerman, K.E.; Blauwet, C.; Constantini, N.; Lebrun, C.; Lundy, B.; Melin, A.K.; Meyer, N.L.; et al. IOC Consensus Statement on Relative Energy Deficiency in Sport (RED-S): 2018 Update. *Br. J. Sports Med.* **2018**, *52*, 687–697. [CrossRef] [PubMed]
20. Melin, A.; Tornberg, Å.B.; Skouby, S.; Møller, S.S.; Faber, J.; Sundgot-Borgen, J.; Sjödin, A. Low-Energy Density and High Fiber Intake Are Dietary Concerns in Female Endurance Athletes. *Scand. J. Med. Sci. Sports* **2016**, *26*, 1060–1071. [CrossRef]
21. Pentz, I.; Nakić Radoš, S. Functional Hypothalamic Amenorrhea and Its Psychological Correlates: A Controlled Comparison. *J. Reprod. Infant. Psychol.* **2017**, *35*, 137–149. [CrossRef]
22. Huhmann, K. Menses Requires Energy: A Review of How Disordered Eating, Excessive Exercise, and High Stress Lead to Menstrual Irregularities. *Clin. Ther.* **2020**, *42*, 401–407. [CrossRef]
23. Berga, S.L.; Loucks, T.L. Use of Cognitive Behavior Therapy for Functional Hypothalamic Amenorrhea. *Ann. N. Y. Acad. Sci.* **2006**, *1092*, 114–129. [CrossRef]
24. Michopoulos, V.; Mancini, F.; Loucks, T.L.; Berga, S.L. Neuroendocrine Recovery Initiated by Cognitive Behavioral Therapy in Women with Functional Hypothalamic Amenorrhea: A Randomized Controlled Trial. *Fertil. Steril.* **2013**, *99*, 2084–2091. [CrossRef]
25. Watrowski, R.; Rohde, A.; Maciejewska-Jeske, M.; Meczekalski, B. Hormonal and Psychosocial Correlates of Psychological Well-Being and Negative Affectivity in Young Gynecological-Endocrinological Patients. *Gynecol. Endocrinol.* **2016**, *32*, 21–24. [CrossRef]
26. Shufelt, C.L.; Torbati, T.; Dutra, E. Hypothalamic Amenorrhea and the Long-Term Health Consequences. *Semin. Reprod. Med.* **2017**, *35*, 256–262. [CrossRef]

27. Tranoulis, A.; Georgiou, D.; Soldatou, A.; Triantafyllidi, V.; Loutradis, D.; Michala, L. Poor Sleep and High Anxiety Levels in Women with Functional Hypothalamic Amenorrhoea: A Wake-up Call for Physicians? *Eur. J. Obstet. Gynecol. Reprod. Biol. X* **2019**, *3*, 100035. [CrossRef] [PubMed]
28. Smith, P.C.; Mong, J.A. Neuroendocrine Control of Sleep. *Neuroendocr. Regul. Behav.* **2019**, *43*, 353–378. [CrossRef]
29. Sanders, K.M.; Kawwass, J.F.; Loucks, T.; Berga, S.L. Heightened Cortisol Response to Exercise Challenge in Women with Functional Hypothalamic Amenorrhea. *Am. J. Obstet. Gynecol.* **2018**, *218*, 230.e1–230.e6. [CrossRef]
30. Lieberman, J.L.; De Souza, M.J.; Wagstaff, D.A.; Williams, N.I. Menstrual Disruption with Exercise Is Not Linked to an Energy Availability Threshold. *Med. Sci. Sports Exerc.* **2018**, *50*, 551–561. [CrossRef]
31. Moskvicheva, Y.B.; Gusev, D.V.; Tabeeva, G.I.; Chernukha, G.E. Evaluation of nutrition, body composition and features of dietetic counseling for patients with functional hypothalamic amenorrhea. *Vopr. Pitan.* **2018**, *87*, 85–91. [CrossRef] [PubMed]
32. Logue, D.; Madigan, S.M.; Delahunt, E.; Heinen, M.; Mc Donnell, S.-J.; Corish, C.A. Low Energy Availability in Athletes: A Review of Prevalence, Dietary Patterns, Physiological Health, and Sports Performance. *Sports Med.* **2018**, *48*, 73–96. [CrossRef] [PubMed]
33. Black, K.; Slater, J.; Brown, R.C.; Cooke, R. Low Energy Availability, Plasma Lipids, and Hormonal Profiles of Recreational Athletes. *J. Strength Cond. Res.* **2018**, *32*, 2816–2824. [CrossRef] [PubMed]
34. Logue, D.M.; Madigan, S.M.; Melin, A.; Delahunt, E.; Heinen, M.; Donnell, S.-J.M.; Corish, C.A. Low Energy Availability in Athletes 2020: An Updated Narrative Review of Prevalence, Risk, Within-Day Energy Balance, Knowledge, and Impact on Sports Performance. *Nutrients* **2020**, *12*, 835. [CrossRef] [PubMed]
35. Slater, J.; Brown, R.; McLay-Cooke, R.; Black, K. Low Energy Availability in Exercising Women: Historical Perspectives and Future Directions. *Sports Med.* **2017**, *47*, 207–220. [CrossRef]
36. Reed, J.L.; De Souza, M.J.; Mallinson, R.J.; Scheid, J.L.; Williams, N.I. Energy Availability Discriminates Clinical Menstrual Status in Exercising Women. *J. Int. Soc. Sports Nutr.* **2015**, *12*, 11. [CrossRef] [PubMed]
37. Loucks, A.B.; Thuma, J.R. Luteinizing Hormone Pulsatility Is Disrupted at a Threshold of Energy Availability in Regularly Menstruating Women. *J. Clin. Endocrinol. Metab.* **2003**, *88*, 297–311. [CrossRef]
38. Fahrenholtz, I.L.; Sjödin, A.; Benardot, D.; Tornberg, Å.B.; Skouby, S.; Faber, J.; Sundgot-Borgen, J.K.; Melin, A.K. Within-Day Energy Deficiency and Reproductive Function in Female Endurance Athletes. *Scand. J. Med. Sci. Sports* **2018**, *28*, 1139–1146. [CrossRef] [PubMed]
39. Cialdella-Kam, L.; Guebels, C.P.; Maddalozzo, G.F.; Manore, M.M. Dietary Intervention Restored Menses in Female Athletes with Exercise-Associated Menstrual Dysfunction with Limited Impact on Bone and Muscle Health. *Nutrients* **2014**, *6*, 3018–3039. [CrossRef]
40. Shahidi, F.; Ambigaipalan, P. Omega-3 Polyunsaturated Fatty Acids and Their Health Benefits. *Ann. Rev. Food Sci. Technol.* **2018**, *9*, 345–381. [CrossRef]
41. Gaskins, A.J.; Chavarro, J.E. Diet and Fertility: A Review. *Am. J. Obstet. Gynecol.* **2018**, *218*, 379–389. [CrossRef]
42. McCabe, D.; Lisy, K.; Lockwood, C.; Colbeck, M. The Impact of Essential Fatty Acid, B Vitamins, Vitamin C, Magnesium and Zinc Supplementation on Stress Levels in Women: A Systematic Review. *JBI Database Syst. Rev. Implement Rep.* **2017**, *15*, 402–453. [CrossRef]
43. Efficacy of Omega-3 PUFAs in Depression: A Meta-Analysis. Available online: https://www.ncbi.nlm.nih.gov/pmc/articles/PMC6683166/ (accessed on 29 January 2021).
44. Omega-3 Polyunsaturated Essential Fatty Acids Are Associated with Depression in Adolescents with Eating Disorders and Weight Loss-Swenne-2011-Acta Paediatrica-Wiley Online Library. Available online: https://onlinelibrary.wiley.com/doi/full/10.1111/j.1651-2227.2011.02400.x (accessed on 29 January 2021).
45. Ackerman, K.E.; Stellingwerff, T.; Elliott-Sale, K.J.; Baltzell, A.; Cain, M.; Goucher, K.; Fleshman, L.; Mountjoy, M.L. #REDS (Relative Energy Deficiency in Sport): Time for a Revolution in Sports Culture and Systems to Improve Athlete Health and Performance. *Br. J. Sports Med.* **2020**, *54*, 369–370. [CrossRef] [PubMed]
46. Torstveit, M.K.; Fahrenholtz, I.; Stenqvist, T.B.; Sylta, Ø.; Melin, A. Within-Day Energy Deficiency and Metabolic Perturbation in Male Endurance Athletes. *Int. J. Sport Nutr. Exerc. Metab.* **2018**, *28*, 419–427. [CrossRef]
47. Brook, E.M.; Tenforde, A.S.; Broad, E.M.; Matzkin, E.G.; Yang, H.Y.; Collins, J.E.; Blauwet, C.A. Low Energy Availability, Menstrual Dysfunction, and Impaired Bone Health: A Survey of Elite Para Athletes. *Scand. J. Med. Sci. Sports* **2019**, *29*, 678–685. [CrossRef]
48. Vitamin D and Depression: Mechanisms, Determination and Application-PubMed. Available online: https://pubmed.ncbi.nlm.nih.gov/31826364/ (accessed on 26 January 2021).
49. McClung, J.P.; Gaffney-Stomberg, E.; Lee, J.J. Female Athletes: A Population at Risk of Vitamin and Mineral Deficiencies Affecting Health and Performance. *J. Trace Elem. Med. Biol.* **2014**, *28*, 388–392. [CrossRef]
50. Jukic, A.M.Z.; Wilcox, A.J.; McConnaughey, D.R.; Weinberg, C.R.; Steiner, A.Z. 25-Hydroxyvitamin D and Long Menstrual Cycles in a Prospective Cohort Study. *Epidemiology* **2018**, *29*, 388–396. [CrossRef]
51. Lopresti, A.L. The Effects of Psychological and Environmental Stress on Micronutrient Concentrations in the Body: A Review of the Evidence. *Adv. Nutr.* **2020**, *11*, 103–112. [CrossRef]
52. Pickering, G.; Mazur, A.; Trousselard, M.; Bienkowski, P.; Yaltsewa, N.; Amessou, M.; Noah, L.; Pouteau, E. Magnesium Status and Stress: The Vicious Circle Concept Revisited. *Nutrients* **2020**, *12*, 3672. [CrossRef]
53. Uwitonze, A.M.; Razzaque, M.S. Role of Magnesium in Vitamin D Activation and Function. *J. Am. Osteopath Assoc.* **2018**, *118*, 181–189. [CrossRef] [PubMed]

54. Mallinson, R.J.; Williams, N.I.; Olmsted, M.P.; Scheid, J.L.; Riddle, E.S.; De Souza, M.J. A Case Report of Recovery of Menstrual Function Following a Nutritional Intervention in Two Exercising Women with Amenorrhea of Varying Duration. *J. Int. Soc. Sports Nutr.* **2013**, *10*, 34. [CrossRef] [PubMed]
55. Twigt, J.M.; Hammiche, F.; Sinclair, K.D.; Beckers, N.G.; Visser, J.A.; Lindemans, J.; de Jong, F.H.; Laven, J.S.E.; Steegers-Theunissen, R.P. Preconception Folic Acid Use Modulates Estradiol and Follicular Responses to Ovarian Stimulation. *J. Clin. Endocrinol. Metab.* **2011**, *96*, E322–E329. [CrossRef] [PubMed]
56. Hecht, S.; Pavlik, R.; Lohse, P.; Noss, U.; Friese, K.; Thaler, C.J. Common 677C→T Mutation of the 5,10-Methylenetetrahydrofolate Reductase Gene Affects Follicular Estradiol Synthesis. *Fertil. Steril.* **2009**, *91*, 56–61. [CrossRef]
57. Effects of the Common 677C>T Mutation of the 5,10-Methylenetetrahydrofolate Reductase (MTHFR) Gene on Ovarian Responsiveness to Recombinant Follicle-Stimulating Hormone-Thaler-2006-American Journal of Reproductive Immunology-Wiley Online Library. Available online: https://onlinelibrary.wiley.com/doi/full/10.1111/j.1600-0897.2005.00357.x?casa_token=MZyBomVJ6rYAAAAA%3AXnOYboJLVNm4GDbDT_2NiAFrXuKhz5IcmCZPciV4A4S3EODHdUisYCyjmA_onuOpoRbzQsPsnLiDXg (accessed on 28 January 2021).
58. Schaal, K.; Van Loan, M.D.; Casazza, G.A. Reduced Catecholamine Response to Exercise in Amenorrheic Athletes. *Med. Sci. Sports Exerc.* **2011**, *43*, 34–43. [CrossRef]
59. Hakimi, O.; Cameron, L.-C. Effect of Exercise on Ovulation: A Systematic Review. *Sports Med.* **2017**, *47*, 1555–1567. [CrossRef]
60. Koehler, K.; De Souza, M.J.; Williams, N.I. Less-than-Expected Weight Loss in Normal-Weight Women Undergoing Caloric Restriction and Exercise Is Accompanied by Preservation of Fat-Free Mass and Metabolic Adaptations. *Eur. J. Clin. Nutr.* **2017**, *71*, 365–371. [CrossRef] [PubMed]
61. Łagowska, K.; Kapczuk, K.; Friebe, Z.; Bajerska, J. Effects of Dietary Intervention in Young Female Athletes with Menstrual Disorders. *J. Int. Soc. Sports Nutr.* **2014**, *11*, 21. [CrossRef]
62. Slater, J.; McLay-Cooke, R.; Brown, R.; Black, K. Female Recreational Exercisers at Risk for Low Energy Availability. *Int. J. Sport Nutr. Exerc. Metab.* **2016**, *26*, 421–427. [CrossRef] [PubMed]
63. Logue, D.M.; Madigan, S.M.; Heinen, M.; McDonnell, S.-J.; Delahunt, E.; Corish, C.A. Screening for Risk of Low Energy Availability in Athletic and Recreationally Active Females in Ireland. *Eur. J. Sport Sci.* **2019**, *19*, 112–122. [CrossRef]
64. Egan, S.J.; Bodill, K.; Watson, H.J.; Valentine, E.; Shu, C.; Hagger, M.S. Compulsive Exercise as a Mediator between Clinical Perfectionism and Eating Pathology. *Eat. Behav.* **2017**, *24*, 11–16. [CrossRef] [PubMed]
65. Lichtenstein, M.B.; Hinze, C.J.; Emborg, B.; Thomsen, F.; Hemmingsen, S.D. Compulsive Exercise: Links, Risks and Challenges Faced. *Psychol. Res. Behav. Manag.* **2017**, *10*, 85–95. [CrossRef]
66. Turton, R.; Goodwin, H.; Meyer, C. Athletic Identity, Compulsive Exercise and Eating Psychopathology in Long-Distance Runners. *Eat. Behav.* **2017**, *26*, 129–132. [CrossRef] [PubMed]
67. Melin, A.K.; Ritz, C.; Faber, J.; Skouby, S.; Pingel, J.; Sundgot-Borgen, J.; Sjodin, A.; Tornberg, A. Impact of Menstrual Function on Hormonal Response to Repeated Bouts of Intense Exercise. *Front. Physiol.* **2019**, *10*, 942. [CrossRef] [PubMed]
68. Williams, N.; Berga, S.; Cameron, J. Synergism between psychosocial and metabolic stressors: Impact on reproductive function in cynomolgus monkeys. *Am. J. Physiol. Endocrinol. Metab.* **2007**, *293*, E270–E276. [CrossRef]
69. Nader, S. Functional Hypothalamic Amenorrhea: Case Presentations and Overview of Literature. *Hormones* **2019**, *18*, 49–54. [CrossRef]
70. Maddalozzo, G.F.; Guebels, C.P.; Kam, L.C.; Manore, M.M. Active Women before/after an Intervention Designed to Restore Menstrual Function: Resting Metabolic Rate and Comparison of Four Methods to Quantify Energy Expenditure and Energy Availability. *Int. J. Sport Nutr. Exerc. Metab.* **2014**, *24*, 37–46. [CrossRef]
71. Parazzini, F.; Di Martino, M.; Pellegrino, P. Magnesium in the Gynecological Practice: A Literature Review. *Magnes. Res.* **2017**, *30*, 1–7. [CrossRef] [PubMed]
72. Ji, X.; Grandner, M.A.; Liu, J. The Relationship between Micronutrient Status and Sleep Patterns: A Systematic Review. *Public Health Nutr.* **2017**, *20*, 687–701. [CrossRef] [PubMed]

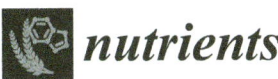

Review

Genistein: Dual Role in Women's Health

Linda Yu, Eddy Rios, Lysandra Castro, Jingli Liu, Yitang Yan and Darlene Dixon *

Molecular Pathogenesis Group, Mechanistic Toxicology Branch (MTB), Division of the National Toxicology Program (DNTP), National Institute of Environmental Health Sciences (NIEHS), National Institutes of Health (NIH), Research Triangle Park, Durham, NC 27709, USA; yu1@niehs.nih.gov (L.Y.); eddy.rios@nih.gov (E.R.); castro@niehs.nih.gov (L.C.); jingli.liu@nih.gov (J.L.); yitang.yan@nih.gov (Y.Y.)
* Correspondence: dixon@niehs.nih.gov

Citation: Yu, L.; Rios, E.; Castro, L.; Liu, J.; Yan, Y.; Dixon, D. Genistein: Dual Role in Women's Health. *Nutrients* **2021**, *13*, 3048. https://doi.org/10.3390/nu13093048

Academic Editor: Pasquapina Ciarmela

Received: 31 July 2021
Accepted: 25 August 2021
Published: 30 August 2021

Publisher's Note: MDPI stays neutral with regard to jurisdictional claims in published maps and institutional affiliations.

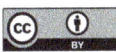

Copyright: © 2021 by the authors. Licensee MDPI, Basel, Switzerland. This article is an open access article distributed under the terms and conditions of the Creative Commons Attribution (CC BY) license (https://creativecommons.org/licenses/by/4.0/).

Abstract: Advanced research in recent years has revealed the important role of nutrients in the protection of women's health and in the prevention of women's diseases. Genistein is a phytoestrogen that belongs to a class of compounds known as isoflavones, which structurally resemble endogenous estrogen. Genistein is most often consumed by humans via soybeans or soya products and is, as an auxiliary medicinal, used to treat women's diseases. In this review, we focused on analyzing the geographic distribution of soybean and soya product consumption, global serum concentrations of genistein, and its metabolism and bioactivity. We also explored genistein's dual effects in women's health through gathering, evaluating, and summarizing evidence from current in vivo and in vitro studies, clinical observations, and epidemiological surveys. The dose-dependent effects of genistein, especially when considering its metabolites and factors that vary by individuals, indicate that consumption of genistein may contribute to beneficial effects in women's health and disease prevention and treatment. However, consumption and exposure levels are nuanced because adverse effects have been observed at lower concentrations in in vitro models. Therefore, this points to the duplicity of genistein as a possible therapeutic agent in some instances and as an endocrine disruptor in others.

Keywords: genistein; soya products; dual role; dose-dependent

1. Introduction

1.1. Genistein in Food

Genistein (5,7-dihydroxy-3-(4-hydroxyphenyl) chromen-4-one) is a phytoestrogen and isoflavone found in soybeans and soy-derived foods [1], including soya products, meat alternatives, edamame, and tempeh [2]. It has been detected in many processed foods [3] and can also be found in other foods [4]. Genistein's content in mature soybean seeds and therefore in soya products, varies by region, from the highest genistein content (>70 mg/100 g food) in soybean seeds from the US, Korea, and Japan, to the lowest from Europe (39.78 mg/g) and Taiwan (45.88 mg/g) [4]. Alongside reporting high genistein concentrations in soybeans, the US is currently leading the world in soybean production and export [5]. Furthermore, the demand for plant-based protein in Western societies is increasing; while dollar sales of all US foods have increased by 17% over the past two years, plant-based food sales have increased by 43% over this same time period [6]. As a compound that is so commonly found in food and specifically in soy products (Table 1), developing our understanding of genistein is paramount in both preserving global health and furthering advancements in women health.

Table 1. Genistein content in consumable products.

Food	Mean Genistein Concentration [a] (mg Genistein/ 100 g Food)	Standard Deviation	References
Textured Soy Flour	89.42	26.96	[7–15]
Instant Beverage Soy Powder	62.18	3.69	[14,16–20]
Soy Protein Isolate	57.28	14.17	[7,14,16,19,21–29]
Meatless Bacon Bits	45.77	0.11	[13]
Kellog's Smart-Start Soy Protein Cereal	41.90	N/A [b] ($n < 3$)	[13]
Natto	37.66	7.85	[30–36]
Uncooked Tempeh	36.15	17.64	[11,14,16,29,31–37–39]
Miso	23.24	8.37	[14,16,17,30,31,33,35,36,40–43]
Sprouted Raw Soybeans	18.77	11.22	[23,32,40,44–49]
Cooked Firm Tofu	10.83	3.98	[30,40,50]
Red Clovers	10.00	0.00	[51]
Worthington FriChik canned meatless chicken nuggets (prepared)	9.35	N/A ($n < 3$)	[31]
American Soy Cheese	8.70	N/A ($n < 3$)	[30]
Kellog's Kashi Go-Lean Cereal	7.70	N/A ($n < 3$)	[13]
Chocolate Power Bar	3.27	N/A ($n < 3$)	[44]
Hoisin Sauce	3.25	N/A ($n < 3$)	[13]
Cake-Type Plain Doughnuts	2.44	1.11	[13,40]
Raw Pistachios	1.75	N/A ($n < 3$)	[40,52]
Reconstituted Infant Formula (Abbot Nutrition)	1.37	0.37	[53,54]
Cooked USDA Commodity Beef Patties	1.09	0.42	[31]
Fat Free Frankfurter Beef	1.00	N/A ($n < 3$)	[13]
Raw Chicken Breast Tenders	0.25	N/A ($n < 3$)	[13]
Raw White Grapefruit	0.03	N/A ($n < 3$)	[44]
Whole Raw Eggs	0.02	N/A ($n < 3$)	[44,45]
Mature Raw Black Beans	0.00	0.00	[44,55,56]

[a] Data summarized from [4] [b] Not Applicable.

1.2. Genistein Levels in Various Populations

Genistein has been found and quantified globally in measures ranging from daily intake to serum concentration. Prominent data from several different studies in populations are outlined in Table 2, which is representative of two larger correlations of serum genistein concentrations.

Table 2. Genistein levels in populations worldwide.

Population	Number of Subjects	Sample Type	Quantified Genistein	References	Year
Healthy infants in Pennsylvania, collected at the Children's Hospital of Philadelphia and its affiliated clinics	165	Blood, urine, and saliva samples from cow- and breast-milk-fed infants Urine (cow-formula-fed infants) Blood (soy-formula-fed infants) Urine (soy-formula-fed infants) Saliva (soy-formula-fed infants)	Large majority, except for cow's milk-formula-fed infants, below LOD (<27 ng/mL in blood, <1.4 ng/mL in saliva, and <0.8 ng/mL in urine) 13.6 ng/mL 890.7 ng/mL (median) 7220 ng/mL (median) 10.9 ng/mL (median)	[57]	2009

Table 2. Cont.

Population	Number of Subjects	Sample Type	Quantified Genistein	References	Year
Cohort of women in Philadelphia, PA, USA	451	Daily consumption	2.4–3.9 mg (average)	[58]	2008
Subgroup of larger cohort of women in Philadelphia, PA, USA	27	Daily urine excretion	136.4 ng genistein/mg creatine (average)		
Adult participants from Ireland, Italy, the Netherlands, and the UK	7312	Daily consumption (Ireland) Daily consumption (Italy) Daily consumption (The Netherlands) Daily consumption (the UK)	0.368 mg/day (average) 0.302 mg/day (average) 0.516 mg/day (average) 0.389 mg/day (average)	[59]	2003
Women of various racial and ethnic groups across the US	1550	Daily consumption (White women)	3.6 µg genistein/day (average)	[60]	2006
	935	Daily consumption (African American women)	1.7 µg genistein/day (Average)		
	286	Daily consumption (Hispanic women)	0 µg genistein/day (average)		
	185	Daily consumption (Chinese women)	3534 µg genistein/day (average)		
	195	Daily consumption (Japanese women)	6788 µg genistein/day (average)		
Adults from various regions of Japan	215	Daily consumption Serum level Daily excretion in urine	14.5–18.3 mg genistein/day 475.3 nmol genistein/liter of serum 14.2 µmol genistein/day	[61]	2001
Chinese men	48	Daily consumption	19.4 ± 12.36 mg/day	[62]	2007
Adult (20–39 years old) women from the UK	20	Plasma genistein concentration of women that rarely consumed soy products	14.3 nmol/L (geometric mean)	[63]	2001
	20	Plasma genistein concentration of women that drank no soy milk but ate some solid soya foods	16.5 nmol/L (Geometric mean)		
	20	Plasma genistein concentration of women that drank 0.25 pints of soy milk daily and ate some solid soya foods	119 nmol/L (geometric mean)		
	20	Plasma genistein concentration of women that drank 0.5+ pints of soy milk daily and ate solid soya foods regularly	378 nmol/L (geometric mean)		

First, Table 2 shows that individuals who consume more soy products or soy-derived foods have higher serum levels of genistein. Supporting data from Verkasalo et al. [63] demonstrated that among four groups of twenty British women consuming increasing amounts of soya products (determined via a food diary method), plasma concentrations of genistein increased in a manner correlated with total soya consumption. In order of lowest to highest soya product consumption, the participant groups' geometric mean plasma concentrations (nmol/L) of genistein were 14.3, 16.5, 119, and 378. The Spearman correlation coefficient a quantitative measure for the strength of this correlation between plasma isoflavone concentrations and estimated dietary intakes was determined to be between 0.66 and 0.80 [63]. This correlation also extends beyond blood serum, as genistein has been shown to be more common in the breast milk of mothers that are consuming vegetarian and especially vegan diets [3]. It was further demonstrated that genistein can cross the placental barrier and potentially affect the developing fetus, as it was detected in similar concentrations in the maternal plasma, umbilical cord plasma, amniotic fluid, and neonate plasma in seven healthy Japanese mother-child pairs [64].

Secondly, the data in Table 2 also shows that both residents of Asian countries and Asian minority populations in Western countries consume significantly more soy products and, therefore, have higher serum genistein levels than other populations. This is further displayed in Figure 1, and validated when considering that China is the world's largest importer of soybeans, consuming roughly one-third of the global annual soybean harvest [65]. However, evidence suggests that eating a soya-rich diet, as vegetarians and vegans commonly do [66], can elevate daily genistein intake levels among individuals to a similar degree. British women who consumed soya regularly were reported to have a daily soya-product consumption that rivals that of Japanese adults consuming a traditional diet [63].

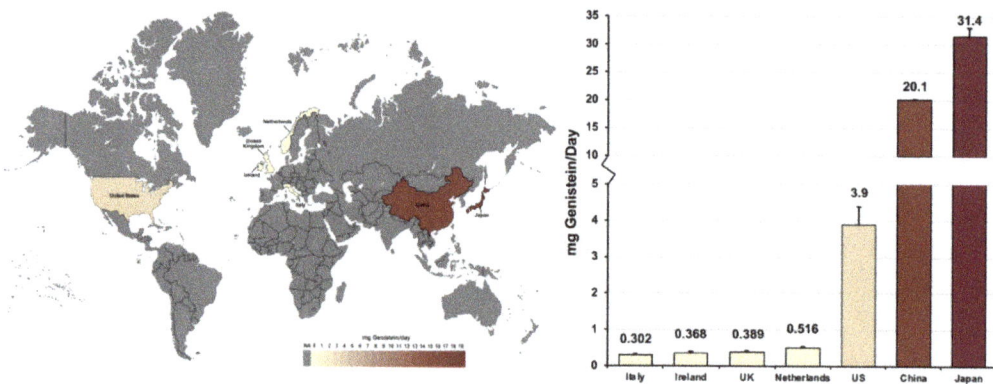

Figure 1. Heatmap showing daily genistein consumption levels across 7 surveyed countries. Data from [58,59,61,62].

Another relevant population in relation to genistein is perimenopausal and postmenopausal aged women. As literature regarding the clinical applications of phytoestrogens has risen to prominence, millions of peri- and postmenopausal women have begun taking genistein and soya supplements, aiming to alleviate their menopausal symptoms [67,68]. Taken in conjunction with the aforementioned populations, it is important to investigate genistein's effects, not only because of increased global soya consumption [69], but because genistein is ubiquitously present in food, breast milk, and human serum and is therefore bioactive in vulnerable, underrepresented, maternal, and neonatal populations.

1.3. Metabolism and Metabolites of Genistein

Genistein is typically ingested from vegetation as the glycoside genistin. Genistin is hydrolyzed by phlorizin hydrolase (a small intestine brush-border lactase) [70] or by enteric microflora [71] into genistein (the bioactive aglycone) before absorption or further modification by enteric microflora [72]. Genistein, like other polyphenols, has an oral bioavailability of roughly 10% [73]. With its low absorption potential, its lipophilic nature, and low molecular weight, genistein can be passively transported into intestinal cells [74], leading to post-absorption metabolism.

Most orally consumed genistein is eliminated by urine within a day of consumption [75]. When absorbed into the bloodstream via the intestinal tract, genistein and all of its metabolites were shown in a mouse model to have a half-life of 46 h [76]. However, in a study of nineteen healthy women, its bioactive life as unconjugated genistein aglycone was shown to be much shorter at just 7.13 h [77] This short bioactive life most commonly ends when genistein is modified by uridine diphosphate-glucuronosyltransferases (UGTs) and sulfotransferases (SULTs) in the intestinal enterocytes and liver [73,78]. Conversion to genistein glucuronide is the most common fate of absorbed genistein [76,79], and though it varies greatly between individuals, it is also less commonly carried out by UGTs in the kidneys [80]. The large majority of the circulating genistein that is not converted to a glucuronide form is converted via enterocytic and hepatic sulfotransferases (SULTs) to a sulfate form [76]. These sulfate and glucuronide groups are added to the 7 and 4′ positions, creating different compounds that can have 1 glucuronide, 1 sulfate, 2 glucuronides, or one of each [79]. It is also important to mention that sufficient expression and localization of UGTs and SULTs in other organs, such as the heart and lungs, allows for minor metabolism of genistein in these organs [78,81]. Furthermore, different cell types, due to the composition of different ratios of UGT:SULT enzymes, may vary in their metabolism of genistein [82].

To a significantly lesser extent [83,84], genistein is also metabolized via cytochrome P450 (CYP) reaction to produce mostly hydroxylated metabolites [84–86]. The enzyme CYP1A2 is the most relevant of the CYP group, converting genistein to orobol (3′-OH-genistein) [86,87]. Less often, other CYP enzymes such as CYP2E1, CYP2D6, and CYP3A4, and CYP2C8 also metabolize genistein via oxidation [86,87]. Figure 2 illustrates ingested genistein's most common metabolic processes and metabolites.

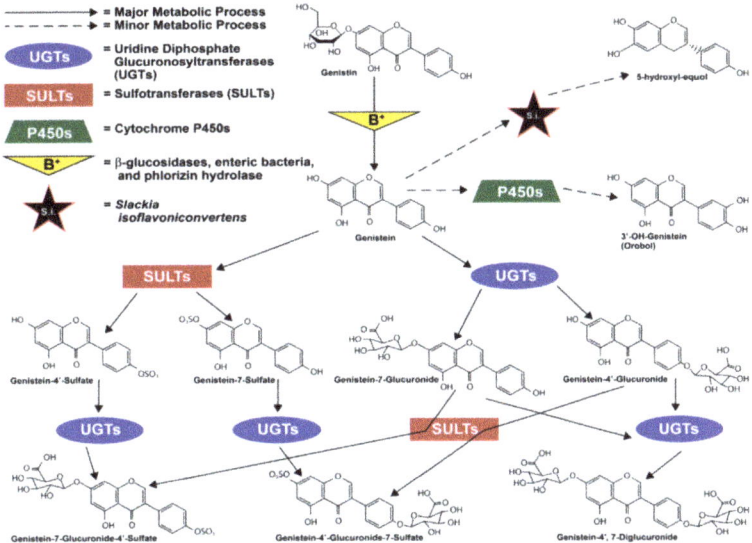

Figure 2. Major genistein metabolites. Data from [79,82,86–89]. Structures from [1,79].

Though enteric bacteria are known to play a prominent role in the uptake and metabolism of genistein [3], Munro et al. [90] reported that its metabolic pathway may be significantly altered by variations in microflora, intestinal transit time, pH, redox potential, and even immune status and diet. There is even a likely temporal aspect to this metabolic plasticity, as data presented in Hoey et al. [91] suggests that the ability to hydrolyze glycosides to aglycones, and therefore genistin to genistein, develops before 4–6 months postnatally and plays an important role in isoflavone metabolic capabilities.

Equol, metabolized from daidzein, another isoflavone found in soybeans, is also relevant when discussing enteric bacteria and genistein because it is an isoflavone metabolite with stronger estrogenic activity than all other known isoflavones and isoflavone metabolites; it also exhibits the strongest antioxidant activity of any isoflavone metabolite [92–94]. Although equol itself is produced when intestinal bacteria metabolize daidzein and its glycoside form daidzin, the human microfloral bacteria *Slackia isoflavoniconvertens* has also been described as capable of converting genistein to 5-hydroxy-equol [88]. However, while this metabolite is slightly altered, 5-hydroxy-equol shares many of equol's chemical properties, exhibiting a greater antioxidant capacity than genistein [95].

It is difficult to quantify the significance of this genistein metabolite in terms of women's health, as most women likely do not have the correct gut bacteria for producing it. Depending on genetic and dietary factors, only 25–50% of people are believed to have gut bacteria that are capable of producing equol from daidzein [96]; this is especially relevant considering multiple different bacteria can catalyze this conversion, and only a fraction of them are known to be concurrently capable of 5-hydroxy-equol formation from genistein.

1.4. Estrogenic Effects of Genistein

Given the structural similarity of genistein and estrogen, genistein may exhibit a litany of possible biological effects while circulating. Many of these effects stem from its status as an isoflavone and therefore an estrogen mimic [75]; it acts on estrogen receptors (ERs), ER alpha and beta, primarily through the classical genomic mechanism [97]. It does differ from estrogen, however, in its preference for ER beta (gene name: ESR2) over ER alpha (gene name: ESR1). In a solid-phase competition experiment, genistein was shown to have a binding affinity for ER alpha that is 4% of that of 17 β-estradiol (E2), and a relative binding affinity for ER beta of 87% [97]. Because of genistein's hydroxyl substituents, these relative binding affinities for both ERs are significantly higher than that of other isoflavones, such as daidzein and formononetin [97]. This, however, is complicated by variation in the presence and distribution of both ERs temporally, between different body tissues and cell types, and even between individuals and populations [98–100].

Genistein has also been shown to exhibit agonistic activity with G protein-coupled estrogen receptor 1 (GPER1) [101], yielding a binding affinity higher than that of E2 but smaller than that of E2 [101,102]. This activity is compounded by results reported in Du et al. [103], in which treatment with genistein induced greater gene and protein expression of GPER while inhibiting MAP kinase activation in mouse microglial cells. Other molecular targets of genistein include topoisomerase I and II [104,105], protein tyrosine kinases [106], and 5α-reductase [107].

2. Biological Effects and Mechanism(s) of Genistein

2.1. In Vivo Experimental and Clinical Findings

Before soy gained widespread usage and more media attention, genistein was thought to be a primarily beneficial chemoprotective compound in vivo. Barnes [108] created a table detailing 29 studies characterizing the effects of genistein and genistein-containing products on carcinogenesis in rats and mice, finding a protective effect of genistein in 21 studies, and no effect in the other 8 studies. In vivo evidence also supports genistein's capability for supporting bone health and suppressing cancer development in tissue. Messing et al. [109] treated pre-operative bladder cancer patients with daily oral genistein (placebo, 300, or 600 mg per day), finding that once excised, the cancerous bladder tissue had significantly lower levels of EGFR phosphorylation. Among its reported antitumor, osteoblastic, and anticarcinogenic abilities, genistein has also been suggested to exhibit antioxidant [110], positive cardiovascular [111], and antilipogenic [112] effects. Although many subsequent reviews have echoed these positive findings, there exists some recent controversy over genistein's net beneficial effects.

Given its strong potential for therapeutic activity, genistein has faced more scrutiny over the past decade; it does have the potential to exhibit adverse effects. Turner et al. [113] found that serum genistein levels that correlate with those found in women consuming a high-soy diet did not affect bone loss in a rat model for postmenopausal osteoporosis; this evidence outright contradicts previous literature on genistein's osteoblastic capabilities [114,115].

Singh et al. [116] demonstrated that a single high dose of genistein (500 and 1000 mg/kg) had hepatotoxic, oxidative stress, and correlative genetic expression effects within 24 h of intraperitoneal administration into male Swiss albino mice. However, this was not the case with lower doses; thus, these negative effects were elicited by levels of circulating genistein that was within the realm of pharmacological treatment [109].

Studies with rats have also demonstrated that peri- and neonatal exposure of rats to genistein can negatively affect their reproductive capabilities. Wisniewski et al. [117] found that exposing male rats to even low doses of genistein during gestation resulted in significantly decreased phallic length, testis size, circulating testosterone, and general reproductive fitness. This is especially concerning considering genistein's ability to cross the human placental barrier [64]. Lewis et al. [118] also demonstrated that near-therapeutic doses of genistein (40 mg/kg subcutaneously) given to neonatal female rats could cause increased uterine weight, advanced onset of puberty, and even permanent estrus. However, these effects were not replicated in females dosed with 4 mg/kg, correlating with the exposure level for human infants drinking soy-based formula [57].

In vivo studies of genistein's effects may be further confounded by the timing and frequency of genistein consumption. Kerrie et al. [119] hypothesized that lifetime soy consumption, if begun early in life, causes epigenetic changes that reduce the occurrence and reoccurrence of breast cancer. Some of the most prominent data supporting this claim come from the work of Korde et al. [120], which found the most consistent reduction in breast cancer risk among Asian American women who had their largest soy intakes during childhood as opposed to adolescence or adulthood (although a decrease in risk was seen across all 3 groups). Kerrie et al. further reported that three other case-control studies on Asian and Asian-American women supported the association between reduction of breast cancer incidence and initiation of soy consumption at an earlier age. Interestingly, Joanne et al. [121] reported that although Caucasian women see the same significant benefits, they show less of a reduction in breast cancer risk. However, the idea that genistein's positive effects are somehow race- or ethnicity-dependent has been mostly discredited, as Asian immigrants to western countries who reduce their soy-intake have a similar cancer incidence as Western individuals [122–124].

2.2. In Vitro Experimental Findings

Genistein is of particular interest in vitro because it exhibits highly variable and often contrasting biological effects, especially in relation to cell proliferation and cancer. Akiyama et al. [125] showed that, in vitro, genistein inhibited tyrosine-specific protein kinase activity of the EGF receptor, pp60^{v-src} and pp110$^{gag-fes}$, and therefore inhibited growth and metastasis, in A-431 epidermoid carcinoma cells. In vivo, genistein was also shown to inhibit serine- and threonine-specific protein kinase activity in the EGF receptor of these cells [125]. Agarwal et al. [126] reported that, in DU145 metastatic prostate carcinoma cells, genistein inhibited the activation of extracellular signal-related protein kinase (ERK) 1/2, a kinase whose overactivation is a fundamental aspect of prostate cancer proliferation. Treatment of the DU145 cells, a prostate cancer cell line, at doses of 100–200 mM of genistein coincidentally resulted in significant cell growth inhibition and induction of apoptosis [126]. In contrast to this inhibition, Chen et al. [127] demonstrated that lower concentrations (1 mM) of genistein increased the proliferation of MCF-7 human breast cancer cells by increasing the protein and mRNA content of the IGF-1 receptor (IGF-IR) and insulin receptor substrate-1 (IRS-1), enhancing tyrosine phosphorylation of IGF-IR and IRS-1.

However, there is a large body of evidence suggesting that genistein's metabolism and biological effects may vary by dosage or exposure levels, even depending on the cell type affected. For example, Chen et al. [127] and Wang et al. [128] showed that MCF-7 breast cancer cell growth was stimulated by low concentrations of genistein (10^{-8}–10^{-6} M) and inhibited by higher concentrations (>10^{-5} M). Moore et al. [129] found that low in vitro concentrations of genistein ($\leq$1 µg/mL; 3.7 µM) elicited proliferation in human uterine leiomyoma cells, while higher exposure levels ($\geq$10 µg/mL; 37 µM) had inhibitory effects. This non-monotonic dose response to genistein was different for the uterine smooth muscle cells, and a similar dose response to genistein on behavioral parameters in rat offspring has been observed in vivo [130]; it is also a hallmark of environmental endocrine disruptors such as BPA [131]. Figure 3 illustrates this point by portraying three different cell lines' non-monotonic responses to genistein between 0.001 and 100+ µM. For reference, the dose response curves on this figure are overlaid with serum genistein levels for three surveyed populations.

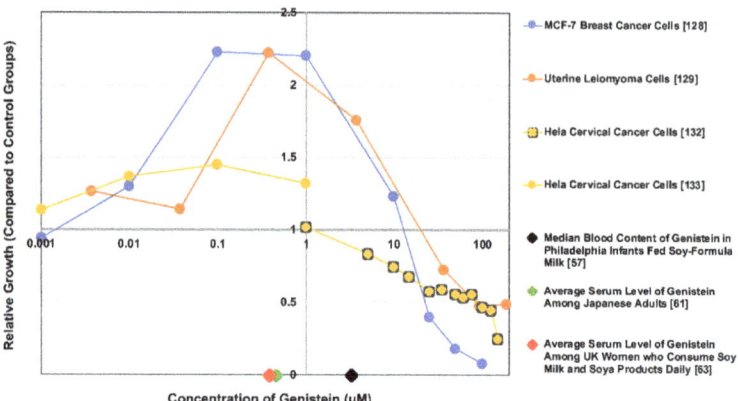

Figure 3. Relative growth of several cell lines at variable concentrations of genistein overlaid with serum levels of genistein for three populations. Data from [57,61,63,128,129,132,133]. Note that no (0) genistein marks a value of 1 relative growth unit. This is considered the control group for all studies. Also, note that none of the cell lines were reported to be prominent metabolizers of genistein. Concurrently, the serum concentration studies only assessed circulating genistein, while its metabolites (likely the most predominant forms in vivo) would presumably also have effects on the cell lines.

However, it is important to note that these in vitro studies and reference values do not account for genistein's metabolites. Given variable bioactivity between genistein and its metabolites, the half-life of genistein and the levels of circulating metabolites may be another pertinent variable in determining the effects of genistein on various tissues in vivo. As such, in vitro studies that treat cells with genistein alone may find significantly different results when compared to studies that used characteristic concentrations of genistein and its metabolites. Further in vitro research should consider genistein metabolites when conducting all forms of exposure assessment, as doing so will provide a more accurate picture of genistein's net effects.

3. Genistein and Women's Diseases

3.1. Genistein and Obesity

Multiple studies purport genistein's ability to combat obesity at various system-wide levels. This is one of the reasons post-menopausal women may supplement their diet with genistein, as studies with ovariectomized mice have shown orally-consumed genistein to be an inhibitor of the increased fat accumulation, weight gain, insulin resistance, and hepatic lipogenesis that is typically associated with post-menopausal estrogen deficiency [134]. Part of this effect was even shown to be a result of genistein inducing apoptosis in inguinal fat [135].

Genistein was further shown to decrease the adipose tissue content of female mice when compared to vehicle treatment groups [136]. However, genistein's mechanism of action for reducing body fat likely differs from its activity in other body tissues. While genistein has a much higher binding affinity for ER beta, this same study found that genistein was incapable of significantly reducing the adipose tissue content of female ER alpha knockout mice (αERKO) when compared to a vehicle control [136]. This suggests genistein's mechanism of action on adipocytes uncharacteristically favors ER alpha rather than ER beta [136], as it did not reproduce this adipose tissue reduction in mice that were lacking ER alpha while expressing ER beta. Further evidence showed that in utero exposures to genistein also potentiates obesity throughout the lives of Agouti mice born to dams consuming high-soy diets during gestation [137], suggesting an expecting dam's genistein intake may play a role in their offspring's predisposition towards obesity. Genistein may also regulate obesity by affecting thyroid peroxidase [138], insulin [139], and leptin activity [140].

These anti-obesity effects are not exclusive to the genistein aglycone. For example, orobol (3'-OH-Genistein), the metabolite from the CYP1A2 enzymatic pathway, has been shown to have a significantly greater inhibitory effect on mouse fibroblast adipogenesis than genistein [141].

It is important to mention that genistein's status as a soy-derived compound means it is generally consumed alongside significant amounts of plant-based protein, and it is well documented that protein is among the most thermogenic and appetite-reducing of the macronutrient groups [142]. Velasquez and Bhathena [143] compiled six human studies, all of which showed that soy-protein was significantly more effective than carbohydrates at increasing metabolic rate and lowering body weight. Though one of these studies did show pork to be more thermogenic than soy [144], three of them showed soy protein to be as or more thermogenic than meat and milk-based proteins [145–147]. This means that supplementing one's diet with genistein from natural sources, and therefore consuming plant-based protein, likely yields many of the thermogenic benefits associated with meat and animal protein consumption. Importantly, one meta-analysis of 24 studies [148] concluded that soy consumption generally elicited either no weight change or weight gain. However, this same review concluded that isoflavone—and therefore genistein—consumption significantly reduced the body mass index (BMI) in postmenopausal women independent of soy protein intake.

3.2. Genistein and Breast Cancer

Breast cancer is the most common cancer in women in the United States, causing thousands of deaths each year. Given results from multiple literature reviews and studies [108,119,120,149,150], genistein has clearly shown a strong potential for breast cancer prevention. Women who eat more genistein, especially earlier in life, have a significantly decreased likelihood of developing breast cancer. These same women also have a lower risk of recurrence of treated breast cancer [119–121]. Genistein also inhibits the growth of human MCF-7 breast cancer cells at a concentration of 10^{-5} M [128], and even potentiates the anticarcinogenic effects of tamoxifen on the growth of ESR1-positive and HER2-overexpressing human breast cancer cells [150].

It is important to mention that genistein's anticarcinogenic property is attenuated based on both the concentration of genistein and the cell surface receptors of the target cells. Although Wang et al. [128] demonstrated genistein's ability to inhibit MCF-7 tumor growth at higher concentrations, at lower concentrations they saw stimulated growth. Furthermore, Pons et al. [151] illustrated that at concentrations representing genistein blood levels of individuals consuming a high-soy diet, genistein's potentiating effects on breast cancer cells were influenced by the ESR1/ESR2 ratio of the cells. In this study, MCF-7 cells, which have a higher ESR1/ESR2 ratio, being treated with cisplatin, paclitaxel, or tamoxifen saw an increase in cell survivability when also treated with genistein. This suggests that genistein may have the potential to elicit counterproductive effects in women already being treated for a high ESR1/ESR2 ratio breast cancer using these common over-the-counter therapeutics [151]. Conversely, genistein was shown to have a harmless or beneficial effect when the procedure was repeated using cells with a low ESR1/ESR2 ratio (including both T47D cells and MCF-7 cells transformed to overexpress ESR2) [151]. Taken in context, this suggests that a genistein-supplemented regimen for treating breast cancer can be beneficial; however, it might be contraindicated for women whose tumors present with a high ESR1/ESR2 ratio.

Because of its numerous dose-dependent and receptor-influenced biological effects and its various metabolic pathways, it is difficult to conclude genistein's role in breast cancer development and treatment. Though sufficient consumption has been shown to prevent breast cancer development [152], the literature is controversial regarding genistein's effects on active cases of breast cancers. For example, a review published in 2000 focusing on genistein and breast cancer stated that the net result of genistein consumption on breast cancer activity or proliferation was inconclusive [119]. Furthermore, a meta-analysis of 164+ relevant studies in 2019 on genistein and breast cancer concluded that "the impact of dietary genistein intake on breast cancer remains unclear" [153]. Like the aforementioned studies, this review stated that variation in mode of intake, metabolism, menopausal status, estrogen receptor expression pattern, and gene mutations among individuals is key to determining the net effect of genistein consumption. These data suggest that further studies focused on the above factors and their interactions may yield more definitive answers and even future treatments for one of the most common cancers that affect women.

3.3. Genistein and Uterine Leiomyoma

Human uterine leiomyomas, also called fibroids, clinically affect about 40% of childbearing aged women in the United States with symptoms of bleeding, dysregulation of the menstrual cycle, belly pain and infertility. Genistein's effects on uterine leiomyomas is a rapidly expanding research subject, also appearing to follow a dose-dependent interaction pattern. Moore et al. [129] found that low in vitro concentrations of genistein (≤ 1 µg/mL) elicited proliferation in human uterine leiomyoma cells but did not do so in human uterine smooth muscle cells. However, higher exposure levels had inhibitory effects on both cell types causing cellular morphological changes, inhibiting cell proliferation, inducing apoptosis, and even causing targeted leiomyoma autophagy [154]. This type of biphasic dose-response is similar to what has been characterized regarding genistein and breast cancer [128]. It is also important to note that leiomyoma cells were more sensitive to the proliferative effects of genistein at a high dose (>1 µg/mL) than the smooth muscle cells, indicating a possible risk factor in terms of genistein consumption and fibroids.

There are many pathways by which genistein has been shown to affect leiomyoma growth; understanding these pathways is a critical step in revealing the mechanisms behind genistein-induced cell proliferation or inhibition and its therapeutic potential. Results from Di et al. [155] suggest that the inhibition described in Moore et al. [129] was the result of a high dose of genistein's down-regulation of the TGF-β pathway, most notably activin A and Smad3. Although outlined in Eker rats, another pathway by which genistein was shown to inhibit leiomyoma cell proliferation was by acting as a ligand for peroxisome proliferator-activated receptor-γ [156]. Wang et al. [128] elaborated on these findings by hypothesizing that genistein's emergent inhibitory effects at higher concentrations (>10^{-5} M) might occur through regulating the estrogen-responsive pS2 in contrast to its proposed activity at low concentrations.

Di et al. [157] demonstrated that low concentrations of genistein increased proliferation of uterine leiomyoma cells by rapidly associating with the IGF-1 receptor, causing interactions between ERα and IGF-IR, and activating the extracellular regulated kinase and MAP kinase pathways. Low concentrations of genistein have also been shown, in human leiomyoma cells, to activate MAPKp44/42, MSK1, and increase phosphorylation of histone H3 at serine10 (H3S10ph) [158]; these effects lead to increased cell proliferation, further demonstrating that genistein can even have epigenetic effects on human leiomyoma cells.

While there is sufficient evidence to conclude genistein can affect fibroids once formed, there is less evidence for associations between genistein consumption and the risk of fibroid incidence. As an example, Simon et al. [159] found that, across 328 women, there was no correlation between fibroid occurrence and urinary output of genistein (used as a proxy for blood genistein content). However, the inhibitory effects of genistein at high doses indicate that a requisite level of soy product consumption might be an important consideration in protecting patients with either predisposition towards or active fibroids.

3.4. Genistein and Endometriosis

Given genistein's ability to mimic estrogen and endometriosis' hormone-responsiveness [160], a reasonable hypothesis might assert that genistein could affect the incidence, severity, or timing of endometriosis that affects thousands of premenopausal women in the United States. Though 54 mg of oral genistein consumed daily has been shown to be an effective alternative treatment for managing endometrial hyperplasia in premenopausal women [161], much of the literature regarding its effects on endometriosis in women is conflicting. A large majority of it appears to be focused on in vivo rodent studies.

Regarding the incidence of endometriosis, it is uncertain as to whether genistein consumption affects a woman's likelihood of developing the condition. One study encompassing over 500 American women found no significant correlation between endometriosis and urine concentration of genistein [162]. The same study further concluded that, among the women with moderate-to-severe endometriosis, there was no correlation between phytoestrogen consumption and disease severity. This study conflicts with results from another study which found that higher levels of urinary genistein were correlated with a reduction in advanced endometriosis risk [163]. However, this study is less generalizable because it only included women that were infertile and nulliparous. One might assume that comparing the prevalence of endometriosis across populations with large discrepancies in genistein consumption may help explain these conflicting results. However, women living in Asia and Japan, populations known to consume significantly more genistein than their Caucasian counterparts, develop endometriosis at a 1.5–3× greater rate than women in Western populations do [164]. Given that peer-reviewed studies have concluded that genistein may be associated with increased, decreased, or unchanged endometriosis risk, further controlled research is needed on a larger scale to explain any confounding variables, potential associations, or lack thereof.

The dispute over genistein's anti-endometriosis effects appears to be less common across rodent studies. For example, Cotroneo and Lamartiniere [165] concluded that genistein's effect on a rat model of endometriosis depended on the method of intake; subcutaneously injected genistein sustained intestinally implanted endometrial tissue, while dietary genistein did not. However, rats given oral genistein in Yavuz et al. [166] saw a significant regression of peritoneal endometriotic implants when compared to the control group. These two studies suggest genistein might have an inhibitory and even regressive effect on endometriotic cells, which is supported by studies showing that genistein inhibits expression of proinflammatory cytokines NF-κB, ESR2 [167], Bcl-2, COX-2, and PGE [168] in rodent models of endometriosis. There does not appear to be thorough research into why rodent studies are more conclusive in supporting genistein's potential for treating endometriosis, but it may be due to several factors ranging from the paucity of human investigations, fundamental physiological differences between humans and rodents, confounding lifestyle variables, and more.

3.5. Genistein and Endometrial Cancer

In 2018, there were 89,929 related deaths and 382,069 new cases of endometrial cancer, globally [169]. The global incidence rate is also projected to pass 573,000 new cases by 2040 [170]. Genistein has been shown to inhibit endometrial cancer through a variety of direct and indirect pathways. For example, genistein was shown to suppress endometrial cancer cell proliferation in ECC-1 and RL-95-2 cell lines by decreasing expression of hTERT and ERα, leading to effects on both the AKT/mTOR and MAPK pathways [171]. Treatment with 5 mM of genistein was also sufficient to significantly affect Ishikawa cell proliferation and initiate downregulation of several prominent oncogenes, including the MAPK pathway-related genes (AA704613, MYC-associated zinc finger protein; and AA829383, mitogen-activated protein kinase), the cell cycle-related genes (AA789328, cyclin-dependent kinase (CDC2-like) 10; and W70051 M-phase phosphoprotein 9), and the cell migration and adhesion-related genes (AA283090 CD44 antigen; and N66616 phosphodiesterase 7A [172]. Further research confirmed a significant negative correlation among breast cancer survivors between consumption of genistein-containing herbal products and endometrial cancer incidence [173]. It appears that a significant body of research on the subject suggests that consumption of genistein has anti-endometrial cancer properties.

Understanding genistein's effects on endometrial cancer-related hormones is critical in assessing genistein's role in endometrial carcinogenesis. Though estrogen has been shown to induce the proliferation of endometrial cancer cells, genistein has been shown to suppress this process. Sampey et al. [174] showed that though genistein itself did not increase Ishikawa cell growth nor affect estrogen's proliferative effects on an Ishikawa monoculture, 10–100 nM of genistein did suppress estrogen's proliferative effects on a coculture including endometrial stromal cells along with Ishikawa cells. The same study further discussed how studies using ESR2-specific agonists yielded similar data. Since estrogen is a naturally occurring hormone in all women, this means that genistein is likely able, in vivo, to suppress endometrial cancer proliferation. This concept is further validated when considering results outlined in Zhang et al. [175] and Lee et al. [176], two literature analyses that discussed multiple epidemiological studies that showed a negative correlation between soya intake and endometrial cancer risk, and genistein and ovarian cancer risk, respectively.

3.6. Genistein and Polycystic Ovarian Syndrome

Given that polycystic ovarian syndrome (PCOS) is considered a possibly heritable disorder whose pathology might be partially hormonal in nature [177], there is a valid interest in genistein as a potential therapeutic for and effector of this disorder. Khani et al. [178] found that women with PCOS treated with a 3 month genistein regimen of 18 mg per 12 h saw decreases in circulating luteinizing hormone, serum triglyceride, LDL cholesterol, and testosterone; all of which are commonly increased in all PCOS patients. This evidence suggests that genistein can significantly improve the hormonal and lipid profile of women with PCOS, thereby reducing their likelihood of developing comorbid cardiovascular or metabolic disorders. This is supported by findings described in Jamilian and Asemi [179], a study that compared isoflavone supplementation to placebo in two groups of 35 women with PCOS. They found that the group that was supplemented daily with 50 mg of soy isoflavone for 12 weeks saw significant improvements in their hormonal and lipid profiles; the same group further showed decreased insulin resistance. Furthermore, another study utilizing a test diet including 35% soy protein found that women with PCOS that adhered to the diet saw improvements in BMI, glycemic control, circulating testosterone, and lipid profiles, alongside significant increases in circulating nitric oxide (NO) and glutathione (GSH) [180].

Using 36 mg/day, Romualdi et al. [181] reported similar findings with regards to cholesterol levels and triglycerides. However, this study was contradicted by both Khani et al. [178] and Jamilian and Asemi [179] in finding no significant changes in hormonal profiles and glycoinsulemic metabolism. However, this difference may be attributable to sample size (n = 12) or the profile of the sample population (all women in Romualdi et al. [181] had both hyperinsulemia and dyslipidemia alongside their PCOS).

Isoflavone supplementation has also been shown to clinically improve the gut health of women with PCOS. For example, after isoflavone intervention, a 50 mg isoflavones/day regimen over just three consecutive days improved predicted stool metagenomic pathways, microbial alpha diversity, and glucose homeostasis in PCOS patients. The effect was so profound that, post-treatment, these variables resembled the profile of the control group at baseline [182]. Though further testing is required, evidence suggests that dietary supplementation of genistein may be a viable natural option for treating many of the symptoms of PCOS [175–179].

3.7. Genistein and Cervical Cancer

Cervical cancer used to be the leading cause of cancer death of women in the United States; however, in the past 40 years, the number of cases of cervical cancer and cancer deaths have decreased significantly because of Pap tests and HPV vaccinations [183]. As with breast cancer, there exists conflicting evidence and controversial conclusions regarding genistein's effects on the viability, incidence, and severity of cervical cancer. For example, while cervical cancer cells of the HeLa [184], CaSki and ME180 [185] lines have been shown to be sensitized to radiation therapy by high doses of genistein (20–40 mM), low concentrations of genistein (0.001–1 µM) have also been shown to promote HeLa cell proliferation and inhibit apoptosis via the PI3K/Akt-NF-κB pathway [133].

These results were directly challenged by Sahin et al. [186], who found that 25 µM genistein sensitized HeLa cells to cisplatin by inhibiting the NF-κB and Akt/mTOR pathways. The same results were also challenged by Hussain et al. [132], who found that genistein inhibited HeLa cell proliferation and promoted both apoptosis and cell cycle arrest at doses as low as 5 µM, becoming more effective with higher doses tested up to 150 µM.

The difference between the conclusions of these studies seems to lie in the concentration of genistein used to expose HeLa cervical cancer cells. Similar to the biphasic concentration-dependent responses observed in uterine leiomyoma [129] and MCF-7 breast cancer cells [128] (noted in Figure 3), HeLa cells appeared to show the same nonmonotonic response to genistein across these three studies; exhibiting proliferation at lower concentrations and suppression at higher concentrations. Most notably, increasing the dosage meant that genistein had the opposite effect on the NF-κB pathway. Though more research is needed—especially in terms of epidemiological and human in vivo evidence—to come to a sound conclusion regarding genistein and cervical cancer, this evidence suggests that using genistein at controlled high concentrations could be an effective treatment for both inhibiting the growth of and radiosensitizing cervical cancer cells for therapy.

3.8. Genistein and Menopause (Hormone Regulation)

Menopause is marked by a series of physiological changes linked to a reduction in bodily estrogen and progesterone production, potentially eliciting symptoms such as hot flashes secondary to vasomotor dysfunction, sweating, thinning of vaginal membranes, mood effects, sleep insufficiency, and more [187]. It occurs in women between ages 40–58, and even older, yet the age of onset can be affected by multiple factors including smoking, contraceptive use, BMI, and more [188]. It is unlikely that genistein influences the timing of menopause onset itself; despite a large disparity in genistein consumption between Asian and Caucasian women, they both typically experience menopause at around the same age [189,190].

Genistein has been thoroughly explored for its potential use in postmenopausal hormonal replacement therapy in alleviating the severity of menopausal symptoms. This is largely because although current hormone-replacement therapies are available, many of them may increase the risk of thromboembolism, cancer, stroke, and other complications [191]. The use of genistein as a form of hormone replacement therapy is common [114], and has been shown to be significantly more effective than a placebo at combatting several of the post-menopausal symptoms and physiological effects in women.

Double-blind studies showed that 54 mg of daily oral genistein reduced hot flashes without negatively affecting endometrial thickness, liver function, or blood physiology in postmenopausal women [192]. The same dosage has also been shown to reduce bone resorption while increasing bone deposition [193], improve brachial arterial vasodilation and perfusion capability [194], enhance endothelium function as effectively as estrogen/progesterone treatment [195], and even showed cardioprotective activity in postmenopausal women [196].

Even considering different populations, those that consume more genistein such as Asian women have a significantly decreased propensity towards postmenopausal hot flashes [114]. Reinforcing this notion, a 2016 meta-analysis of 62 clinical trials across 6653 postmenopausal women found that phytoestrogen supplementation was significantly correlated with reductions in the number of daily hot flashes and general vaginal dryness [197].

The literature appears to mostly support genistein supplementation as a viable option for reducing many of the symptoms of menopause (Table 3).

Table 3. Summary of 62 human studies and literature reviews of human studies on genistein's effects on women's health—both in vivo and in vitro studies are included.

Category of Studies' Conclusions Regarding Genistein/Whole Isoflavones/Genistein Metabolites	Total Number of Studies (Number Included in the Exposure Testing Range/Daily Dosage Column In Vivo) [a]	Exposure Testing Range In Vitro (µM)	Daily Dosage Testing Range In Vivo (mg)	References
Evidence suggests effects are primarily beneficial	42 (27)	Genistein: 2.0–370	Genistein: 36–600 (all doses above 54 were in one study) Genistein Mode: 54 (7 studies) Whole Isoflavones: 40–165 Soy Intakes/Week: 0.76–12.0	[67,68,95,108–112,120,121,125,132,143–147,149,150,152,161,171–173,175,176,178–180,182,184–186,192–200]
Evidence suggests effects are debated/inconclusive, but does suggest potential benefits	11 (9)	Genistein: 0.0037–185	Genistein: 30–54 Whole Isoflavones: 45	[108,114,119,128,129,151,154,155,163,174,181]
Evidence suggests effects are debated/inconclusive, and does not show any potential for benefits	4 (2)	Genistein: 1–10	Whole Isoflavones: 33.3–300	[148,153,159,162]
Evidence suggests effects are primarily detrimental	5 (5)	Genistein: 0.001–3.7	N/A [b]	[127,133,157,158,201]

[a] Omitted studies include those which reported measures that could not be converted to fit this table. [b] Not applicable.

4. Clinical Therapeutic Options

Because of its numerous positive biological effects, genistein has begun to see widespread medicinal use. Over the counter genistein supplements are marketed to the general public using buzzwords such as "life extension, wellbeing, health supplement," and more [202]; however, even "Amazon's Choice" genistein supplement lacks citations, instead stating that these claims have not been validated by the FDA in the fine print [203]. While there is a large body of evidence suggesting the numerous health benefits of genistein for nearly all populations, it is important that the public also be informed of the risks associated with supplementation. This is especially relevant and concerning considering many of these marketed supplements are individual pills containing 125+ mg pure genistein aglycone each [202], greater than 5× the total daily average whole genistin and genistein consumption values for Chinese [62] and Japanese adults [61]. Values in this range are within the realm of doses given in genistein's clinical trials [109]. Despite the therapeutic potential of these significantly larger dosages, they also carry increased risks [116–118]. Given the need for further investigation into maximizing the benefits and minimizing the potential side effects, genistein supplementation is currently not recommended without first consulting a pharmacist or physician [204]. Across much of the literature, the most consistent and safe results appear to be found at genistein consumption levels similar to those found in traditional Asian diets [108,110,112,120,121,193,205].

As previously mentioned, genistein has been used in human clinical trials for purposes such as restricting growth and growth factor activity in cancer cells [109]; a 2008 literature review [149] reported that across 20+ studies, genistein has been shown to be a strong potentiator of antitumor chemotherapeutics, including tamoxifen [150]. Genistein was even found to increase the sensitivity of renal [198], prostate [206], esophageal [199], and cervical cancers [185] to radiation therapy. Genistein therapies show great potential; they utilize genistein's dual effects that are cell- and organ-specific, hormone receptor content-mediated, and concentration-dependent to improve the clinical outlook of a broad range of women's diseases.

5. Conclusions

The geographic distribution of soya product consumption has resulted in differential serum concentrations of genistein globally. We have evaluated and summarized research evidence from current in vivo and in vitro studies, clinical observations, and epidemiological surveys to show that genistein has been reported to have dual effects in women's health when all data are taken under consideration. The effects of genistein appear to be dose-dependent and varies by individuals and suggests that genistein's effects may be dependent on the levels of consumption, serum concentrations, and other factors that may contribute to its beneficial effects in women's health, disease prevention, and treatment. However, there have been inconclusive beneficial effects of genistein reported in women and in in vivo animal studies; conversely, even adverse effects have been observed at lower concentrations in in vitro and in in vivo animal models. Therefore, the duplicity of genistein in women's health is that it has been reported to serve as a possible beneficial or therapeutic agent in some instances and as an endocrine disruptor in other situations.

Author Contributions: All authors have read and agreed to the published version of the manuscript.

Funding: This work was funded by the Intramural Research Program of the NIH, NIEHS and DNTP (ES021196-27).

Institutional Review Board Statement: Not applicable.

Informed Consent Statement: Not applicable.

Data Availability Statement: Not Applicable.

Acknowledgments: The authors sincerely thank Yin Li and Hong Li for their critical review of the manuscript.

Conflicts of Interest: The authors declare no conflict of interest.

References

1. National Center for Biotechnology Information. Compound Summary for CID 5280961, Genistein. Available online: https://pubchem.ncbi.nlm.nih.gov/compound/Genistein (accessed on 17 December 2020).
2. UCSF Health. A Guide to Foods Rich in Soy. Available online: https://www.ucsfhealth.org/education/a-guide-to-foods-rich-in-soy (accessed on 17 December 2020).
3. The Scientific Advisory Committee on Nutrition (SACN). *Statement on the Potential Risks from High Levels of Soya Phytoestrogens in the Infant Diet*; Committee on Toxicity of Chemicals in Food, Consumer Products and the Environment: London, UK, 2003.
4. Bhagwat, S.; Hayowitz, D.B.; Holden, J.M. *USDA Database for the Isoflavone Content of Selected Foods, Release 2.0*; US Department of Agriculture: Washington, DC, USA, 2008. [CrossRef]
5. Economic Research Service. ERS Charts of Note: Soybeans & Oil Crops. Available online: https://www.ers.usda.gov/data-products/charts-of-note/charts-of-note/?topicId=14851#:~:text=Brazil%20is%20a%20leading%20global,the%202018%2F19%20marketing%20year (accessed on 17 December 2020).
6. The Good Food Institute. Plant-Based Market Overview. Available online: https://www.gfi.org/marketresearch (accessed on 17 December 2020).
7. Coward, L.; Smith, M.; Kirk, M.; Barnes, S. Chemical modification of isoflavones in soyfoods during cooking and processing. *Am. J. Clin. Nutr.* **1998**, *68*, 1486S–1491S. [CrossRef]
8. King, R.; Bignell, C.M. Concentrations of isoflavone phytoestrogens and their glucosides in Australian soya beans and soya foods. *Aust. J. Nutr. Dietics* **2000**, *57*, 70–78.
9. Liggins, J.; Bluck, L.J.C.; Runswick, S.; Atkinson, C.; Coward, W.A.; Bingham, S.A. Daidzein and genistein contents of vegetables. *Br. J. Nutr.* **2007**, *84*, 717–725. [CrossRef]
10. Murphy, P.A.; Barua, K.; Hauck, C.C. Solvent extraction selection in the determination of isoflavones in soy foods. *J. Chromatogr. B Anal. Technol. Biomed. Life Sci.* **2002**, *777*, 129–138. [CrossRef]
11. Nguyenle, T.; Wang, E.; Cheung, A.P. An investigation on the extraction and concentration of isoflavones in soy-based products. *J. Pharm. Biomed. Anal.* **1995**, *14*, 221–232. [CrossRef]
12. Rostagno, M.A.; Palma, M.; Barroso, C.G. Fast analysis of soy isoflavones by high-performance liquid chromatography with monolithic columns. *Anal. Chim. Acta* **2007**, *582*, 243–249. [CrossRef] [PubMed]
13. Umphress, S.T.; Murphy, S.P.; Franke, A.A.; Custer, L.J.; Blitz, C.L. Isoflavone content of foods with soy additives. *J. Food Compos. Anal.* **2005**, *18*, 533–550. [CrossRef]
14. Wang, H.; Murphy, P.A. Isoflavone Content in Commercial Soybean Foods. *J. Agric. Food Chem.* **1994**, *42*, 1666–1673. [CrossRef]

15. Genovese, M.I.; Hassimoto, N.M.A.; Lajolo, F.M. Isoflavone profile and antioxidant activity of Brazilian soybean varieties. *Food Sci. Technol. Int.* **2005**, *11*, 205–211. [CrossRef]
16. Coward, L.; Barnes, N.C.; Setchell, K.D.R.; Barnes, S. Genistein, daidzein, and their beta-glycoside conjugates: Antitumor isoflavones in soybean foods from American and Asian diets. *J. Agric. Food Chem.* **1993**, *41*, 1961–1967. [CrossRef]
17. Chiou, R.Y.; Cheng, S.L. Isoflavone transformation during soybean koji preparation and subsequent miso fermentation supplemented with ethanol and NaCl. *J. Agric. Food Chem.* **2001**, *49*, 3656–3660. [CrossRef]
18. Charron, C.S.; Allen, F.L.; Johnson, R.D.; Pantalone, V.R.; Sams, C.E. Correlations of oil and protein with isoflavone concentration in soybean [*Glycine max* (L.) Merr.]. *J. Agric. Food Chem.* **2005**, *53*, 7128–7135. [CrossRef]
19. Murphy, P.A.; Barua, K.; Song, T. *Soy Isoflavones in Foods: Database Development*; American Chemical Society Symposium Series; American Chemical Society: Washington, DC, USA, 1998; pp. 138–149.
20. Xu, X.; Wang, H.J.; Murphy, P.A.; Cook, L.; Hendrich, S. Daidzein is a more bioavailable soymilk isoflavone than is genistein in adult women. *J. Nutr.* **1994**, *124*, 825–832. [CrossRef]
21. Achouri, A.; Boye, J.I.; Belanger, D. Soybean isoflavones: Efficacy of extraction conditions and effect of food type on extractability. *Food Res. Int.* **2005**, *38*, 1199–1204. [CrossRef]
22. Barnes, S.; Kirk, M.; Coward, L. Isoflavones and their conjugates in soy foods: Extraction conditions and analysis by HPLC-mass spectrometry. *J. Agric. Food Chem.* **1994**, *42*, 2466–2474. [CrossRef]
23. Franke, A.A.; Custer, L.J.; Wang, W.; Shi, C.Y. HPLC analysis of isoflavonoids and other phenolic agents from foods and from human fluids. *Proc. Soc. Exp. Biol. Med.* **1998**, *217*, 263–273. [CrossRef] [PubMed]
24. Coward, L.; Kirk, M.; Albin, N.; Barnes, S. Analysis of plasma isoflavones by reversed-phase HPLC-multiple reaction ion monitoring-mass spectrometry. *Clin. Chim. Acta* **1996**, *247*, 121–142. [CrossRef]
25. Downing, J.M.; Chung, O.K.; Seib, P.A.; Hubbard, J.D. Pressurized Solvent Extraction of Genistein and Its β-Glucoside Conjugates from Soybean Flours and Soy-Based Foods. *Cereal Chem.* **2007**, *84*, 44–47. [CrossRef]
26. Fang, N.; Yu, S.; Badger, T.M. Comprehensive Phytochemical Profile of Soy Protein Isolate. *J. Agric. Food Chem.* **2004**, *52*, 4012–4020. [CrossRef]
27. Seo, A.; Morr, C.V. Improved high-performance liquid chromatographic analysis of phenolic acids and isoflavonoids from soybean protein products. *J. Agric. Food Chem.* **1984**, *32*, 530–533. [CrossRef]
28. Wang, C.; Ma, Q.; Pagadala, S.; Sherrard, M.S.; Krishnan, P.G. Changes of isoflavones during processing of soy protein isolates. *J. Am. Oil Chem. Soc.* **1998**, *75*, 337–341. [CrossRef]
29. Wang, H.-J.; Murphy, P.A. Mass Balance Study of Isoflavones during Soybean Processing. *J. Agric. Food Chem.* **1996**, *44*, 2377–2383. [CrossRef]
30. Franke, A.A.; Hankin, J.H.; Yu, M.C.; Maskarinec, G.; Low, S.H.; Custer, L.J. Isoflavone levels in soy foods consumed by multiethnic populations in Singapore and Hawaii. *J. Agric. Food Chem.* **1999**, *47*, 977–986. [CrossRef] [PubMed]
31. Murphy, P.A.; Song, T.; Buseman, G.; Barua, K.; Beecher, G.R.; Trainer, D.; Holden, J. Isoflavones in Retail and Institutional Soy Foods. *J. Agric. Food Chem.* **1999**, *47*, 2697–2704. [CrossRef] [PubMed]
32. Choi, Y.S.; Lee, B.H.; Kim, J.H.; Kim, N.S. Concentration of phytoestrogens in soybeans and soybean products in Korea. *J. Sci. Food Agric.* **2000**, *80*, 1709–1712. [CrossRef]
33. Fukutake, M.; Takahashi, M.; Ishida, K.; Kawamura, H.; Sugimura, T.; Wakabayashi, K. Quantification of genistein and genistin in soybeans and soybean products. *Food Chem. Toxicol.* **1996**, *34*, 457–461. [CrossRef]
34. Murphy, P.A. Green soy beans (Edame, dry), Soy beans (small Jade Black), Natto (DHA), Natto (fermented soy beans), Soy bean butter (full fat), Natto Kibun, Soy nuts (full fat), Soy nuts (plain halves), Soy flakes (white, not roasted), Green soy beans (Edame, fresh). Daidzein, Genistein, Glycitein. Unpublished data.
35. Nakamura, Y.; Tsuji, S.; Tonogai, Y. Determination of the levels of isoflavonoids in soybeans and soy-derived foods and estimation of isoflavonoids in the Japanese daily intake. *J. AOAC Int.* **2000**, *83*, 635–650. [CrossRef]
36. Toda, T.; Sakamoto, A.; Takayanagi, T.; Yokotsuka, K. Changes in Isoflavone Compositions of Sobean Foods during Cooking Process. *Food Sci. Technol. Res.* **2000**, *6*, 314–319. [CrossRef]
37. Hutabarat, L.S.; Greenfield, H.; Mulholland, M. Isoflavones and Coumestrol in Soybeans and Soybean Products from Australia and Indonesia. *J. Food Compos. Anal.* **2001**, *14*, 43–58. [CrossRef]
38. Hutchins, A.M.; Slavin, J.L.; Lampe, J.W. Urinary isoflavonoid phytoestrogen and lignan Excretion After Consumption of Fermented and Unfermented Soy Products. *J. Am. Diet. Assoc.* **1995**, *95*, 545–551. [CrossRef]
39. Nakajima, N.; Nozaki, N.; Ishihara, K.; Ishikawa, A.; Tsuji, H. Analysis of isoflavone content in tempeh, a fermented soybean, and preparation of a new isoflavone-enriched tempeh. *J. Biosci. Bioeng.* **2005**, *100*, 685–687. [CrossRef] [PubMed]
40. Thompson, L.U.; Boucher, B.A.; Liu, Z.; Cotterchio, M.; Kreiger, N. Phytoestrogen Content of Foods Consumed in Canada, Including Isoflavones, Lignans, and Coumestan. *Nutr. Cancer* **2006**, *54*, 184–201. [CrossRef] [PubMed]
41. Lu, L.J.; Broemeling, L.D.; Marshall, M.V.; Ramanujam, V.M. A simplified method to quantify isoflavones in commercial soybean diets and human urine after legume consumption. *Cancer Epidemiol. Biomark. Prev.* **1995**, *4*, 497–503.
42. Mitani, K.; Narimatsu, S.; Kataoka, H. Determination of daidzein and genistein in soybean foods by automated on-line in-tube solid-phase microextraction coupled to high-performance liquid chromatography. *J. Chromatogr. A* **2003**, *986*, 169–177. [CrossRef]
43. Yamabe, S.; Kobayashi-Hattori, K.; Kaneko, K.; Endo, H.; Takita, T. Effect of soybean varieties on the content and composition of isoflavone in rice-koji miso. *Food Chem.* **2007**, *100*, 369–374. [CrossRef]

44. Pamela, L.H.-R.; Stephen, B.; Marion, L.; Lori, C.; Mandel, J.E.; Jocelyn, K.; Esther, M.J.; Michelle, S. Assessing Phytoestrogen Exposure in Epidemiologic Studies: Development of a Database (United States). *Cancer Causes Control* **2000**, *11*, 289–298. [CrossRef]
45. Lin, P.-Y.; Lai, H.-M. Bioactive Compounds in Legumes and Their Germinated Products. *J. Agric. Food Chem.* **2006**, *54*, 3807–3814. [CrossRef]
46. Müllner, C.; Sontag, G. Determination of some phytoestrogens in soybeans and their processed products with HPLC and coulometric electrode array detection. *Fresenius' J. Anal. Chem.* **1999**, *364*, 261–265. [CrossRef]
47. Nakamura, Y.; Kaihara, A.; Yoshii, K.; Tsumura, Y.; Ishimitsu, S.; Tonogai, Y. Content and Composition of Isoflavonoids in Mature or Immature Beans and Bean Sprouts Consumed in Japan. *J. Health Sci.* **2001**, *47*, 394–406. [CrossRef]
48. Plaza, L.; de Ancos, B.; Cano, P.M. Nutritional and health-related compounds in sprouts and seeds of soybean (*Glycine max*), wheat (*Triticum aestivum.L*) and alfalfa (*Medicago sativa*) treated by a new drying method. *Eur. Food Res. Technol.* **2003**, *216*, 138–144. [CrossRef]
49. Wang, G.; Kuan, S.S.; Francis, O.J.; Ware, G.M.; Carman, A.S. A simplified HPLC method for the determination of phytoestrogens in soybean and its processed products. *J. Agric. Food Chem.* **1990**, *38*, 185–190. [CrossRef]
50. Grün, I.U.; Adhikari, K.; Li, C.; Li, Y.; Lin, B.; Zhang, J.; Fernando, L.N. Changes in the Profile of Genistein, Daidzein, and Their Conjugates during Thermal Processing of Tofu. *J. Agric. Food Chem.* **2001**, *49*, 2839–2843. [CrossRef] [PubMed]
51. Krenn, L.; Unterrieder, I.; Ruprechter, R. Quantification of isoflavones in red clover by high-performance liquid chromatography. *J. Chromatogr. B Anal. Technol. Biomed. Life Sci.* **2002**, *777*, 123–128. [CrossRef]
52. Gentile, C.; Tesoriere, L.; Butera, D.; Fazzari, M.; Monastero, M.; Allegra, M.; Livrea, M.A. Antioxidant Activity of Sicilian Pistachio (Pistacia vera L. Var. Bronte) Nut Extract and Its Bioactive Components. *J. Agric. Food Chem.* **2007**, *55*, 643–648. [CrossRef]
53. Johns, P.; Dowlati, L.; Wargo, W. Determination of isoflavones in ready-to-feed soy-based infant formula. *J. AOAC Int.* **2003**, *86*, 72–78. [CrossRef]
54. Setchell, K.D.R.; Welsh, M.B.; Lim, C.K. High-performance liquid chromatographic analysis of phytoestrogens in soy protein preparations with ultraviolet, electrochemical and thermospray mass spectrometric detection. *J. Chromatogr. A* **1987**, *386*, 315–323. [CrossRef]
55. Franke, A.A.; Custer, L.J.; Cerna, C.M.; Narala, K. Rapid HPLC analysis of dietary phytoestrogens from legumes and from human urine. *Proc. Soc. Exp. Biol. Med.* **1995**, *208*, 18–26. [CrossRef]
56. Antonelli, M.L.; Faberi, A.; Pastorini, E.; Samperi, R.; Lagana, A. Simultaneous quantitation of free and conjugated phytoestrogens in Leguminosae by liquid chromatography-tandem mass spectrometry. *Talanta* **2005**, *66*, 1025–1033. [CrossRef]
57. Cao, Y.; Calafat, A.M.; Doerge, D.R.; Umbach, D.M.; Bernbaum, J.C.; Twaddle, N.C.; Ye, X.; Rogan, W.J. Isoflavones in urine, saliva, and blood of infants: Data from a pilot study on the estrogenic activity of soy formula. *J. Expo. Sci. Environ. Epidemiol.* **2008**, *19*, 223–234. [CrossRef]
58. Tseng, M.; Olufade, T.; Kurzer, M.S.; Wähälä, K.; Fang, C.Y.; van der Schouw, Y.T.; Daly, M.B. Food Frequency Questionnaires and Overnight Urines Are Valid Indicators of Daidzein and Genistein Intake in U.S. Women Relative to Multiple 24-h Urine Samples. *Nutr. Cancer* **2008**, *60*, 619–626. [CrossRef]
59. Van Erp-Baart, M.-A.J.; Brants, H.A.M.; Kiely, M.; Mulligan, A.; Turrini, A.; Sermoneta, C.; Kilkkinen, A.; Valsta, L.M. Isoflavone intake in four different European countries: The VENUS approach. *Br. J. Nutr.* **2003**, *89*, S25–S30. [CrossRef]
60. Huang, M.-H.; Luetters, C.; Buckwalter, G.J.; Seeman, T.E.; Gold, E.B.; Sternfeld, B.; Greendale, G.A. Dietary genistein intake and cognitive performance in a multiethnic cohort of midlife women. *Menopause* **2006**, *13*, 621–630. [CrossRef]
61. Yamamoto, S.; Sobue, T.; Sasaki, S.; Kobayashi, M.; Arai, Y.; Uehara, M.; Adlercreutz, H.; Watanabe, S.; Takahashi, T.; Iitoi, Y.; et al. Validity and reproducibility of a self-administered food-frequency questionnaire to assess isoflavone intake in a japanese population in comparison with dietary records and blood and urine isoflavones. *J. Nutr.* **2001**, *131*, 2741–2747. [CrossRef] [PubMed]
62. Lee, S.A.; Wen, W.; Xiang, Y.B.; Barnes, S.; Liu, D.; Cai, Q.; Zheng, W.; Shu, X.O. Assessment of dietary isoflavone intake among middle-aged Chinese men. *J. Nutr.* **2007**, *137*, 1011–1016. [CrossRef]
63. Verkasalo, P.K.; Appleby, P.N.; Allen, N.E.; Davey, G.; Adlercreutz, H.; Key, T.J. Soya intake and plasma concentrations of daidzein and genistein: Validity of dietary assessment among eighty British women (Oxford arm of the European Prospective Investigation into Cancer and Nutrition). *Br. J. Nutr.* **2001**, *86*, 415–421. [CrossRef] [PubMed]
64. Adlercreutz, H.; Yamada, T.; Wähälä, K.; Watanabe, S. Maternal and neonatal phytoestrogens in Japanese women during birth. *Am. J. Obstet. Gynecol.* **1999**, *180*, 737–743. [CrossRef]
65. Newton, J.; Nelson, M. China Uses One-Third of World's Soybeans. Available online: https://www.fb.org/market-intel/china-uses-one-third-of-worlds-soybeans (accessed on 17 December 2020).
66. Rosell, M.S.; Appleby, P.N.; Spencer, E.A.; Key, T.J. Soy intake and blood cholesterol concentrations: A cross-sectional study of 1033 pre- and postmenopausal women in the Oxford arm of the European Prospective Investigation into Cancer and Nutrition. *Am. J. Clin. Nutr.* **2004**, *80*, 1391–1396. [CrossRef] [PubMed]
67. Tempfer, C.B.M.D.; Bentz, E.-K.M.D.; Leodolter, S.M.D.; Tscherne, G.M.D.; Reuss, F.M.D.; Cross, H.S.; Huber, J.C. Phytoestrogens in clinical practice: A review of the literature. *Fertil. Steril.* **2007**, *87*, 1243–1249. [CrossRef]
68. Kurzer, M.S.; Xu, X. Dietary Phytoestrogens. *Annu. Rev. Nutr.* **1997**, *17*, 353–381. [CrossRef]

69. Barrett, A. Long-Term World Soybean Outlook. Available online: https://ussoy.org/long-term-world-soybean-outlook/#:~:text=The%20increase%20in%20world%20meat,of%20coarse%20grains%20and%20soybeans.&text=Global%20soybean%20utilization%20is%20estimated,in%20second%20at%2061%20MMT (accessed on 17 December 2020).
70. Walsh, K.R.; Haak, S.J.; Bohn, T.; Tian, Q.; Schwartz, S.J.; Failla, M.L. Isoflavonoid glucosides are deconjugated and absorbed in the small intestine of human subjects with ileostomies. *Am. J. Clin. Nutr.* **2007**, *85*, 1050–1056. [CrossRef]
71. Bokkenheuser, V.D.; Shackleton, C.H.L.; Winter, J. Hydrolysis of dietary flavonoid glycosides by strains of intestinal Bacteroides from humans. *Biochem. J.* **1987**, *248*, 953–956. [CrossRef]
72. Mattison, D.R.; Karyakina, N.; Goodman, M.; LaKind, J.S. Pharmaco- and toxicokinetics of selected exogenous and endogenous estrogens: A review of the data and identification of knowledge gaps. *Crit. Rev. Toxicol.* **2014**, *44*, 696–724. [CrossRef]
73. Hu, M. Commentary: Bioavailability of Flavonoids and Polyphenols: Call to Arms. *Mol. Pharm.* **2007**, *4*, 803–806. [CrossRef] [PubMed]
74. Liu, Y.; Hu, M. Absorption and metabolism of flavonoids in the caco-2 cell culture model and a perused rat intestinal model. *Drug Metab. Dispos.* **2002**, *30*, 370–377. [CrossRef]
75. Rozman, K.K.; Bhatia, J.; Calafat, A.M.; Chambers, C.; Culty, M.; Etzel, R.A.; Flaws, J.A.; Hansen, D.K.; Hoyer, P.B.; Jeffery, E.H.; et al. NTP-CERHR expert panel report on the reproductive and developmental toxicity of genistein. *Birth Defects Res. Part. B Dev. Reprod. Toxicol.* **2006**, *77*, 485–638. [CrossRef]
76. Yang, Z.; Zhu, W.; Gao, S.; Xu, H.; Wu, B.; Kulkarni, K.; Singh, R.; Tang, L.; Hu, M. Simultaneous determination of genistein and its four phase II metabolites in blood by a sensitive and robust UPLC–MS/MS method: Application to an oral bioavailability study of genistein in mice. *J. Pharm. Biomed. Anal.* **2010**, *53*, 81–89. [CrossRef]
77. Setchell, K.D.R.; Brown, N.M.; Desai, P.; Zimmer-Nechemias, L.; Wolfe, B.E.; Brashear, W.T.; Kirschner, A.S.; Cassidy, A.; Heubi, J.E. Bioavailability of Pure Isoflavones in Healthy Humans and Analysis of Commercial Soy Isoflavone Supplements. *J. Nutr.* **2001**, *131*, 1362S–1375S. [CrossRef]
78. Riches, Z.; Stanley, E.L.; Bloomer, J.C.; Coughtrie, M.W.H. Quantitative Evaluation of the Expression and Activity of Five Major Sulfotransferases (SULTs) in Human Tissues: The SULT "Pie". *Drug Metab. Dispos.* **2009**, *37*, 2255–2261. [CrossRef]
79. Boonpawa, R.; Spenkelink, A.; Punt, A.; Rietjens, I.M.C.M. In vitro-in silico-based analysis of the dose-dependent *in vivo* oestrogenicity of the soy phytoestrogen genistein in humans. *Br. J. Pharmacol.* **2017**, *174*, 2739–2757. [CrossRef]
80. Liu, J.; Yu, X.; Zhong, S.; Han, W.; Liang, Z.; Ye, L.; Zhao, J.; Liu, M.; Liu, S.; Wei, Q.; et al. Hepatic and renal metabolism of genistein: An individual-based model to predict glucuronidation behavior of genistein in different organs. *J. Pharm. Biomed. Anal.* **2017**, *139*, 252–262. [CrossRef]
81. Kurkela, M.; Garcia-Horsmant, J.A.; Luukkanen, L.; Mörsky, S.; Taskinen, J.; Baumann, M.; Kostiainen, R.; Hirvonen, J.; Finel, M. Expression and characterization of recombinant human UDP-glucuronosyltransferases (UGTs): UGT1A9 is more resistant to detergent inhibition than the other UGTs and was purified as an active dimeric enzyme. *J. Biol. Chem.* **2003**, *278*, 3536–3544. [CrossRef]
82. Yuan, B.; Zhen, H.; Jin, Y.; Xu, L.; Jiang, X.; Sun, S.; Li, C.; Xu, H. Absorption and Plasma Disposition of Genistin Differ from Those of Genistein in Healthy Women. *J. Agric. Food Chem.* **2012**, *60*, 1428–1436. [CrossRef] [PubMed]
83. Chang, Y.-C.; Nair, M.G. Metabolism of Daidzein and Genistein by Intestinal Bacteria. *J. Nat. Prod.* **1995**, *58*, 1892–1896. [CrossRef] [PubMed]
84. Kulling, S.E.; Honig, D.M.; Metzler, M. Oxidative Metabolism of the Soy Isoflavones Daidzein and Genistein in Humans *in Vitro* and *in Vivo*. *J. Agric. Food Chem.* **2001**, *49*, 3024–3033. [CrossRef]
85. Bursztyka, J.; Perdu, E.; Tulliez, J.; Debrauwer, L.; Delous, G.; Canlet, C.; De Sousa, G.; Rahmani, R.; Benfenati, E.; Cravedi, J.-P. Comparison of genistein metabolism in rats and humans using liver microsomes and hepatocytes. *Food Chem. Toxicol.* **2008**, *46*, 939–948. [CrossRef]
86. Breinholt, V.M.; Rasmussen, S.E.; Brosen, K.; Friedberg, T.H. *In vitro* Metabolism of Genistein and Tangeretin by Human and Murine Cytochrome P450s. *Pharmacol. Toxicol.* **2003**, *93*, 14–22. [CrossRef]
87. Hu, M.; Krausz, K.; Chen, J.; Ge, X.; Li, J.; Gelboin, H.L.; Gonzalez, F.J. Identification of cyp1a2 as the main isoform for the phase i hydroxylated metabolism of genistein and a prodrug converting enzyme of methylated isoflavones. *Drug Metab. Dispos.* **2003**, *31*, 924–931. [CrossRef]
88. Matthies, A.; Blaut, M.; Braune, A. Isolation of a human intestinal bacterium capable of daidzein and genistein conversion. *Appl. Environ. Microbiol.* **2009**, *75*, 1740–1744. [CrossRef]
89. Hosoda, K.; Furuta, T.; Yokokawa, A.; Ishii, K. Identification and quantification of daidzein-7-glucuronide-4′-sulfate, genistein-7-glucuronide-4′-sulfate and genistein-4′,7-diglucuronide as major metabolites in human plasma after administration of kinako. *Anal. Bioanal. Chem.* **2010**, *397*, 1563–1572. [CrossRef]
90. Munro, I.C.; Harwood, M.; Hlywka, J.J.; Stephen, A.M.; Doull, J.; Flamm, W.G.; Adlercreutz, H. Soy Isoflavones: A Safety Review. *Nutr. Rev.* **2003**, *61*, 1–33. [CrossRef]
91. Hoey, L.; Rowland, I.R.; Lloyd, A.S.; Clarke, D.B.; Wiseman, H. Influence of soya-based infant formula consumption on isoflavone and gut microflora metabolite concentrations in urine and on faecal microflora composition and metabolic activity in infants and children. *Br. J. Nutr.* **2004**, *91*, 607–616. [CrossRef] [PubMed]
92. Jackson, R.L.; Greiwe, J.S.; Schwen, R.J. Emerging evidence of the health benefits of S-equol, an estrogen receptor beta agonist. *Nutr. Rev.* **2011**, *69*, 432–448. [CrossRef]

93. Choi, E.J.; Kim, G.H. The antioxidant activity of daidzein metabolites, Odesmethylangolensin and equol, in HepG2 cells. *Mol. Med. Rep.* **2014**, *9*, 328–332. [CrossRef]
94. Wei, X.J.; Wu, J.; Ni, Y.D.; Lu, L.Z.; Zhao, R.Q. Antioxidant effect of a phytoestrogen equol on cultured muscle cells of embryonic broilers. *Vitr. Cell Dev. Biol. Anim.* **2011**, *47*, 735–741. [CrossRef]
95. Arora, A.; Nair, M.G.; Strasburg, G.M. Antioxidant Activities of Isoflavones and Their Biological Metabolites in a Liposomal System. *Arch. Biochem. Biophys.* **1998**, *356*, 133–141. [CrossRef]
96. Mayo, B.; Vazquez, L.; Belen Florez, A. Equol: A Bacterial Metabolite from The Daidzein Isoflavone and Its Presumed Beneficial Health Effects. *Nutrients* **2019**, *11*, 2231. [CrossRef] [PubMed]
97. Kuiper, G.G.J.M.; Lemmen, J.G.; Carlsson, B.; Corton, J.C.; Safe, S.H.; van der Saag, P.T.; van der Burg, B.; Gustafsson, J.-Å. Interaction of Estrogenic Chemicals and Phytoestrogens with Estrogen Receptor β. *Endocrinology* **1998**, *139*, 4252–4263. [CrossRef] [PubMed]
98. Koenig, A.; Buskiewicz, I.; Huber, S.A. Age-associated changes in estrogen receptor ratios correlate with increased female susceptibility to coxsackievirus B3-induced myocarditis. *Front. Immunol.* **2017**, *8*, 1585. [CrossRef] [PubMed]
99. Qing, X.; Zhihong, L.; You-Hong, C.; Chiang-Ching, H.; Erica, M.; Ping, Y.; Magdy, P.M.; Edmond, C.; Scott, R.; Joy, I.; et al. Promoter Methylation Regulates Estrogen Receptor 2 in Human Endometrium and Endometriosis. *Biol. Reprod.* **2007**, *77*, 681–687. [CrossRef]
100. Abbasi, S. Estrogen Receptor-Beta Gene Polymorphism in women with Breast Cancer at the Imam Khomeini Hospital Complex, Iran. *BMC Med. Genet.* **2010**, *11*, 109. [CrossRef]
101. Maggiolini, M.; Vivacqua, A.; Fasanella, G.; Recchia, A.G.; Sisci, D.; Pezzi, V.; Montanaro, D.; Musti, A.M.; Picard, D.; Ando, S. The G protein-coupled receptor GPR30 mediates c-fos up-regulation by 17beta-estradiol and phytoestrogens in breast cancer cells. *J. Biol. Chem.* **2004**, *279*, 27008–27016. [CrossRef] [PubMed]
102. Thomas, P.; Pang, Y.; Filardo, E.J.; Dong, J. Identity of an estrogen membrane receptor coupled to a G protein in human breast cancer cells. *Endocrinology* **2005**, *146*, 624–632. [CrossRef] [PubMed]
103. Du, Z.-R.; Feng, X.-Q.; Li, N.; Qu, J.-X.; Feng, L.; Chen, L.; Chen, W.-F. G protein-coupled estrogen receptor is involved in the anti-inflammatory effects of genistein in microglia. *Phytomedicine* **2018**, *43*, 11–20. [CrossRef]
104. Okura, A.; Arakawa, H.; Oka, H.; Yoshinari, T.; Monden, Y. Effect of genistein on topoisomerase activity and on the growth of [VAL 12]Ha- ras-transformed NIH 3T3 cells. *Biochem. Biophys. Res. Commun.* **1988**, *157*, 183–189. [CrossRef]
105. Johnson, A.; Roberts, L.; Elkins, G. Complementary and Alternative Medicine for Menopause. *J. Evid. Based Integr. Med.* **2019**, *24*, 2515690X19829380. [CrossRef]
106. Sobhy, M.M.K.; Mahmoud, S.S.; El-Sayed, S.H.; Rizk, E.M.A.; Raafat, A.; Negm, M.S.I. Impact of treatment with a Protein Tyrosine Kinase Inhibitor (Genistein) on acute and chronic experimental Schistosoma mansoni infection. *Exp. Parasitol.* **2018**, *185*, 115–123. [CrossRef]
107. Evans, B.A.; Griffiths, K.; Morton, M.S. Inhibition of 5 alpha-reductase in genital skin fibroblasts and prostate tissue by dietary lignans and isoflavonoids. *J. Endocrinol.* **1995**, *147*, 295–302. [CrossRef]
108. Barnes, S. Effect of genistein on *in vitro* and *in vivo* models of cancer. *J. Nutr.* **1995**, *125*, 777S–783S. [CrossRef]
109. Messing, E.; Gee, J.R.; Saltzstein, D.R.; Kim, K.; DiSant'Agnese, A.; Kolesar, J.; Harris, L.; Faerber, A.; Havighurst, T.; Young, J.M.; et al. A phase 2 cancer chemoprevention biomarker trial of isoflavone G-2535 (genistein) in presurgical bladder cancer patients. *Cancer Prev. Res.* **2012**, *5*, 621–630. [CrossRef]
110. Rüfer, C.E.; Kulling, S.E. Antioxidant Activity of Isoflavones and Their Major Metabolites Using Different *in Vitro* Assays. *J. Agric. Food Chem.* **2006**, *54*, 2926–2931. [CrossRef]
111. De Gregorio, C.; Marini, H.; Alibrandi, A.; Di Benedetto, A.; Bitto, A.; Adamo, E.B.; Altavilla, D.; Irace, C.; Di Vieste, G.; Pancaldo, D.; et al. Genistein supplementation and cardiac function in postmenopausal women with metabolic syndrome: Results from a pilot strain-echo study. *Nutrients* **2017**, *9*, 584. [CrossRef]
112. Borradaile, N.M.; De Dreu, L.E.; Wilcox, L.J.; Edwards, J.Y.; Huff, M.W. Soya phytoestrogens, genistein and daidzein, decrease apolipoprotein B secretion from HepG2 cells through multiple mechanisms. *Biochem. J.* **2002**, *366*, 531–539. [CrossRef]
113. Turner, R.T.; Iwaniec, U.T.; Andrade, J.E.; Branscum, A.J.; Neese, S.L.; Olson, D.A.; Wagner, L.; Wang, V.C.; Schantz, S.L.; Helferich, W.G. Genistein administered as a once-daily oral supplement had no beneficial effect on the tibia in rat models for postmenopausal bone loss. *Menopause* **2013**, *20*, 677–686. [CrossRef]
114. Thangavel, P.; Puga-Olguín, A.; Rodríguez-Landa, J.F.; Zepeda, R.C. Genistein as Potential Therapeutic Candidate for Menopausal Symptoms and Other Related Diseases. *Molecules* **2019**, *24*, 3892. [CrossRef]
115. Odle, B.; Dennison, N.; Al-Nakkash, L.; Broderick, T.L.; Plochocki, J.H. Genistein treatment improves fracture resistance in obese diabetic mice. *BMC Endocr. Disord.* **2017**, *17*, 55. [CrossRef]
116. Singh, P.; Sharma, S.; Kumar Rath, S. Genistein Induces Deleterious Effects during Its Acute Exposure in Swiss Mice. *Biomed. Res. Int.* **2014**, *2014*, 619617. [CrossRef] [PubMed]
117. Wisniewski, A.B.; Klein, S.L.; Lakshmanan, Y.; Gearhart, J.P. Exposure to Genistein During Gestation and Lactation Demasculinizes the Reproductive System in Rats. *J. Urol.* **2003**, *169*, 1582–1586. [CrossRef]
118. Lewis, R.W.; Brooks, N.; Milburn, G.M.; Soames, A.; Stone, S.; Hall, M.; Ashby, J. The effects of the phytoestrogen genistein on the postnatal development of the rat. *Toxicol. Sci.* **2003**, *71*, 74–83. [CrossRef] [PubMed]

119. Kerrie, B.B.; Leena, H.-C. Genistein: Does It Prevent or Promote Breast Cancer? *Environ. Health Perspect.* **2000**, *108*, 701–708. [CrossRef]
120. Korde, L.A.; Wu, A.H.; Fears, T.; Nomura, A.M.Y.; West, D.W.; Kolonel, L.N.; Pike, M.C.; Hoover, R.N.; Ziegler, R.G. Childhood Soy Intake and Breast Cancer Risk in Asian American Women. *Cancer Epidemiol. Biomark. Prev.* **2009**, *18*, 1050–1059. [CrossRef] [PubMed]
121. Joanne, T.; Michelle, C.; Beatrice, A.B.; Nancy, K.; Lilian, U.T. Adolescent Dietary Phytoestrogen Intake and Breast Cancer Risk (Canada). *Cancer Causes Control* **2006**, *17*, 1253–1261. [CrossRef]
122. Yatani, R.; Chigusa, I.; Akazaki, K.; Stemmermann, G.N.; Welsh, R.A.; Correa, P. Geographic pathology of latent prostatic carcinoma. *Int. J. Cancer* **1982**, *29*, 611–616. [CrossRef]
123. Messina, M.; Nagata, C.; Wu, A.H. Estimated Asian Adult Soy Protein and Isoflavone Intakes. *Nutr. Cancer* **2006**, *55*, 1–12. [CrossRef]
124. Tham, D.M.; Gardner, C.D.; Haskell, W.L. Clinical review 97-Potential health benefits of dietary phytoestrogens: A review of the clinical, epidemiological, and mechanistic evidence. *J. Clin. Endocrinol. Metab.* **1998**, *83*, 2223–2235. [CrossRef] [PubMed]
125. Akiyama, T.; Ishida, J.; Nakagawa, S.; Ogawara, H.; Watanabe, S.; Itoh, N.; Shibuya, M.; Fukami, Y. Genistein, a specific inhibitor of tyrosine-specific protein kinases. *J. Biol. Chem.* **1987**, *262*, 5592–5595. [CrossRef]
126. Agarwal, R. Cell signaling and regulators of cell cycle as molecular targets for prostate cancer prevention by dietary agents. *Biochem. Pharmacol.* **2000**, *60*, 1051–1059. [CrossRef]
127. Chen, W.-F.; Wong, M.-S. Genistein Enhances Insulin-Like Growth Factor Signaling Pathway in Human Breast Cancer (MCF-7) Cells. *J. Clin. Endocrinol. Metab.* **2004**, *89*, 2351–2359. [CrossRef] [PubMed]
128. Wang, T.T.Y.; Sathyamoorthy, N.; Phang, J.M. Molecular effects of genistein on estrogen receptor mediated pathways. *Carcinogenesis* **1996**, *17*, 271–275. [CrossRef] [PubMed]
129. Moore, A.B.; Castro, L.; Yu, L.; Zheng, X.; Di, X.; Sifre, M.I.; Kissling, G.E.; Newbold, R.R.; Bortner, C.D.; Dixon, D. Stimulatory and inhibitory effects of genistein on human uterine leiomyoma cell proliferation are influenced by the concentration. *Hum. Reprod.* **2007**, *22*, 2623–2631. [CrossRef] [PubMed]
130. Kohara, Y.; Kuwahara, R.; Kawaguchi, S.; Jojima, T.; Yamashita, K. Perinatal exposure to genistein, a soy phytoestrogen, improves spatial learning and memory but impairs passive avoidance learning and memory in offspring. *Physiol. Behav.* **2014**, *130*, 40–46. [CrossRef] [PubMed]
131. Vandenberg, L.N. Non-Monotonic Dose Responses in Studies of Endocrine Disrupting Chemicals: Bisphenol a as a Case Study. *Dose-Response* **2013**, *12*, 259–276. [CrossRef] [PubMed]
132. Hussain, A.; Harish, G.; Prabhu, S.A.; Mohsin, J.; Khan, M.A.; Rizvi, T.A.; Sharma, C. Inhibitory effect of genistein on the invasive potential of human cervical cancer cells via modulation of matrix metalloproteinase-9 and tissue inhibitiors of matrix metalloproteinase-1 expression. *Cancer Epidemiol.* **2012**, *36*, e387–e393. [CrossRef]
133. Chen, H.-H.; Chen, S.-P.; Zheng, Q.-L.; Nie, S.-P.; Li, W.-J.; Hu, X.-J.; Xie, M.-Y. Genistein promotes proliferation of human cervical cancer cells through estrogen receptor-mediated PI3K/Akt-NF-κB pathway. *J. Cancer* **2018**, *9*, 288–295. [CrossRef]
134. Shen, H.-H.; Huang, S.-Y.; Kung, C.-W.; Chen, S.-Y.; Chen, Y.-F.; Cheng, P.-Y.; Lam, K.-K.; Lee, Y.-M. Genistein ameliorated obesity accompanied with adipose tissue browning and attenuation of hepatic lipogenesis in ovariectomized rats with high-fat diet. *J. Nutr. Biochem.* **2019**, *67*, 111–122. [CrossRef] [PubMed]
135. Kim, H.K.; Nelson-Dooley, C.; Della-Fera, M.A.; Yang, J.Y.; Zhang, W.; Duan, J.; Hartzell, D.L.; Hamrick, M.W.; Baile, C.A. Genistein decreases food intake, body weight, and fat pad weight and causes adipose tissue apoptosis in ovariectomized female mice. *J. Nutr.* **2006**, *136*, 409–414. [CrossRef] [PubMed]
136. Naaz, A.; Yellayi, S.; Zakroczymski, M.A.; Bunick, D.; Doerge, D.R.; Lubahn, D.B.; Helferich, W.G.; Cooke, P.S. The Soy Isoflavone Genistein Decreases Adipose Deposition in Mice. *Endocrinology* **2003**, *144*, 3315–3320. [CrossRef]
137. Dolinoy, D.C.; Weidman, J.R.; Waterland, R.A.; Jirtle, R.L. Maternal genistein alters coat color and protects A(vy) mouse offspring from obesity by modifying the fetal epigenome. *Environ. Health Perspect.* **2006**, *114*, 567–572. [CrossRef]
138. Chang, H.C.; Doerge, D.R. Dietary genistein inactivates rat thyroid peroxidase *in vivo* without an apparent hypothyroid effect. *Toxicol. Appl. Pharm.* **2000**, *168*, 244–252. [CrossRef] [PubMed]
139. Nogowski, L.; Nowak, K.W.; Kaczmarek, P.; Mackowiak, P. The influence of coumestrol, zearalenone, and genistein administration on insulin receptors and insulin secretion in ovariectomized rats. *J. Recept. Signal. Transduct. Res.* **2002**, *22*, 449–457. [CrossRef] [PubMed]
140. Tsai, Y.C.; Leu, S.Y.; Peng, Y.J.; Lee, Y.M.; Hsu, C.H.; Chou, S.C.; Yen, M.H.; Cheng, P.Y. Genistein suppresses leptin-induced proliferation and migration of vascular smooth muscle cells and neointima formation. *J. Cell. Mol. Med.* **2017**, *21*, 422–431. [CrossRef] [PubMed]
141. Yang, H.; Lee, S.H.; Ji, H.; Kim, J.-E.; Yoo, R.; Kim, J.H.; Suk, S.; Huh, C.S.; Park, J.H.Y.; Heo, Y.-S.; et al. Orobol, an Enzyme-Convertible Product of Genistein, exerts Anti-Obesity Effects by Targeting Casein Kinase 1 Epsilon. *Sci. Rep.* **2019**, *9*, 8942. [CrossRef]
142. Skov, A.R.; Toubro, S.; Ronn, B.; Holm, L.; Astrup, A. Randomized trial on protein vs carbohydrate in ad libitum fat reduced diet for the treatment of obesity. *Int. J. Obes. Relat. Metab. Disord.* **1999**, *23*, 528–536. [CrossRef]
143. Velasquez, M.T.; Bhathena, S.J. Role of Dietary Soy Protein in Obesity. *Int. J. Med. Sci.* **2007**, *4*, 72–82. [CrossRef]

144. Mikkelsen, P.B.; Toubro, S.; Astrup, A. Effect of fat-reduced diets on 24-h energy expenditure: Comparisons between animal protein, vegetable protein, and carbohydrate. *Am. J. Clin. Nutr.* **2000**, *72*, 1135–1141. [CrossRef]
145. Bosello, O.; Cominacini, L.; Zocca, I.; Garbin, U.; Compri, R.; Davoli, A.; Brunetti, L. Short- and long-term effects of hypocaloric diets containing proteins of different sources on plasma lipids and apoproteins of obese subjects. *Ann. Nutr. Metab.* **1988**, *32*, 206–214. [CrossRef]
146. Yamashita, T.; Sasahara, T.; Pomeroy, S.E.; Collier, G.; Nestel, P.J. Arterial compliance, blood pressure, plasma leptin, and plasma lipids in women are improved with weight reduction equally with a meat-based diet and a plant-based diet. *Metabolism* **1998**, *47*, 1308–1314. [CrossRef]
147. Anderson, J.W.; Hoie, L.H. Weight loss and lipid changes with low-energy diets: Comparator study of milk-based versus soy-based liquid meal replacement interventions. *J. Am. Coll. Nutr.* **2005**, *24*, 210–216. [CrossRef]
148. Akhlaghi, M.; Zare, M.; Nouripour, F. Effect of Soy and Soy Isoflavones on Obesity-Related Anthropometric Measures: A Systematic Review and Meta-analysis of Randomized Controlled Clinical Trials. *Adv. Nutr.* **2017**, *8*, 705–717. [CrossRef] [PubMed]
149. Banerjee, S.; Li, Y.; Wang, Z.; Sarkar, F.H. Multi-targeted therapy of cancer by genistein. *Cancer Lett.* **2008**, *269*, 226–242. [CrossRef] [PubMed]
150. Mai, Z.; Blackburn, G.L.; Zhou, J.R. Genistein sensitizes inhibitory effect of tamoxifen on the growth of estrogen receptor-positive and HER2-overexpressing human breast cancer cells. *Mol. Carcinog.* **2007**, *46*, 534–542. [CrossRef]
151. Pons, D.G.; Nadal-Serrano, M.; Torrens-Mas, M.; Oliver, J.; Roca, P. The Phytoestrogen Genistein Affects Breast Cancer Cells Treatment Depending on the ERα/ERβ Ratio. *J. Cell. Biochem.* **2016**, *117*, 218–229. [CrossRef] [PubMed]
152. Hilakivi-Clarke, L.; Andrade, J.E.; Helferich, W. Is Soy Consumption Good or Bad for the Breast? *J. Nutr.* **2010**, *140*, 2326S–2334S. [CrossRef]
153. Liu, R.; Yu, X.; Chen, X.; Zhong, H.; Liang, C.; Xu, X.; Xu, W.; Cheng, Y.; Wang, W.; Yu, L.; et al. Individual factors define the overall effects of dietary genistein exposure on breast cancer patients. *Nutr. Res.* **2019**, *67*, 1–16. [CrossRef]
154. Castro, L.; Gao, X.; Moore, A.B.; Yu, L.; Di, X.; Kissling, G.E.; Dixon, D. A High Concentration of Genistein Induces Cell Death in Human Uterine Leiomyoma Cells by Autophagy. *Expert Opin. Environ. Biol.* **2016**, *5* (Suppl. 1), 10.4172/2325-9655.S1-003. [CrossRef] [PubMed]
155. Di, X.; Andrews, D.M.K.; Tucker, C.J.; Yu, L.; Moore, A.B.; Zheng, X.; Castro, L.; Hermon, T.; Xiao, H.; Dixon, D. A high concentration of genistein down-regulates activin A, Smad3 and other TGF-β pathway genes in human uterine leiomyoma cells. *Exp. Mol. Med.* **2012**, *44*, 281–292. [CrossRef]
156. Miyake, A.; Takeda, T.; Isobe, A.; Wakabayashi, A.; Nishimoto, F.; Morishige, K.-I.; Sakata, M.; Kimura, T. Repressive effect of the phytoestrogen genistein on estradiol-induced uterine leiomyoma cell proliferation. *Gynecol. Endocrinol.* **2009**, *25*, 403–409. [CrossRef] [PubMed]
157. Di, X.; Yu, L.; Moore, A.B.; Castro, L.; Zheng, X.; Hermon, T.; Dixon, D. A low concentration of genistein induces estrogen receptor-alpha and insulin-like growth factor-I receptor interactions and proliferation in uterine leiomyoma cells. *Hum. Reprod.* **2008**, *23*, 1873–1883. [CrossRef]
158. Yu, L.; Ham, K.; Gao, X.; Castro, L.; Yan, Y.; Kissling, G.E.; Tucker, C.J.; Flagler, N.; Dong, R.; Archer, T.K.; et al. Epigenetic regulation of transcription factor promoter regions by low-dose genistein through mitogen-activated protein kinase and mitogen-and-stress activated kinase 1 nongenomic signaling. *Cell Commun. Signal.* **2016**, *14*, 18. [CrossRef]
159. Simon, G.A.; Fletcher, H.M.; Golden, K.; McFarlane-Anderson, N.D. Urinary isoflavone and lignan phytoestrogen levels and risk of uterine fibroid in Jamaican women. *Maturitas* **2015**, *82*, 170–175. [CrossRef] [PubMed]
160. Kennedy, S.; Bergqvist, A.; Chapron, C.; D'Hooghe, T.; Dunselman, G.; Greb, R.; Hummelshoj, L.; Prentice, A.; Saridogan, E. ESHRE guideline for the diagnosis and treatment of endometriosis. *Hum. Reprod.* **2005**, *20*, 2698–2704. [CrossRef]
161. Bitto, A.; Granese, R.; Polito, F.; Triolo, O.; Giordano, D.; Squadrito, F.; D'Anna, R.; Santamaria, A. Genistein reduces angiogenesis and apoptosis in women with endometrial hyperplasia. *Botanics* **2015**, *5*, 27–32. [CrossRef]
162. Mumford, S.L.; Weck, J.; Kannan, K.; Louis, G.M.B. Urinary phytoestrogen concentrations are not associated with incident endometriosis in premenopausal women. *J. Nutr.* **2017**, *147*, 227–234. [CrossRef]
163. Tsuchiya, M.; Miura, T.; Hanaoka, T.; Iwasaki, M.; Sasaki, H.; Tanaka, T.; Nakao, H.; Katoh, T.; Ikenoue, T.; Kabuto, M.; et al. Effect of soy isoflavones on endometriosis: Interaction with estrogen receptor 2 gene polymorphism. *Epidemiology* **2007**, *18*, 402–408. [CrossRef]
164. Yen, C.F.; Kim, M.R.; Lee, C.L. Epidemiologic Factors Associated with Endometriosis in East Asia. *Gynecol. Minim. Invasive* **2019**, *8*, 4–11. [CrossRef]
165. Cotronero, M.S.; Lamartiniere, C.A. Pharmacologic, but not dietary, genistein supports endometriosis in a rat model. *Toxicol. Sci.* **2001**, *61*, 68–75. [CrossRef]
166. Yavuz, E.M.D.; Oktem, M.M.D.; Esinler, I.M.D.; Toru, S.A.M.D.; Zeyneloglu, H.B.M.D. Genistein causes regression of endometriotic implants in the rat model. *Fertil. Steril.* **2007**, *88*, 1129–1134. [CrossRef] [PubMed]
167. Sutrisno, S.; Wulandari, R.R.C.L.; Sulistyowati, D.W.W.; Wulandari, R.F.; Wahyuni, E.S.; Yueniwati, Y.; Santoso, S. Effect of genistein on proinflammatory cytokines and estrogen receptor-β in mice model of endometriosis. *Asian Pac. J. Reprod.* **2015**, *4*, 96–99. [CrossRef]

168. Sutrisno, S.; Sulistyorini, C.; Manungkalit, E.M.; Winarsih, L.; Noorhamdani, N.; Winarsih, S. The effect of genistein on TGF-β signal, dysregulation of apoptosis, cyclooxygenase-2 pathway, and NF-kB pathway in mice peritoneum of endometriosis model. *Middle East. Fertil. Soc. J.* **2017**, *22*, 295–299. [CrossRef]
169. Bray, F.; Ferlay, J.; Soerjomataram, I.; Siegel, R.L.; Torre, L.A.; Jemal, A. Global cancer statistics 2018: GLOBOCAN estimates of incidence and mortality worldwide for 36 cancers in 185 countries. *CA Cancer J. Clin.* **2018**, *68*, 394–424. [CrossRef] [PubMed]
170. Morice, P.D.P.; Leary, A.M.D.; Creutzberg, C.P.; Abu-Rustum, N.P.; Darai, E.P. Endometrial cancer. *Lancet* **2015**, *387*, 1094–1108. [CrossRef]
171. Malloy, K.M.; Wang, J.; Clark, L.H.; Fang, Z.; Sun, W.; Yin, Y.; Kong, W.; Zhou, C.X.; Bae-Jump, V.L. Novasoy and genistein inhibit endometrial cancer cell proliferation through disruption of the AKT/mTOR and MAPK signaling pathways. *Am. J. Transl. Res.* **2018**, *10*, 784–795. [PubMed]
172. Konstantakopoulos, N.; Montgomery, K.G.; Chamberlain, N.; Quinn, M.A.; Baker, M.S.; Rice, G.E.; Georgiou, H.M.; Campbell, I.G. Changes in gene expressions elicited by physiological concentrations of genistein on human endometrial cancer cells. *Mol. Carcinog.* **2006**, *45*, 752–763. [CrossRef]
173. Hu, Y.-C.; Wu, C.-T.; Lai, J.-N.; Tsai, Y.-T. Detection of a negative correlation between prescription of Chinese herbal products containing coumestrol, genistein or daidzein and risk of subsequent endometrial cancer among tamoxifen-treated female breast cancer survivors in Taiwan between 1998 and 2008: A population-based study. *J. Ethnopharmacol.* **2015**, *169*, 356–362. [CrossRef]
174. Sampey, B.P.; Lewis, T.D.; Barbier, C.S.; Makowski, L.; Kaufman, D.G. Genistein effects on stromal cells determines epithelial proliferation in endometrial co-cultures. *Exp. Mol. Pathol.* **2011**, *90*, 257–263. [CrossRef]
175. Zhang, G.Q.; Chen, J.L.; Liu, Q.; Zhang, Y.; Zeng, H.; Zhao, Y. Soy Intake Is Associated With Lower Endometrial Cancer Risk: A Systematic Review and Meta-Analysis of Observational Studies. *Medicine* **2015**, *94*, e2281. [CrossRef]
176. Lee, J.Y.; Kim, H.S.; Song, Y.S. Genistein as a Potential Anticancer Agent against Ovarian Cancer. *J. Tradit. Complement. Med.* **2012**, *2*, 96–104. [CrossRef]
177. Sirmans, S.M.; Pate, K.A. Epidemiology, diagnosis, and management of polycystic ovary syndrome. *Clin. Epidemiol.* **2013**, *6*, 1–13. [CrossRef] [PubMed]
178. Khani, B.; Mehrabian, F.; Khalesi, E.; Eshraghi, A. Effect of soy phytoestrogen on metabolic and hormonal disturbance of women with polycystic ovary syndrome. *J. Res. Med. Sci.* **2011**, *16*, 297–302. [PubMed]
179. Jamilian, M.; Asemi, Z. The Effects of Soy Isoflavones on Metabolic Status of Patients With Polycystic Ovary Syndrome. *J. Clin. Endocrinol. Metab.* **2016**, *101*, 3386–3394. [CrossRef] [PubMed]
180. Karamali, M.; Kashanian, M.; Alaeinasab, S.; Asemi, Z. The effect of dietary soy intake on weight loss, glycaemic control, lipid profiles and biomarkers of inflammation and oxidative stress in women with polycystic ovary syndrome: A randomised clinical trial. *J. Hum. Nutr. Diet.* **2018**, *31*, 533–543. [CrossRef]
181. Romualdi, D.; Costantini, B.; Campagna, G.; Lanzone, A.; Guido, M. Is there a role for soy isoflavones in the therapeutic approach to polycystic ovary syndrome? Results from a pilot study. *Fertil. Steril.* **2008**, *90*, 1826–1833. [CrossRef]
182. Haudum, C.; Lindheim, L.; Ascani, A.; Trummer, C.; Horvath, A.; Muenzker, J.; Obermayer-Pietsch, B. Impact of Short-Term Isoflavone Intervention in Polycystic Ovary Syndrome (PCOS) Patients on Microbiota Composition and Metagenomics. *Nutrients* **2020**, *12*, 1622. [CrossRef] [PubMed]
183. Fontham, E.T.H.; Wolf, A.M.D.; Church, T.R.; Etzioni, R.; Flowers, C.R.; Herzig, A.; Guerra, C.E.; Oeffinger, K.C.; Shih, Y.C.T.; Walter, L.C.; et al. Cervical cancer screening for individuals at average risk: 2020 guideline update from the American Cancer Society. *CA Cancer J. Clin.* **2020**, *70*, 321–346. [CrossRef] [PubMed]
184. Zhang, B.; Liu, J.; Pan, J.; Han, S.; Yin, X.; Wang, B.; Hu, G. Combined Treatment of Ionizing Radiation With Genistein on Cervical Cancer HeLa Cells. *J. Pharmacol. Sci.* **2006**, *102*, 129–135. [CrossRef] [PubMed]
185. Yashar, C.M.; Spanos, W.J.; Taylor, D.D.; Gercel-Taylor, C. Potentiation of the radiation effect with genistein in cervical cancer cells. *Gynecol. Oncol.* **2005**, *99*, 199–205. [CrossRef] [PubMed]
186. Sahin, K.; Tuzcu, M.; Basak, N.; Caglayan, B.; Kilic, U.; Sahin, F.; Kucuk, O. Sensitization of Cervical Cancer Cells to Cisplatin by Genistein: The Role of NFκB and Akt/mTOR Signaling Pathways. *J. Oncol.* **2012**, *2012*, 461562. [CrossRef]
187. Nelson, H.D. Menopause. *Lancet* **2008**, *371*, 760–770. [CrossRef]
188. Melby, M.K.; Lock, M.; Kaufert, P. Culture and symptom reporting at menopause. *Hum. Reprod. Update* **2005**, *11*, 495–512. [CrossRef]
189. Gold, E.B. Factors Associated with Age at Natural Menopause in a Multiethnic Sample of Midlife Women. *Am. J. Epidemiol.* **2001**, *153*, 865–874. [CrossRef]
190. Boulet, M.J.; Oddens, B.J.; Lehert, P.; Vemer, H.M.; Visser, A. Climacteric and menopause in seven south-east Asian countries. *Maturitas* **2008**, *61*, 34–53. [CrossRef]
191. Mintziori, G.; Lambrinoudaki, I.; Goulis, D.G.; Ceausu, I.; Depypere, H.; Erel, C.T.; Perez-Lopez, F.R.; Schenck-Gustafsson, K.; Simoncini, T.; Tremollieres, F.; et al. EMAS position statement: Non-hormonal management of menopausal vasomotor symptoms. *Maturitas* **2015**, *81*, 410–413. [CrossRef]
192. Crisafulli, A.; Marini, H.; Bitto, A.; Altavilla, D.; Squadrito, G.; Romeo, A.; Adamo, E.B.; Marini, R.; D'Anna, R.; Corrado, F.; et al. Effects of genistein on hot flushes in early postmenopausal women: A randomized, double-blind EPT- and placebo-controlled study. *Menopause* **2004**, *11*, 400–404. [CrossRef]

193. Morabito, N.; Crisafulli, A.; Vergara, C.; Gaudio, A.; Lasco, A.; Frisina, N.; D'Anna, R.; Corrado, F.; Pizzoleo, M.A.; Cincotta, M.; et al. Effects of Genistein and Hormone-Replacement Therapy on Bone Loss in Early Postmenopausal Women: A Randomized Double-Blind Placebo-Controlled Study. *J. Bone Miner. Res.* **2002**, *17*, 1904–1912. [CrossRef] [PubMed]
194. Squadrito, F.; Altavilla, D.; Morabito, N.; Crisafulli, A.; D'Anna, R.; Corrado, F.; Ruggeri, P.; Campo, G.M.; Calapai, G.; Caputi, A.P.; et al. The effect of the phytoestrogen genistein on plasma nitric oxide concentrations, endothelin-1 levels and endothelium dependent vasodilation in postmenopausal women. *Atherosclerosis* **2002**, *163*, 339–347. [CrossRef]
195. Squadrito, F.; Altavilla, D.; Crisafulli, A.; Saitta, A.; Cucinotta, D.; Morabito, N.; D'Anna, R.; Corrado, F.; Ruggeri, P.; Frisina, N.; et al. Effect of genistein on endothelial function in postmenopausal women: A randomized, double-blind, controlled study. *Am. J. Med.* **2003**, *114*, 470–476. [CrossRef]
196. Crisafulli, A.; Altavilla, D.; Marini, H.; Bitto, A.; Cucinotta, D.; Frisina, N.; Corrado, F.; D'Anna, R.; Squadrito, G.; Adamo, E.B.; et al. Effects of the phytoestrogen genistein on cardiovascular risk factors in postmenopausal women. *Menopause* **2005**, *12*, 186–192. [CrossRef] [PubMed]
197. Franco, O.H.; Chowdhury, R.; Troup, J.; Voortman, T.; Kunutsor, S.; Kavousi, M.; Oliver-Williams, C.; Muka, T. Use of Plant-Based Therapies and Menopausal Symptoms: A Systematic Review and Meta-analysis. *JAMA J. Am. Med. Assoc.* **2016**, *315*, 2554–2563. [CrossRef] [PubMed]
198. Hillman, G.G.; Wang, Y.; Che, M.; Raffoul, J.J.; Yudelev, M.; Kucuk, O.; Sarkar, F.H. Progression of renal cell carcinoma is inhibited by genistein and radiation in an orthotopic model. *BMC Cancer* **2007**, *7*, 4. [CrossRef] [PubMed]
199. Akimoto, T.; Nonaka, T.; Ishikawa, H.; Sakurai, H.; Saitoh, J.-I.; Takahashi, T.; Mitsuhashi, N. Genistein, a tyrosine kinase inhibitor, enhanced radiosensitivity in human esophageal cancer cell lines *in vitro*: Possible involvement of inhibition of survival signal transduction pathways. *Int. J. Radiat. Oncol. Biol. Phys.* **2001**, *50*, 195–201. [CrossRef]
200. Takaoka, O.; Mori, T.; Ito, F.; Okimura, H.; Kataoka, H.; Tanaka, Y.; Koshiba, A.; Kusuki, I.; Shigehiro, S.; Amami, T.; et al. Daidzein-rich isoflavone aglycones inhibit cell growth and inflammation in endometriosis. *J. Steroid Biochem. Mol. Biol.* **2018**, *181*, 125–132. [CrossRef] [PubMed]
201. Brahmbhatt, S.; Brahmbhatt, R.M.; Boyages, S.C. Thyroid ultrasound is the best prevalence indicator for assessment of iodine deficiency disorders: A study in rural/tribal schoolchildren from Gujarat (Western India). *Eur. J. Endocrinol.* **2000**, *143*, 37–46. [CrossRef] [PubMed]
202. Amazon. Search: "Genistein Supplements". Available online: https://www.amazon.com/s?k=genistein+supplements&crid=27YEIAKQM5YCZ&sprefix=Genistein+supple%2Caps%2C185&ref=nb_sb_ss_ts-da-p_1_16 (accessed on 17 December 2020).
203. Vital Nutrients. Genistein 125 mg Supplement. Available online: https://www.vitalnutrients.net/genistein.html (accessed on 20 December 2020).
204. WebMD. Genistein Combined Polysaccharide. Available online: https://www.webmd.com/vitamins/ai/ingredientmono-1088/genistein-combined-polysaccharide (accessed on 17 December 2020).
205. Susan, R.; Loretta, P.M.; Patricia, B.H.; Charles, H.T.; Stephen, B.; Connie, M.W. A Longitudinal Study of the Effect of Genistein on Bone in Two Different Murine Models of Diminished Estrogen-Producing Capacity. *J. Osteoporos.* **2010**, *2010*, 145170. [CrossRef]
206. Gilda, G.H.; Jeffrey, D.F.; Omer, K.; Mark, Y.; Richard, L.M.; Johanna, R.; Andrey, L.; Samuel, T.-M.; Judith, A.; Fazlul, H.S. Genistein Potentiates the Radiation Effect on Prostate Carcinoma Cells. *Clin. Cancer Res.* **2001**, *7*, 382–390.

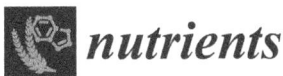

Article

The Role of Cell Proliferation and Extracellular Matrix Accumulation Induced by Food Additive Butylated Hydroxytoluene in Uterine Leiomyoma

Yi-Fen Chiang [1], Hsin-Yuan Chen [1,2], Mohamed Ali [3], Tzong-Ming Shieh [4], Yun-Ju Huang [1,5], Kai-Lee Wang [6], Hsin-Yi Chang [7], Tsui-Chin Huang [8], Yong-Han Hong [2] and Shih-Min Hsia [1,7,9,10,*]

1. School of Nutrition and Health Sciences, College of Nutrition, Taipei Medical University, Taipei 11031, Taiwan; yvonne840828@gmail.com (Y.-F.C.); hsin246@gmail.com (H.-Y.C.); yjhunag@stust.edu.tw (Y.-J.H.)
2. Department of Nutrition, I-Shou University, Kaohsiung 84001, Taiwan; yonghan@isu.edu.tw
3. Clinical Pharmacy Department, Faculty of Pharmacy, Ain Shams University, Cairo 11566, Egypt; mohamed.aboouf@pharma.asu.edu.eg
4. School of Dentistry, College of Dentistry, China Medical University, Taichung 40402, Taiwan; tmshieh@mail.cmu.edu.tw
5. Department of Biotechnology and Food Technology, Southern Taiwan University of Science and Technology, Tainan 71005, Taiwan
6. Department of Nursing, Ching Kuo Institute of Management and Health, Keelung 20301, Taiwan; kellywang@tmu.edu.tw
7. Graduate Institute of Metabolism and Obesity Sciences, College of Nutrition, Taipei Medical University, Taipei 11031, Taiwan; hsinyi.chang@tmu.edu.tw
8. Graduate Institute of Cancer Biology and Drug Discovery, College of Medical Science and Technology, Taipei Medical University, Taipei 11031, Taiwan; tsuichin@tmu.edu.tw
9. School of Food and Safety, Taipei Medical University, Taipei 11031, Taiwan
10. Nutrition Research Center, Taipei Medical University Hospital, Taipei 11031, Taiwan
* Correspondence: bryanhsia@tmu.edu.tw; Tel.: +886-273-61661-6558

Abstract: Leiomyoma is the most common benign uterine tumor in reproductive-age women. Increasing numbers of studies are focusing on the effects of environmental exposure on the incidence and progression of tumors. One major step taken in the food industry is the addition of food preservatives to maintain freshness. Butylated hydroxytoluene (BHT) is a synthetic phenolic antioxidant, which is widely used as an additive to develop fat-soluble characteristics, as well as in cosmetics and rubber. Previous studies also highlighted that BHT may be related to increased fibrosis capacity and carcinogenic effects. In this study, we explored the effects of the commonly used food additive BHT on leiomyoma progression, and the related mechanism. The exposure of the ELT-3 leiomyoma cell line to BHT for 48 h increased the proliferative effect. Since leiomyoma progression is related to increases in extracellular matrix (ECM) accumulation and matrix metalloproteinase (MMP), BHT could effectively increase ECM-related protein expression, as well as MMP-2 and MMP-9 protein expression. This increase in ECM, in response to BHT, may be linked to the activation of the phosphoinositide 3-kinase (PI3K)/Akt and mitogen-activated protein kinase (MAPK) signaling pathway. Through PI3K inhibition, BHT's effect on leiomyoma progression could be partially modulated. These results suggest the harmful effect of BHT exposure on leiomyoma progression may relate to PI3K modulation. However, an in vivo study is necessary to confirm these findings.

Keywords: butylated hydroxytoluene; leiomyoma; uterine fibroids; extracellular matrix; matrix metalloproteinase; environmental exposure

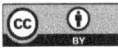

1. Introduction

Leiomyoma (aka uterine fibroids) are the most common benign uterine tumors in reproductive-age women, with an incidence rate of more than 70% [1,2]. Clinically, the leiomyoma is categorized according to its location. The International Federation of Gynecology and Obstetrics (FIGO) classified the definition, submucosal myomas (FIGO type 0, 1, 2) and intramural myomas (FIGO type 3, 4, 5). Submucosal myomas were located below the endometrium, and intramural myomas were located within the uterine wall [3,4]. The main symptoms of leiomyoma are abnormal vaginal bleeding, lower abdominal pain, and bulk symptoms [5]. Recently, studies have reported links between leiomyoma and recurrent miscarriage and infertility [5,6].

Although the pathogenesis of uterine leiomyoma is still not entirely clear, one of the most commonly accepted hypotheses is the accumulation of extracellular matrix (ECM) [7,8]. Extracellular matrix deposition contributes to the amassing of symptoms and the firmness of the tumors, and studies have shown that ECM can enhance the excessive proliferation [9] of the uterine myometrium in a process called mechanotransduction [10]. The components of the ECM include collagen (COL1A1), fibronectin, and proteoglycan.

Leiomyoma cells express significantly higher levels of ECM components than normal uterine smooth muscle cells [11]. Under normal conditions, the ECM is degraded by matrix metalloproteinases (MMPs), of which MMP-2 and MMP-9 are enzymes that mainly degrade collagen [12,13]. In turn, the activity of MMPs is regulated via tissue inhibitors of metalloproteinase (TIMPs) [13,14]; therefore, the balance between MMPs and TIMPs regulates the remodeling of ECM.

With the progression of ECM deposition, intracellular signaling pathways are triggered, such as the mitogen-activated protein kinase (MAPK) and PI3K/Akt (protein kinase B (PKB)) pathways, which increase proliferation and cell survival and maintain the ECM's deposition microenvironment in leiomyoma [15,16].

Considering the rapidly increasing consumption of food additives, more and more studies are revealing their potentially harmful and toxic effects. To preserve food freshness, antioxidant additives are widely used. Butylated hydroxytoluene (BHT) is one of the most commonly used antioxidant additives, which can improve the stability of fat-soluble vitamins and cosmetics and prevent spoilage [17]. As food antioxidants, the Joint Committee of Experts from FAO/WHO point out the consumption of BHT, its acceptable daily intake (ADI) should not be higher than 0.5 mg/kg body weight [18]. In cosmetics formulations, BHT was used in a wide range, from 0.0002% to 0.5% [19]. In the pulmonary fibrosis animal model, BHT was used as a successful model, with significant endothelial injury and fibrosis phenomenon [20,21]. Additionally, BHT was found to have a systemic effect on the lung, reproductive system, liver, and kidney [17]. However, previous studies have shown that the consumption of BHT could induce lung carcinogenesis [22]. Notably, BHT's role in leiomyoma is still not clear. The aim and the novelty of this study were to investigate the role of BHT in leiomyoma progression.

2. Materials and Methods

2.1. Cell Culture and Treatments

The Eker rat-derived uterine leiomyoma ELT3 cell line was provided by Dr. Lin-Hung Wei (Department of Oncology, National Taiwan University Hospital, Taipei, Taiwan). Cells were cultured in Dulbecco's modified Eagle medium/Ham's F-12 Medium in a 1:1 ratio (CAISSON Labs, Smithfield, UT, USA), supplemented with 10% fetal bovine serum (FBS; GIBCO, Grand Island, NY, USA), 100 units/mL penicillin (CORNING; Manassas, VA, USA), 100 µg/mL streptomycin, sodium bicarbonate (2.438 g/L, BioShop, Burlington, ON, Canada), and 4-(2-Hydroxyethyl)piperazine-1-ethanesulfonic acid (HEPES; 5.986 g/L; BioShop) under cultured conditions (37 °C, 5% CO_2) [23].

The cells were starved in serum-free medium for 24 hours and then treated with BHT in 1% FBS medium for 24, 48, and 72 h.

2.2. Cell Viability Assay

The effect of BHT (Sigma-Aldrich, St. Louis, MO, USA) on cell viability was analyzed using the MTT (3-[4,5-dimethyl-2-thiazolyl]-2,5-diphenyl-2H-tetrazolium bromide; Abcam,

Cambridge, MA, USA) assay. After treatments, 1 mg/mL MTT in phosphate-buffered saline was added and incubated for an additional 3 h. The formazan crystals were dissolved in 100 μL dimethyl sulfoxide (DMSO; ECHO Chemical Co. Ltd., Taipei, Taiwan). The optical density was measured using a VERSA Max microplate reader (Molecular Devices, San Jose, CA, USA) at 570 nm and 630 nm. We used the absorbance of the control group as the denominator to calculate the cell viability percentage.

2.3. Colony Formation

Cells were seeded in 6-well plates (500 cells/well) and treated with different concentrations of BHT for 48 h. After 48 h, we removed the medium and replaced it with a completed medium, which we then cultured for 1 week. The colonies were fixed with methanol (Echo Chemical Co. Ltd.) and stained with 0.5% crystal violet (Sigma-Aldrich) [24]. We then added DMSO to dissolve the crystal violet and used a VERSA Max microplate reader to measure the absorbance (595 nm). We used the absorbance of the control group as the denominator to calculate the percentage changes.

2.4. Immunofluorescence

After the treatments, the cells were fixed in 4% paraformaldehyde (Sigma-Aldrich) for 10 minutes at room temperature, treated with 0.5% Triton X-100 in PBS for 10 minutes, and then blocked with 5% bovine serum albumin (BSA for 30 minutes at room temperature), following with previous study [25]. The cells were then incubated with anti-MMP-2 (1:200, Abcam) or anti-MMP-9 (1:200, Santa Cruz Biotechnology, Santa Cruz, CA, USA) diluted in 5% BSA overnight at 4 °C, followed by Alexa Fluor 448-goat anti-rabbit Immunoglobulin or Alexa Fluor 546-goat anti-mouse Immunoglobulin antibodies (Thermo Fisher Scientific, Waltham, MA, USA) for 1 h at room temperature. Photographs were taken under a fluorescence microscope, then Image J was used to quantify the fluorescence intensity.

2.5. Protein Preparation and Western Blot

Cell lysates were homogenized with ice-cold RIPA buffer containing protease (Roche, Basel, Switzerland) and phosphatase inhibitor (Roche, Basel, Switzerland). Following quantification, 30 μg of protein was boiled for 5 minutes, then separated using 10% or 15% SDS–polyacrylamide gel electrophoresis and transferred to polyvinylidene fluoride membranes (0.22 μm). Nonspecific binding sites were blocked with blocking buffer (5% BSA) for 1 h at room temperature, and the membranes were incubated with the primary antibodies for proliferating cell nuclear antigen (PCNA) (1:1000, Cell signaling), matrix metallopeptidase 9 (MMP-9) (1:1000, Santa Cruz Biotechnology), MMP-2 (1:1000, Abcam), collagen type I (COL1A1) (1:1000, Genetex), alpha-smooth muscle actin (α-SMA) (1:1000, Genetex (Irvine, CA, USA), PI3K (1:1000, Cell Signaling Technology, Danvers, MA, USA), p-Akt (1:1000, Cell Signaling), Akt (1:1000, Cell Signaling), extracellular-signal-regulated kinase (ERK) (1:1000, Cell signaling), p-ERK (1:1000, Cell signaling), p38 MAPKinase (1:1000, Cell signaling), p-p38 (1:1000, Cell signaling), and glyceraldehyde-3-phosphate dehydrogenase (GAPDH) (1:10000, Proteintech, Rosemont, IL, USA) at 4 °C overnight. The membranes were washed and incubated for 2 h with anti-rabbit/mouse IgG coupled with alkaline phosphatase (1: 10,000) and then washed with TBST buffer. The bands were detected using ECL and visualized with the eBlot Touch Imager tm (eBlot Photoelectric Technology, Shanghai, China). The values shown were normalized to the internal control GAPDH and analyzed via the ImageJ software.

2.6. Statistical Analysis

Data are expressed as mean ± standard deviation. Statistical analysis was performed with Graphpad Prism version 9 (GraphPad Software, Inc., San Diego, CA, USA), using Student's t-test and one-way analysis of variance (ANOVA), and we used Tukey's test for post-mortem analysis. $p < 0.05$ indicates a statistically significant difference

3. Results
3.1. Effects of BHT on Leiomyoma Proliferation
3.1.1. Proliferative Effect

We used MTT as the cell proliferation assay to evaluate the changes in cell viability following BHT exposure in ELT-3 cells. The ELT-3 cells were seeded in a 96-well plate for 24 h. After starvation for 24 h, they were treated with a graded concentration of BHT (0.1–25 µM) for 24 and 48 h. All the concentrations used for the 48 h treatments could significantly increase leiomyoma cell viability (Figure 1A,B), indicating the potential role of BHT in leiomyoma cell viability. The doubling time of BHT treatments significantly decreased the doubling time (Figure 1C); moreover, the PCNA expression (Figure 1D) would increase after BHT treatments, showing that BHT could increase the ELT-3 cell proliferation.

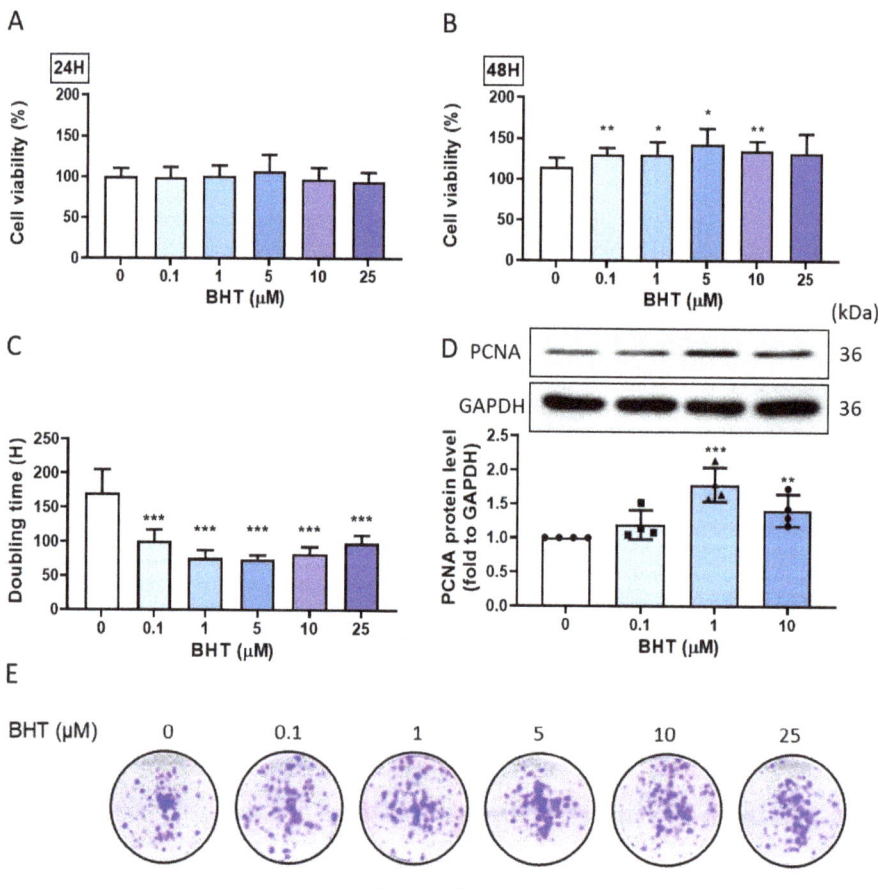

Figure 1. *Cont.*

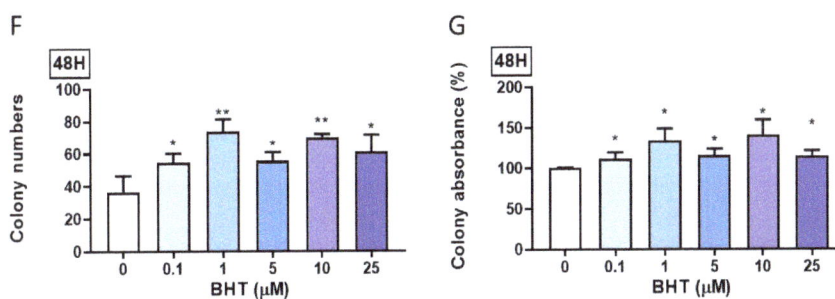

Figure 1. Butylated hydroxytoluene (BHT) effects on leiomyoma proliferation. ELT-3 cells were cultured in a 96-well plate (3000 cells/well) after starvation with a serum-free medium for 24 h. They were then treated with different concentrations of BHT for 24 and 48 h, and we performed the following assays: (**A**) MTT assay to evaluate the cell viability for 24 h and (**B**) 48 h, used doubling time formula to calculate the (**C**) doubling time and Western blot for (**D**) proliferating cell nuclear antigen (PCNA) expression; (**E**) colony formation assay, following culturing in a 6-well plate for the analysis of the long-term effect of different concentrations of BHT; (**F**) graphical representation of colony numbers and (**G**) absorbance percentage following BHT exposure at different concentrations. ImageJ was used to determine the colony number. *, $p < 0.05$; **, $p < 0.01$; and ***, $p < 0.001$, compared with the control group. Doubling time = duration * log (2)/(log (final concentration) − log (initial concentration)).

3.1.2. Colony Formation

To investigate the long-term effect of BHT on ELT-3 cell proliferation and its ability to stimulate stem cell characteristics, such as colony formation, a colony formation assay was performed after BHT exposure for 48 h and the replacement of the complete medium. The results show that BHT could significantly increase colony formation (Figure 1E), as evidenced by the increased colony count assessed via image J (Figure 1F). Furthermore, we used DMSO to dissolve the staining and measure the absorbance (Figure 1G). Overall, BHT exposure could significantly enhance colony progression and leiomyoma's proliferation potential.

3.2. Effects of BHT on MMP Modulation

3.2.1. Effects of BHT on MMP-9 and MMP-2 Protein Expression Using Immunofluorescence

Immunofluorescence was used to measure the protein expression of MMP-9 and MMP-2 following 48 h of BHT exposure. The intensity of fluorescence was significantly increased in both MMP-9 and MMP-2, indicating that BHT enhanced the levels in live cells (Figure 2A–C).

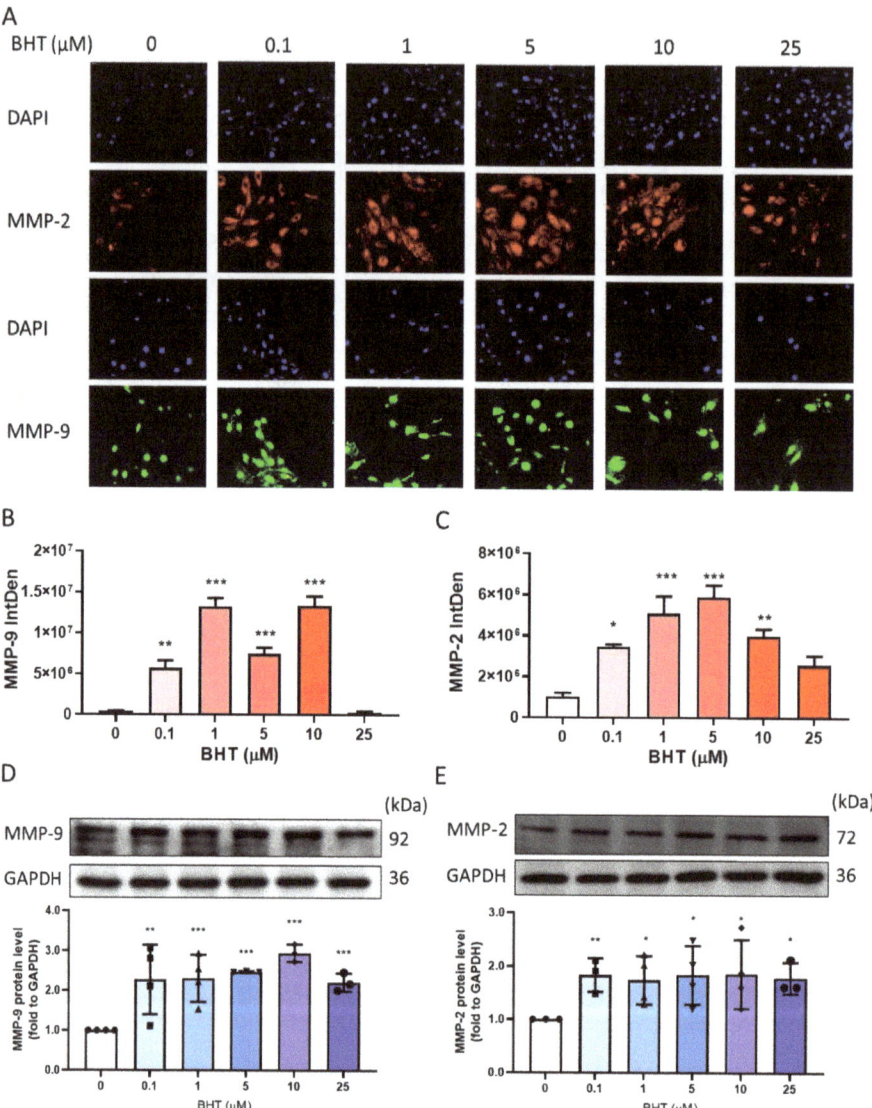

Figure 2. Effects of BHT on MMP modulation. ELT-3 cells were cultured in DMEM/F12 medium. After serum-free starvation for 24 h, cells were treated with different concentrations of BHT for 48 h, and the following experiments were performed: (**A**) immunofluorescence to measure expression changes, employing graphical representations of the fluorescence intensity levels of (**B**) MMP-9 and (**C**) MMP-2. Additionally, increased (**D**) MMP-9 and (**E**) MMP-2 protein expression ($n = 3$–4) are shown. *, $p < 0.05$; **, $p < 0.01$; ***, $p < 0.001$, compared with the control group. We used a fluorescent microscope at 40× magnification. IntDen: integrated density.

3.2.2. Effects of BHT on MMP-9 and MMP-2 Protein Expression Using Western Blot

Matrix metalloproteinases act as a regulator of ECM accumulation. Western blot analysis confirmed that BHT exposure could significantly increase MMP-9 (Figure 2D) and MMP-2 (Figure 2E) protein expression.

3.3. Effect of BHT on Extracellular Matrix Related Proteins

3.3.1. Effects of BHT on ECM Related Protein Expression Using Immunofluorescence

Immunofluorescence was used to measure the protein expression of α-SMA and COL1A1 following 48 h of BHT treatment. The intensity of fluorescence was significantly increased in both α-SMA and COL1A1 (Figure 3A–C).

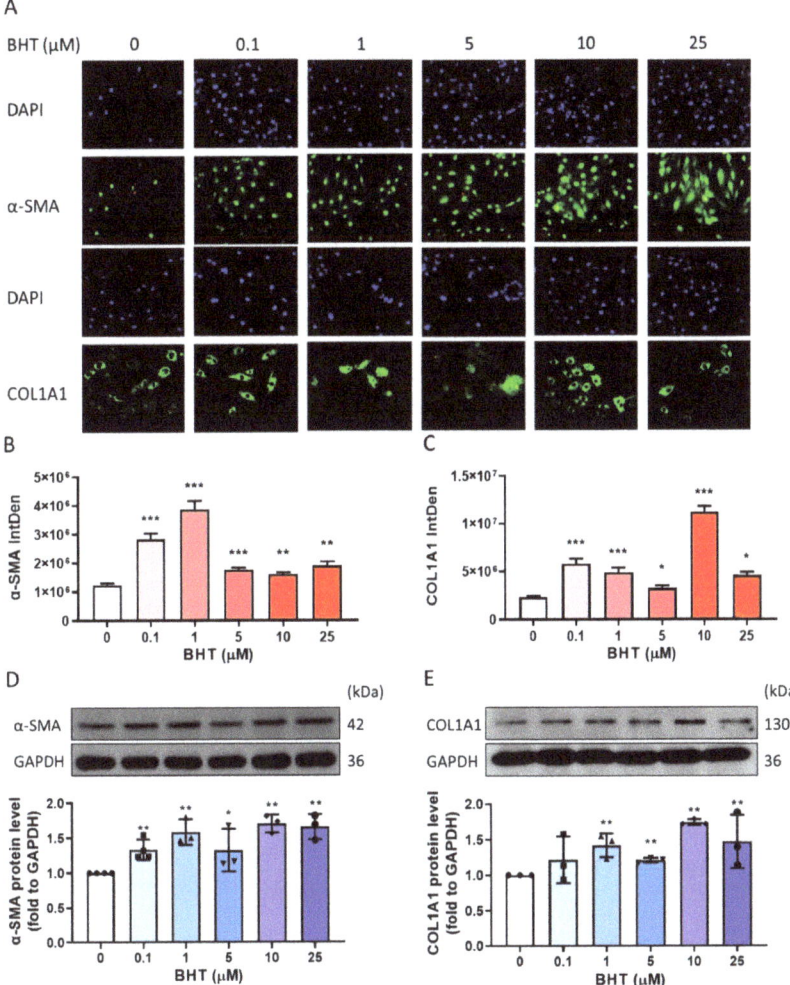

Figure 3. Effect of BHT on extracellular protein expression change. ELT-3 cells were cultured in DMEM/F12 medium. After serum-free starvation for 24 h, cells were treated with different concentrations of BHT for 48 h, and the following experiments were performed: (**A**) immunofluorescence to measure expression changes, employing graphical representations of the fluorescence intensity levels of (**B**) α-SMA and (**C**) COL1A1. Additionally, increased (**D**) α-SMA and (**E**) COL1A1 protein expression (n = 3–4) are shown. *, $p < 0.05$; **, $p < 0.01$; ***, $p < 0.001$, compared with the control group. We used a fluorescent microscope at 40× magnification. IntDen: integrated density.

3.3.2. Effects of BHT on ECM Related Protein Expression Using Western Blot

The overexpression of extracellular matrix-related proteins contributes to leiomyoma progression. Therefore, we explored ECM-related protein expression in response to BHT treatments, including COL1A1 and α-SMA as confirmation for previous immunofluorescence results. Our results were consistent with the fluorescence intensity results. Moreover, BHT exposure induced the significant protein expression of COL1A1 and α-SMA (Figure 3D,E). Collectively, these results indicate that the BHT exposure could enhance ECM accumulation in leiomyoma.

3.4. PI3K/Akt and MAPK Signaling Related Protein Expression Change in BHT Induced ECM Accumulation

One of the well-known triggering factors that regulate extracellular–intracellular signaling is ECM [15]. Studies showed that activation of PI3K/Akt and MAPK signaling pathways could modulate ECM progression [26]. Therefore, we sought to explore whether BHT mediated ECM induction is accompanied by activation of the PI3K/Akt pathway. ELT-3 cells exposure with BHT for 48 h resulted in an increase in PI3K and p-Akt/Akt protein expression (Figure 4A,B), and in low doses, BHT could activate MAPK signaling transduction (Figure 4C,D), indicating that BHT exposure could activate PI3K/Akt and MAPK signaling pathway to increase the ECM accumulation.

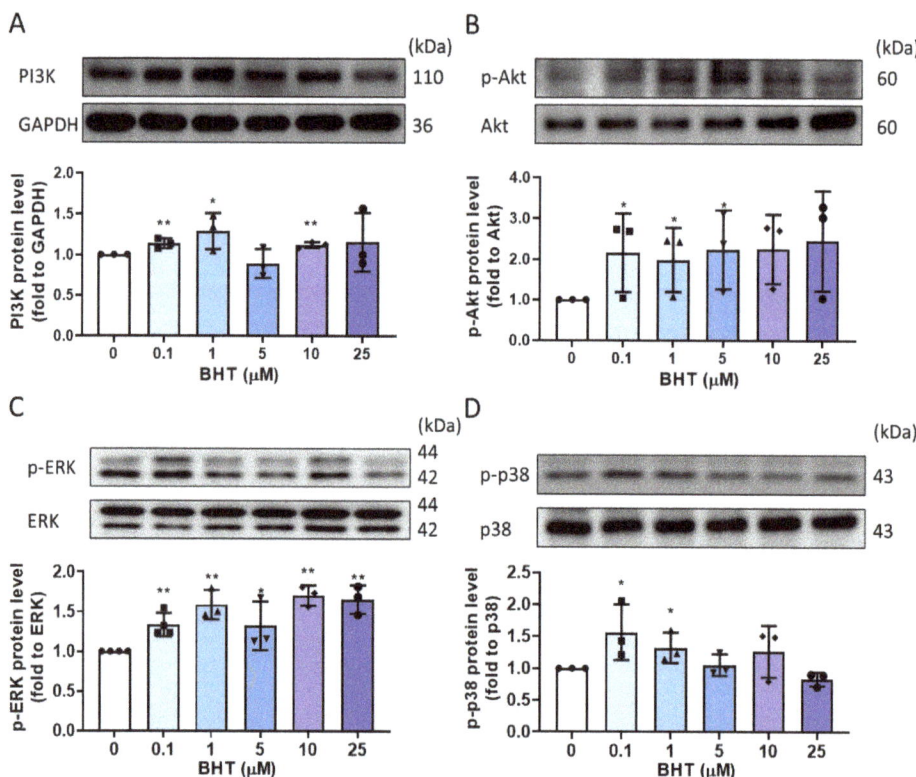

Figure 4. The PI3K/Akt and MAPK signaling pathway involved in BHT-induced ECM accumulation. ELT-3 cells were cultured in DMEM/F12, followed by serum-free starvation for 24 h. Cells were treated with different concentrations of BHT for 48 h. Western blotting was used to explore the protein expression of (**A**) PI3K (**B**) p-Akt/Akt (**C**) p-ERK/ERK, and (**D**) p-p38/p38 protein expression ($n = 3$). *, $p < 0.05$; **, $p < 0.01$; and ***, $p < 0.001$ compared with the control group. GAPDH was used as loading control.

3.5. The Potential Modulative Signaling Pathway in BHT Induced ECM Accumulation

PI3K inhibitor, wortmannin, was used to investigate the potential modulator of BHT on ECM accumulation. According to a previous study, PI3K acts as the important modulator of MMP-2 [27]. By using wortmannin, the results indicated that the PI3K inhibition could reverse the BHT's effect on ECM accumulation (Figure 5).

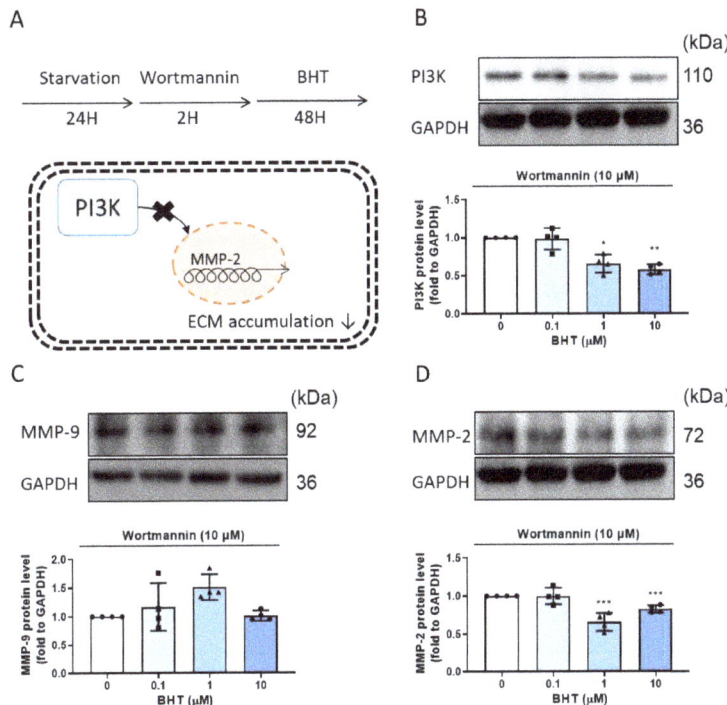

Figure 5. The potential modulative signaling pathway in BHT0induced ECM accumulation: (**A**) the flowchart shows that treated with PI3K inhibitor wortmannin for 2 h and treated with BHT for 48 h to evaluate the PI3K modulated BHT's effect in ECM accumulation. After treatment, Western blot analysis was used to evaluate the (**B**) PI3K, (**C**) MMP-9, and (**D**) MMP-2 protein expression. *, $p < 0.05$; **, $p < 0.01$; and ***, $p < 0.001$ compared with the control group. GAPDH was used as loading control.

4. Discussion

In this study, BHT exposure showed its ability on the progression of uterine leiomyoma by increasing the proliferation and extracellular matrix accumulation effect through PI3K/Akt and MAPK signaling modulation.

The extracellular matrix is engaged in a complex interaction with the surrounding microenvironment while providing structural support to the cell and tissue [11]. Moreover, ECM could induce signaling networks, which, in turn, induce further ECM synthesis and deposition [11]. In leiomyoma, ECM turnover and remodeling are disrupted, with the overexpression of related proteins, such as collagen, fibronectin, and α-SMA [7]. The key modulator of ECM accumulation is the matrix metalloproteinase, which participates in tissue remodeling and modulated the tissue inhibitor of metalloproteinases (TIMPs) in leiomyoma [28]. Leiomyoma pathogenesis involves growth factor stimulation, with subsequent cell proliferation, inflammation, and fibrosis [29]. Several signaling pathways are involved in leiomyoma progression, including the MAPK signaling pathway, the phosphorylation of extracellular signal-regulated kinases (ERK), the phosphoinositide 3-kinase (PI3K)/Akt pathway, and the wingless-type (Wnt)/β-catenin signaling pathway [30].

The PI3K/Akt pathway participates in the regulation of mammalian target of rapamycin (mTOR), and modulates cancer cell survival, proliferation, and apoptosis, therefore playing an important role in cancer progression [24] and in leiomyoma [31].

The pathogenesis of uterine leiomyoma is still not clear, but leiomyoma growth is estrogen- and progesterone dependent, which indicated hormone dependence plays an important role in leiomyoma progression [32,33]. Studies have shown that early exposure to environmental endocrine-disrupting chemicals (EDCs) increases the risk of leiomyoma development later in life [32,34,35]. EDCs are found in sweeteners, preserved food, and food additives [36]. EDCs impart steroidogenesis [37], estrogen-like effects, and promote the development of gynecological tumors.

Food additives maintain quality, taste, and freshness [38]. For food spoilage prevention, these food antioxidant agents are one of the major classes of food additives [39]. The most commonly used category is synthetic phenolic antioxidants, such as butylated hydroxytoluene (BHT) and butylated hydroxyanisole (BHA). These food additives were approved by the US Food and Drug Administration. However, their side effects for humans are still being debated; for example, their consumption increases oxidative stress, carcinogenicity, reproductive toxicity, and DNA repair defects [40,41]. Therefore, BHT has been restricted in some food additives, but females can still be exposed via cosmetics and medicine consumption [19], in addition to exposure to rubber, plastics, and even the environment [42], with long-term effects.

Studies exploring the toxicity of BHT have been inconsistent. One study highlighted its positive effects based on its antioxidant activity, ability to increase intracellular antioxidant enzyme levels [43], and anti-cancer effects [19], while several other studies have indicated that BHT may induce kidney and liver damage [19]. Notably, BHT metabolites are related to toxicity, as shown in a study that used gas chromatography coupled to mass spectrometry (GC-MS) [44]. Based on BHT's structure, it has a greater ability to accumulate in adipose tissue and affect hormone regulation in mammary glands, as well as being transferred through the placenta [45].

BHT was found to be harmful to metabolic- and reproductive-related diseases. In reproductive disorders, the exposure of mouse Leydig cells (TM3) with BHT suppressed cellular proliferation, altered the cell cycle, and changed the cytosolic and mitochondria calcium homeostasis [46]. In addition to causing endoplasmic reticulum (ER) stress and increasing DNA damage, it further triggered the apoptosis signaling pathway, which, in turn, activated the PI3K/Akt and MAPK signaling pathways, eventually promoting carcinogenesis [46].

Antioxidant enzymes could eliminate oxidative stress. Manganese superoxide dismutase (MnSOD), on the other hand, could act as a tumor suppressor [47] and promotor [48]. MnSOD, a highly antioxidative compound, promoted metastatic effects through the upregulation of MMP-2 [49]. In lung cancer patients, MnSOD-positive tumors were related to higher MMP-2 expression and caused tumorigenesis, including proliferation and fibrosis progression [50]. Anti-oxidation or oxidative stress would regulate MMP activation [51]. High doses of MnSOD, with its ability to eliminate oxidative stress, had a tumor-suppressor effect in several cancers [52], while low doses caused no changes in oxidative stress, leading to the accumulation of reactive oxygen species (ROS) and stimulating cancer progression through increased MMP activity [49]. Incomplete ROS degradation may trigger MMP-2 activation [53], and therefore, the different effects of the antioxidant and the additive antioxidant should be considered. Our results also revealed that BHTs' effect on ECM-related protein expression may vary with different dosages—in low dosage exposures, they are most effective.

Studies showed that BHT interacts with PI3K/Akt and MAPK signaling modulation and enhances fibrosis [54]. An injection of 400 mg/kg BHT in BALB/C mice resulted in significant intestinal fibrosis and lung fibrosis within 14 days [55]. Additionally, BHT could induce lung carcinogens and lung damage, as shown in transgenic mice with the rasH2 gene that underwent exposure with BHT for 9 weeks [56]. BHT exposure also increased collagen I, III, and V expressions and altered both the telomerase and apoptosis-related expressions, along with further epithelial cell injury. Collectively, these studies indicate that BHT potentially affects fibrosis progression [57].

In the current study, BHT's role in leiomyoma progression was explored for the first time. BHT increased proliferative effect, increased ECM-related protein expression, and induced ECM accumulation, which is essential to leiomyoma progression. Additionally, in vitro experiments showed that BHT exposure could alter protein expression, in addition to activating the PI3K/Akt and MAPK signaling pathway. The study shows, for the first time, that BHT exposure could increase the leiomyoma progression, indicating that it may participate in PI3K and MAPK signaling pathways. However, the in vitro study used could not fully explain the role of BHT in leiomyoma. The metabolites of BHT may play different roles in leiomyoma progression; therefore, further animal studies are needed to realize its effect in the future.

5. Conclusions

Environmental exposure to BHT could be associated with several disease disorders and disadvantages. Using the ELT-3 rat leiomyoma cell model, the results shed light on BHT's potential in enhancing leiomyoma cell proliferation, colony formation, and ECM accumulation in a mechanism that might involve modulation of PI3K/Akt and MAPK signaling pathways (Figure 6). It is the first study to explore the effect of food additives on leiomyoma progression. Further studies will be needed in the future to investigate the pro-fibroid effects of BHT metabolites in animal studies.

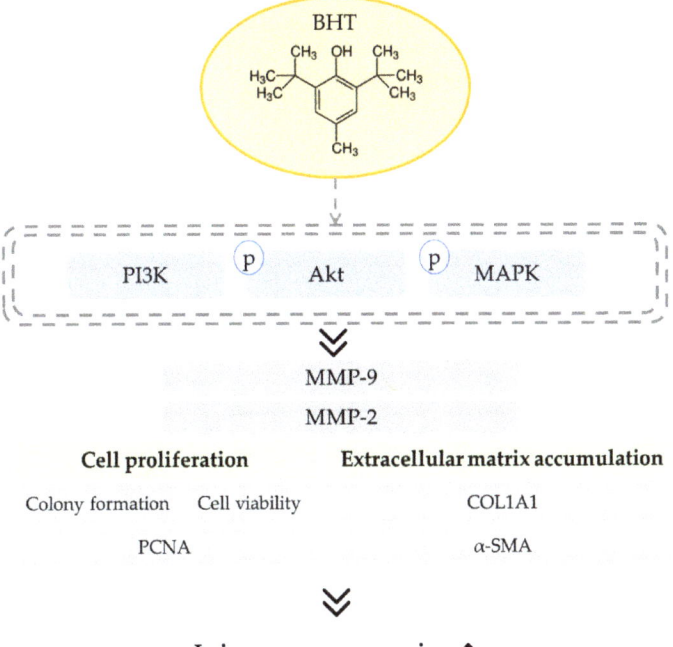

Figure 6. Schematic representation of the potential effects of BHT in leiomyoma progression. BHT could increase cell proliferative effect, modulate PI3K/Akt and MAPK signaling pathways, increase MMP enzyme and protein expression, and increase the ECM-related protein expression.

Author Contributions: Conceptualization, Y.-F.C. and S.-M.H.; experimentation, Y.-F.C. and H.-Y.C. (Hsin-Yuan Chen); data analysis and figure preparation, Y.-F.C.; methodology and resources, Y.-F.C., T.-M.S., Y.-J.H., Y.-H.H., K.-L.W., H.-Y.C. (Hsin-Yi Chang) and T.-C.H.; writing—original draft preparation, Y.-F.C.; writing—review and editing, Y.-F.C., M.A. and S.-M.H.; editing and approval of the final version of the manuscript, S.-M.H. All authors have read and agreed to the published version of the manuscript.

Funding: This study was supported by the grants (MOST 110-2628-B-038-018, MOST 109-2314-B-038-059, MOST 109-2628-B-038-015, MOST 109-2320-B-254-001 and MOST 109-2811-B-038-523) from the Ministry of Science and Technology, Taiwan, as well as grants (MOE-RSC-108RSN0005) from the Ministry of Education, Taiwan.

Data Availability Statement: The data presented in this study are available on request from the corresponding author.

Conflicts of Interest: The authors declare no conflict of interest.

Abbreviations

α-SMA	Alpha smooth muscle actin
BHA	Butylated hydroxyanisole
BHT	Butylated hydroxytoluene
BSA	Bovine serum albumin
COL1A1	Collagen, type I
ECM	Extracellular matrix
EDCs	Environmental endocrine-disrupting chemicals
h	Hours
MAPK	Mitogen-activated protein kinase
MMP	Matrix metalloproteinase
MnSOD	Manganese superoxide dismutase
MTT	(3-(4,5-dimethylthiazol-2-yl)-2,5-diphenyltetrazolium bromide)
PCNA	Proliferating cell nuclear antigen
PI3K	Phosphoinositide 3-kinase
PKB	Protein kinase B
ROS	Reactive oxygen species
TIMPs	Tissue inhibitor of metalloproteinase

References

1. Sabry, M.; Al-Hendy, A. Medical treatment of uterine leiomyoma. *Reprod. Sci.* **2012**, *19*, 339–353. [CrossRef] [PubMed]
2. Sparic, R.; Mirkovic, L.; Malvasi, A.; Tinelli, A. Epidemiology of Uterine Myomas: A Review. *Int. J. Fertil. Steril.* **2016**, *9*, 424–435. [PubMed]
3. Frascà, C.; Tuzzato, G.; Arena, A.; Degli Esposti, E.; Zanello, M.; Raimondo, D.; Seracchioli, R. The Role of Pelvic Ultrasound in Preoperative Evaluation for Laparoscopic Myomectomy. *J. Minim. Invasive Gynecol.* **2018**, *25*, 679–683. [CrossRef] [PubMed]
4. Munro, M.G.; Critchley, H.O.; Broder, M.S.; Fraser, I.S. FIGO classification system (PALM-COEIN) for causes of abnormal uterine bleeding in nongravid women of reproductive age. *Int. J. Gynaecol. Obs.* **2011**, *113*, 3–13. [CrossRef]
5. Barjon, K.; Mikhail, L.N. Uterine Leiomyomata (Fibroids). In *StatPearls*; StatPearls Publishing LLC.: Treasure Island, FL, USA, 2019.
6. Ali, M.; Al-Hendy, A. Selective progesterone receptor modulators for fertility preservation in women with symptomatic uterine fibroids. *Biol. Reprod.* **2017**, *97*, 337–352. [CrossRef] [PubMed]
7. Islam, M.S.; Ciavattini, A.; Petraglia, F.; Castellucci, M.; Ciarmela, P. Extracellular matrix in uterine leiomyoma pathogenesis: A potential target for future therapeutics. *Hum. Reprod. Update* **2018**, *24*, 59–85. [CrossRef]
8. Greco, S.; Islam, M.S.; Zannotti, A.; Delli Carpini, G.; Giannubilo, S.R.; Ciavattini, A.; Petraglia, F.; Ciarmela, P. Quercetin and indole-3-carbinol inhibit extracellular matrix expression in human primary uterine leiomyoma cells. *Reprod. Biomed. Online* **2020**, *40*, 593–602. [CrossRef]
9. Bulun, S.E. Uterine fibroids. *N. Engl. J. Med.* **2013**, *369*, 1344–1355. [CrossRef]
10. Leppert, P.C.; Jayes, F.L.; Segars, J.H. The extracellular matrix contributes to mechanotransduction in uterine fibroids. *Obstet. Gynecol. Int.* **2014**, *2014*, 783289. [CrossRef] [PubMed]
11. Wight, T.N.; Potter-Perigo, S. The extracellular matrix: An active or passive player in fibrosis? *Am. J. Physiol.-Gastrointest. Liver Physiol.* **2011**, *301*, 950–955. [CrossRef]

12. Bogusiewicz, M.; Stryjecka-Zimmer, M.; Postawski, K.; Jakimiuk, A.J.; Rechberger, T. Activity of matrix metalloproteinase-2 and -9 and contents of their tissue inhibitors in uterine leiomyoma and corresponding myometrium. *Gynecol. Endocrinol.* **2007**, *23*, 541–546. [CrossRef]
13. Lin, P.-H.; Kung, H.-L.; Chen, H.-Y.; Huang, K.-C.; Hsia, S.-M. Isoliquiritigenin Suppresses E2-Induced Uterine Leiomyoma Growth through the Modulation of Cell Death Program and the Repression of ECM Accumulation. *Cancers* **2019**, *11*, 1131. [CrossRef]
14. Korompelis, P.; Piperi, C.; Adamopoulos, C.; Dalagiorgou, G.; Korkolopoulou, P.; Sepsa, A.; Antsaklis, A.; Papavassiliou, A.G. Expression of vascular endothelial factor-A, gelatinases (MMP-2, MMP-9) and TIMP-1 in uterine leiomyomas. *Clin. Chem. Lab. Med.* **2015**, *53*, 1415–1424. [CrossRef]
15. Hastings, J.F.; Skhinas, J.N.; Fey, D.; Croucher, D.R.; Cox, T.R. The extracellular matrix as a key regulator of intracellular signalling networks. *Br. J. Pharm.* **2019**, *176*, 82–92. [CrossRef]
16. Lin, P.-H.; Tung, Y.-T.; Chen, H.-Y.; Chiang, Y.-F.; Hong, H.-C.; Huang, K.-C.; Hsu, S.-P.; Huang, T.-C.; Hsia, S.-M. Melatonin activates cell death programs for the suppression of uterine leiomyoma cell proliferation. *J. Pineal Res.* **2019**, *68*, e12620. [CrossRef]
17. Yehye, W.A.; Rahman, N.A.; Ariffin, A.; Abd Hamid, S.B.; Alhadi, A.A.; Kadir, F.A.; Yaeghoobi, M. Understanding the chemistry behind the antioxidant activities of butylated hydroxytoluene (BHT): A review. *Eur. J. Med. Chem.* **2015**, *101*, 295–312. [CrossRef] [PubMed]
18. Lobo, V.; Patil, A.; Phatak, A.; Chandra, N. Free radicals, antioxidants and functional foods: Impact on human health. *Pharm. Rev.* **2010**, *4*, 118–126. [CrossRef] [PubMed]
19. Lanigan, R.S.; Yamarik, T.A. Final report on the safety assessment of BHT(1). *Int. J. Toxicol.* **2002**, *21* (Suppl. S2), 19–94.
20. Martins, V.; Teodoro, W.R.; Velosa, A.P.P.; Andrade, P.; Farhat, C.; Fabro, A.T.; Capelozzi, V.L. Butylated hydroxytoluene induces type-V collagen and overexpression of remodeling genes/proteins in experimental lung fibrosis. *Histol. Histopathol.* **2018**, *33*, 1111–1123.
21. Fujita, M.; Shannon, J.M.; Morikawa, O.; Gauldie, J.; Hara, N.; Mason, R.J. Overexpression of tumor necrosis factor-alpha diminishes pulmonary fibrosis induced by bleomycin or transforming growth factor-beta. *Am. J. Respir. Cell Mol. Biol.* **2003**, *29*, 669–676. [CrossRef] [PubMed]
22. Bauer, A.K.; Dwyer-Nield, L.D. Two-stage 3-methylcholanthrene and butylated hydroxytoluene-induced lung carcinogenesis in mice. *Methods Cell Biol.* **2021**, *163*, 153–173. [PubMed]
23. Chen, H.Y.; Huang, T.C.; Lin, L.C.; Shieh, T.M.; Wu, C.H.; Wang, K.L.; Hong, Y.H.; Hsia, S.M. Fucoidan Inhibits the Proliferation of Leiomyoma Cells and Decreases Extracellular Matrix-Associated Protein Expression. *Cell Physiol. Biochem.* **2018**, *49*, 1970–1986. [CrossRef]
24. Chiang, Y.-F.; Chen, H.-Y.; Huang, K.-C.; Lin, P.-H.; Hsia, S.-M. Dietary Antioxidant Trans-Cinnamaldehyde Reduced Visfatin-Induced Breast Cancer Progression: In Vivo and In Vitro Study. *Antioxidants* **2019**, *8*, 625. [CrossRef] [PubMed]
25. Chiang, Y.-F.; Chen, H.-Y.; Chang, Y.-J.; Shih, Y.-H.; Shieh, T.-M.; Wang, K.-L.; Hsia, S.-M. Protective Effects of Fucoxanthin on High Glucose- and 4-Hydroxynonenal (4-HNE)-Induced Injury in Human Retinal Pigment Epithelial Cells. *Antioxidants* **2020**, *9*, 1176. [CrossRef]
26. Donnini, S.; Morbidelli, L.; Taraboletti, G.; Ziche, M. ERK1-2 and p38 MAPK regulate MMP/TIMP balance and function in response to thrombospondin-1 fragments in the microvascular endothelium. *Life Sci.* **2004**, *74*, 2975–2985. [CrossRef]
27. Wang, G.; Yin, L.; Peng, Y.; Gao, Y.; Gao, H.; Zhang, J.; Lv, N.; Miao, Y.; Lu, Z. Insulin promotes invasion and migration of KRAS(G12D) mutant HPNE cells by upregulating MMP-2 gelatinolytic activity via ERK- and PI3K-dependent signalling. *Cell Prolif.* **2019**, *52*, e12575. [CrossRef] [PubMed]
28. Shin, S.J.; Kim, J.; Lee, S.; Baek, J.; Lee, J.E.; Cho, C.; Ha, E. Ulipristal acetate induces cell cycle delay and remodeling of extracellular matrix. *Int. J. Mol. Med.* **2018**, *42*, 1857–1864. [CrossRef]
29. Ali, M.; Shahin, S.M.; Sabri, N.A.; Al-Hendy, A.; Yang, Q. 1,25 Dihydroxyvitamin D3 Enhances the Antifibroid Effects of Ulipristal Acetate in Human Uterine Fibroids. *Reprod. Sci.* **2019**, *26*, 812–828. [CrossRef]
30. Borahay, M.A.; Al-Hendy, A.; Kilic, G.S.; Boehning, D. Signaling Pathways in Leiomyoma: Understanding Pathobiology and Implications for Therapy. *Mol. Med.* **2015**, *21*, 242–256. [CrossRef]
31. Islam, M.S.; Greco, S.; Janjusevic, M.; Ciavattini, A.; Giannubilo, S.R.; D'Adderio, A.; Biagini, A.; Fiorini, R.; Castellucci, M.; Ciarmela, P. Growth factors and pathogenesis. *Best Pract. Res. Clin. Obs. Gynaecol.* **2016**, *34*, 25–36. [CrossRef]
32. Bariani, M.V.; Rangaswamy, R.; Siblini, H.; Yang, Q.; Al-Hendy, A.; Zota, A.R. The role of endocrine-disrupting chemicals in uterine fibroid pathogenesis. *Curr. Opin. Endocrinol. Diabetes Obes.* **2020**, *27*, 380–387. [CrossRef]
33. Ishikawa, H.; Ishi, K.; Serna, V.A.; Kakazu, R.; Bulun, S.E.; Kurita, T. Progesterone is essential for maintenance and growth of uterine leiomyoma. *Endocrinology* **2010**, *151*, 2433–2442. [CrossRef] [PubMed]
34. Shen, Y.; Xu, Q.; Xu, J.; Ren, M.L.; Cai, Y.L. Environmental exposure and risk of uterine leiomyoma: An epidemiologic survey. *Eur. Rev. Med. Pharm. Sci.* **2013**, *17*, 3249–3256.
35. Katz, T.A.; Yang, Q.; Treviño, L.S.; Walker, C.L.; Al-Hendy, A. Endocrine-disrupting chemicals and uterine fibroids. *Fertil. Steril.* **2016**, *106*, 967–977. [CrossRef] [PubMed]
36. Nagata, C.; Nakamura, K.; Oba, S.; Hayashi, M.; Takeda, N.; Yasuda, K. Association of intakes of fat, dietary fibre, soya isoflavones and alcohol with uterine fibroids in Japanese women. *Br. J. Nutr.* **2009**, *101*, 1427–1431. [CrossRef]

37. Krawczyk, K.; Marynowicz, W.; Gogola-Mruk, J.; Jakubowska, K.; Tworzydło, W.; Opydo-Chanek, M.; Ptak, A. A mixture of persistent organic pollutants detected in human follicular fluid increases progesterone secretion and mitochondrial activity in human granulosa HGrC1 cells. *Reprod. Toxicol.* **2021**, *104*, 114–124. [CrossRef] [PubMed]
38. Lourenço, S.C.; Moldão-Martins, M.; Alves, V.D. Antioxidants of Natural Plant Origins: From Sources to Food Industry Applications. *Molecules* **2019**, *24*, 4132. [CrossRef]
39. Union ECJOJE: *Regulation (EC) No 1333/2008 of the European Parliament and of the Council of 16 December 2008 on Food Additives*; 2008; Volume 354, pp. 16–33. Available online: http://data.europa.eu/eli/reg/2008/1333/oj (accessed on 30 August 2021).
40. Vandghanooni, S.; Forouharmehr, A.; Eskandani, M.; Barzegari, A.; Kafil, V.; Kashanian, S.; Ezzati Nazhad Dolatabadi, J. Cytotoxicity and DNA fragmentation properties of butylated hydroxyanisole. *DNA Cell Biol.* **2013**, *32*, 98–103. [CrossRef]
41. Jeong, S.H.; Kim, B.Y.; Kang, H.G.; Ku, H.O.; Cho, J.H. Effects of butylated hydroxyanisole on the development and functions of reproductive system in rats. *Toxicology* **2005**, *208*, 49–62. [CrossRef] [PubMed]
42. Liang, X.; Zhao, Y.; Liu, W.; Li, Z.; Souders, C.L., 2nd; Martyniuk, C.J. Butylated hydroxytoluene induces hyperactivity and alters dopamine-related gene expression in larval zebrafish (Danio rerio). *Environ. Pollut.* **2020**, *257*, 113624. [CrossRef] [PubMed]
43. Fasihnia, S.H.; Peighambardoust, S.H.; Peighambardoust, S.J.; Oromiehie, A.; Soltanzadeh, M.; Peressini, D. Migration analysis, antioxidant, and mechanical characterization of polypropylene-based active food packaging films loaded with BHA, BHT, and TBHQ. *J. Food Sci.* **2020**, *85*, 2317–2328. [CrossRef]
44. Ousji, O.; Sleno, L. Identification of In Vitro Metabolites of Synthetic Phenolic Antioxidants BHT, BHA, and TBHQ by LC-HRMS/MS. *Int. J. Mol. Sci.* **2020**, *21*, 9525. [CrossRef]
45. Pop, A.; Drugan, T.; Gutleb, A.C.; Lupu, D.; Cherfan, J.; Loghin, F.; Kiss, B. Estrogenic and anti-estrogenic activity of butylparaben, butylated hydroxyanisole, butylated hydroxytoluene and propyl gallate and their binary mixtures on two estrogen responsive cell lines (T47D-Kbluc, MCF-7). *J. Appl. Toxicol.* **2018**, *38*, 944–957. [CrossRef]
46. Ham, J.; Lim, W.; Whang, K.Y.; Song, G. Butylated hydroxytoluene induces dysregulation of calcium homeostasis and endoplasmic reticulum stress resulting in mouse Leydig cell death. *Environ. Pollut.* **2020**, *256*, 113421. [CrossRef] [PubMed]
47. Ough, M.; Lewis, A.; Zhang, Y.; Hinkhouse, M.M.; Ritchie, J.M.; Oberley, L.W.; Cullen, J.J. Inhibition of cell growth by overexpression of manganese superoxide dismutase (MnSOD) in human pancreatic carcinoma. *Free Radic. Res.* **2004**, *38*, 1223–1233. [CrossRef] [PubMed]
48. Kim, J.J.; Chae, S.W.; Hur, G.C.; Cho, S.J.; Kim, M.K.; Choi, J.; Nam, S.Y.; Kim, W.H.; Yang, H.K.; Lee, B.L. Manganese superoxide dismutase expression correlates with a poor prognosis in gastric cancer. *Pathobiology* **2002**, *70*, 353–360. [CrossRef] [PubMed]
49. Zhang, H.J.; Zhao, W.; Venkataraman, S.; Robbins, M.E.; Buettner, G.R.; Kregel, K.C.; Oberley, L.W. Activation of matrix metalloproteinase-2 by overexpression of manganese superoxide dismutase in human breast cancer MCF-7 cells involves reactive oxygen species. *J. Biol. Chem.* **2002**, *277*, 20919–20926. [CrossRef]
50. Chen, P.M.; Wu, T.C.; Shieh, S.H.; Wu, Y.H.; Li, M.C.; Sheu, G.T.; Cheng, Y.W.; Chen, C.Y.; Lee, H. MnSOD promotes tumor invasion via upregulation of FoxM1-MMP2 axis and related with poor survival and relapse in lung adenocarcinomas. *Mol. Cancer Res.* **2013**, *11*, 261–271. [CrossRef]
51. Siwik, D.A.; Pagano, P.J.; Colucci, W.S. Oxidative stress regulates collagen synthesis and matrix metalloproteinase activity in cardiac fibroblasts. *Am. J. Physiol. Cell Physiol.* **2001**, *280*, C53–C60. [CrossRef]
52. Cirigliano, M. Bioidentical hormone therapy: A review of the evidence. *J. Women's Health* **2007**, *16*, 600–631. [CrossRef] [PubMed]
53. Qian, Q.; Wang, Q.; Zhan, P.; Peng, L.; Wei, S.Z.; Shi, Y.; Song, Y. The role of matrix metalloproteinase 2 on the survival of patients with non-small cell lung cancer: A systematic review with meta-analysis. *Cancer Investig.* **2010**, *28*, 661–669. [CrossRef]
54. Yamaki, K.; Taneda, S.; Yanagisawa, R.; Inoue, K.; Takano, H.; Yoshino, S. Enhancement of allergic responses in vivo and in vitro by butylated hydroxytoluene. *Toxicol. Appl. Pharm.* **2007**, *223*, 164–172. [CrossRef] [PubMed]
55. Parra, E.R.; Boufelli, G.; Bertanha, F.; Samorano Lde, P.; Aguiar, A.C., Jr.; Costa, F.M.; Capelozzi, V.L.; Barbas-Filho, J.V. Temporal evolution of epithelial, vascular and interstitial lung injury in an experimental model of idiopathic pulmonary fibrosis induced by butyl-hydroxytoluene. *Int. J. Exp. Pathol.* **2008**, *89*, 350–357. [CrossRef] [PubMed]
56. Umemura, T.; Kodama, Y.; Hioki, K.; Inoue, T.; Nomura, T.; Kurokawa, Y. Butylhydroxytoluene (BHT) increases susceptibility of transgenic rasH2 mice to lung carcinogenesis. *J. Cancer Res. Clin. Oncol.* **2001**, *127*, 583–590. [CrossRef]
57. Parra, E.R.; Pincelli, M.S.; Teodoro, W.R.; Velosa, A.P.P.; Martins, V.; Rangel, M.P.; Barbas-Filho, J.V.; Capelozzi, V.L. Modeling pulmonary fibrosis by abnormal expression of telomerase/apoptosis/collagen V in experimental usual interstitial pneumonia. *Braz. J. Med Biol. Res.* **2014**, *47*, 567–575. [CrossRef] [PubMed]

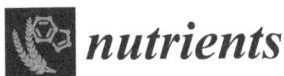

Article

Supplementation with *Spirulina platensis* Prevents Uterine Diseases Related to Muscle Reactivity and Oxidative Stress in Rats Undergoing Strength Training

Paula Benvindo Ferreira [1], Anderson Fellyp Avelino Diniz [1], Francisco Fernandes Lacerda Júnior [1], Maria da Conceição Correia Silva [1], Glêbia Alexa Cardoso [2], Alexandre Sérgio Silva [2] and Bagnólia Araújo da Silva [3],*

[1] Programa de Pós-graduação em Produtos Naturais e Sintéticos Bioativos, Universidade Federal da Paraíba, João Pessoa 58051-970, Brazil; paulabenvindo92@hotmail.com (P.B.F.); andersonfellyp@gmail.com (A.F.A.D.); lacerdafar17@gmail.com (F.F.L.J.); ceicafarma@gmail.com (M.d.C.C.S.)
[2] Departamento de Educação Física, Centro de Ciências da Saúde, Laboratório de Estudos de Treinamento Físico Aplicado à Performance e à Saúde, Universidade Federal da Paraíba, JoãoPessoa 58051-900, Brazil; gacbrasil@hotmail.com (G.A.C.); alexandresergiosilva@yahoo.com.br (A.S.S.)
[3] Departamento de Ciências Farmacêuticas, Centro de Ciências da Saúde, Universidade Federal da Paraíba, João Pessoa 58051-900, Brazil
* Correspondence: bagnolia@ltf.ufpb.br; Tel.: +55-83-99352-5995

Abstract: Strength training increases systemic oxygen consumption, causing the excessive generation of reactive oxygen species, which in turn, provokes oxidative stress reactions and cellular processes that induce uterine contraction. The aim of this study was to evaluate the possible protective effect of *Spirulina platensis* (SP), an antioxidant blue algae, on the contractile and relaxation reactivity of rat uterus and the balance of oxidative stress/antioxidant defenses. Female Wistar rats were divided into sedentary (CG), trained (TG), and T + supplemented (TG50, TG100) groups. Reactivity was analyzed by AQCAD, oxidative stress was evaluated by the malondialdehyde (MDA) formation, and the antioxidant capacity was measured by the 2,2-diphenyl-1-picrylhydrazyl (DPPH) method. Strength training increased contractile reactivity and decreased the pharmaco-mechanical component of relaxing reactivity in rat uterus. In addition, training decreased oxidation inhibition in the plasma and exercise increased oxidative stress in the uterine tissue; however, supplementation with algae prevented this effect and potentiated the increase in antioxidant capacity. Therefore, this study demonstrated that food supplementation prevents changes in reactivity and oxidative stress induced by strength training in a rat uterus, showing for the first time, that the uterus is a target for this exercise modality and antioxidant supplementation with *S. platensis* is an alternative means of preventing uterine dysfunction.

Keywords: *Spirulina platensis*; physical exercise; uterus; oxidative stress; muscle reactivity

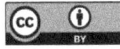

1. Introduction

Regular training has numerous beneficial effects on human health through the induction of homeostatic adaptations in different physiological systems such as the cardiorespiratory and muscle systems [1]. However, the magnitude of the effect of a specific training regime can vary significantly between individuals, as well as in individuals undergoing training who may not respond as expected [2]. This is due to factors such as the characteristics of the training regime, environmental conditions and individual factors, such as habitual physical activity, previous physical fitness level, genetics, psychological factors, age and sex [3].

In the past few decades, women have become increasingly physically active and evidence demonstrates that physical training can increase self-esteem, cardiorespiratory fitness, ovulation, and menstrual regularity while decreasing insulin resistance and body fat [4]. Despite this, several studies have reported that the female reproductive system is highly sensitive to physiological stress, and training with excessive loads is related to diseases such as osteoporosis and reproductive disorders including late menarche, primary and secondary amenorrhea and oligomenorrhea, which occur in 6% to 79% of women involved in athletic activities [5,6].

Additionally, free radicals have a dual role in the reproductive system; they function as key signaling molecules that modulate various reproductive functions and can directly influence the quality of oocytes, the oocyte–sperm interaction, the implant and initial embryonic development in their microenvironments [7]. The extent to which reactive species are useful or harmful is determined by factors such as the duration of exercise, the intensity, physical conditioning and the nutritional status of the individual [8]. Thus, the uterus should definitely be considered an important organ, making it an attractive target for exercise.

Oxidative stress has been widely studied within the scope of aerobic exercise. However, responses to anaerobic exercise, such as strength training have hardly been explored and the main focus has been on the muscles involved with exercise while the consequences for other types of muscles have been neglected. Thus, it is important to investigate the changes in the smooth muscles as a result of the practice of physical exercise since these muscles are mainly responsible for the control of most of the hollow organs in the body systems, including the uterus [9]. Different stages of molecular mechanisms related to muscle contraction have been shown to be susceptible to redox modulation, including the regulation of Ca^{2+} channels in the sarcoplasmic reticulum and myofibrillar sensitivity to Ca^{2+} [10–12].

Considering the important role of oxidative stress in the pathophysiology of several diseases, including some uterine disorders, and that poorly managed training loads can promote oxidative stress, there has recently been an increase in the consumption of nutrients that can act beneficially, either in isolation or in association with physical training, to improve the redox balance [13]. Food intake or antioxidant supplements are used as a non-invasive tool to decrease muscle damage, improve exercise performance, prevent or reduce oxidative stress, and improve lifespan with fewer of the specific risks that strenuous exercise can cause in athletes [14,15]. The benefits of antioxidant supplements may be related to an improvement in the cellular redox state, and in turn, a decrease in oxidative changes in DNA, lipids and proteins [16].

In this context, marine organisms, especially algae-derived compounds, play an important role among natural products due to the presence of secondary metabolites with great chemical diversity [17]. One marine organism that deserves to be highlighted is *Spirulina platensis* (Oscillatoriaceae), a blue-green algae that has been attracting attention due to its medicinal and nutritional properties, because of its antioxidant properties [18] and its effects on the smooth muscles of the aorta [19], trachea [20], ileum [21] and cavernous body [22].

Therefore, experimental models of strength training are considered to be a viable way to investigate the effects of organic dysfunctions induced by exercise on uterine contractility. Assuming that algae promotes beneficial effects in models of intestinal smooth muscle [23] and the vascular system [24] of animals submitted to intense strength training, it was hypothesized that strength exercise alters the contractile and relaxing reactivity of the Wistar rat uterus, and that food supplementation with *S. platensis* prevents uterine dysfunctions caused by exercise.

2. Materials and Methods

2.1. Substances

The salts used for the Locke Ringer's solution were purchased from Vetec (Rio de Janeiro, Brazil), Nuclear (Porto Alegre, Brazil) and Dinâmica (Diadema, Brazil). MDA, 1,1-diphenyl-2-picryl hydrazil (DPPH), methane hydroxymethylamine (tris), phenyl-methyl-sulfonyl fluoride (PMSF), aprotinin, dithiothreitol (DTT), Tween 20 and albumin were purchased from Sigma Aldrich (Rio De Janeiro, Brazil). Distilled water was used to dilute the substances and prepare the stock solutions and the diethylstilbestrol was dissolved in absolute alcohol (96° GL). The carbogen mixture (95% O_2 and 5% CO_2) was obtained from White Martins (Rio De Janeiro, Brazil). All substances were weighed on analytical scales, GEHAKA model AG 200 (São Paulo, Brazil).

2.2. Animals

Two-month-old virgin Wistar female rats (*Rattusnorvegicus*) weighing approximately 150–250 g, were purchased from the Animal Production Unit of the Instituto de Pesquisaem Fármacos e Medicamentos (IPeFarM). The animals were maintained under controlled ventilation and temperature (21 ± 1 °C) with water ad libitum in a 12 h light-dark cycle (lights on from 6 a.m. to 6 p.m.). Female rats were treated 24 h before euthanasia with diethylstilbestrol (1 mg/kg, s.c.) for estrus induction. The experiments were carried out from 7 a.m. to 11 p.m. The euthanasia of the rats was performed during the light period of this cycle. The experimental procedures (Ethics Committee on Animal Use of UFPB: 0211/2014) were performed following the guidelines for the ethical use of animals in applied etiology studies [25], and those of the National Council for Animal Experimentation Control (in Brazil) [26].

2.3. Preparation and Supplementationwith Spirulina platensis

Spirulina platensis in powder form was purchased from the INFINITY Pharma laboratory (Hong Kong, China) (Lot No. 17J11-B004-02504). The powder was prepared at the Royal Manipulation Pharmacy (João Pessoa, Brazil) (Lot No. 20121025). The *S. platensis* powder was prepared and dissolved daily in saline solution (NaCl 0.9%) and a solution was obtained at the dose to be used in the study (50 and 100 mg/kg) and administered to the rats after its preparation [19]. Supplementation occurred for a period of eight weeks [27] and algae was administered orally, thirty minutes before the exercise session [28] with the aid of stainless-steel needles for gavage (BD-12, Insight, Ribeirão Preto, Brazil) and 5 mL disposable syringes with 0.2 mL precision (BD, João Pessoa, Brazil).

2.4. Experimental Groups

Female rats were randomly divided into a sedentary group, or submitted to a strength training protocol and supplemented with *S. platensis* (50 and 100 mg/kg). Thus, the study consisted of the following groups with 28 rats each: sedentary group (CG, control), a group trained for 8 weeks (TG), a group trained and supplemented with algae 50 mg/kg (TG50), and a group trained and supplemented with *S. platensis* 100 mg/kg (TG100).

2.5. Strength Training Program

Female rats belonging to the strength training group were submitted to a training program that consisted of jumping in a liquid medium in a cylindrical PVC container (dimensions: 30 cm in diameter and 70 cm in length). The depth of water in the tanks was 50 cm, equivalent to twice the length of the mouse to prevent them from climbing to the edge of the cylinder. The water was previously heated to a temperature of 32 °C, as this was considered neutral in relation to the rat's body temperature [29].

Strength training was performed according to the protocol developed by Marqueti et al. (2006) for jumping in liquid medium [29]. The protocol consisted of 4 sets of 10 to 12 repetitions with an interval of 30 s between sets, and with progressive overload being adjusted according to the animal's weight (Scheme 1). The overload was applied to the animals' chest through a fabric vest that allowed the jumps to be performed without the load disconnecting from the body or impeding their movements. An overload corresponding to the weight of the vest when wet (25 g) was considered and charged to the specific load corresponding to the animal's body mass for better training accuracy

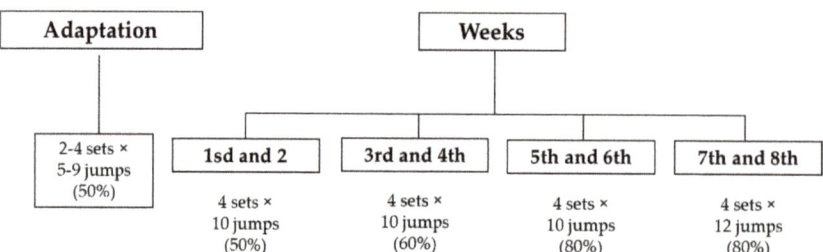

Scheme 1. Strength training program. Adaptation week—three alternate days of exercise sessions with a load of 50% of the animal's body weight, number of sets and repetitions adjusted for each session (1st day: 2 sets × 5 jumps; 2nd day: 4 sets × 5 jumps; and 3rd day: 4 sets × 9 jumps). 1st and 2nd weeks—4 sets of 10 jumps and an overload of 50% of the animal's body weight. 3rd and 4th weeks—4 sets of 10 jumps and load of 60% of body weight. 5th and 6th weeks—the 4 sets of 10 jumps and an overload of 80% of the animal's body weight. 7th and 8th weeks—continue the 4 sets of 12 jumps and load 80% of body weight. A rest period of 30 s was given between all sets.

After the end of the training protocols, the animals in the training group were euthanized by anesthesia with ketamine 100 mg/kg (i.p.) and xylazine 10 mg/kg (i.p.), followed by a complementary method of decapitation with the aid of a guillotine. They were euthanized 48 h after the last exercise session in order to eliminate the acute effect of the exercise on the reactivity (MOURA et al., 2012) [30].

2.6. Isolating the Uterus of Female Rats

Female rats were treated 24 h before euthanasia with diethylstilbestrol (1 mg/kg, s.c.) for estrus induction. The abdominal cavity was opened, and the uterus was dissected and placed in Locke Ringer's nutrient solution at 32 °C gassed with a mixture of carbogen. Then, the 2 uterine horns were separated by incision, opened longitudinally and suspended vertically by cotton thread in baths of isolated organs (6 mL), under tension of 1 g and kept at rest for at least 40 min. The solution was changed to every 15 min [31].

Uterus and plasma fragments were obtained for the biochemical measurements. These samples were quickly removed and stored in a freezer at −80 °C until the moment of analysis.

Locke Ringer's solution (adjusted to pH 7.4 with NaOH or 1N HCl) was carbonated with carbon and kept at 32 °C, and its composition (mM) was: NaCl (154.0); KCl (5.6); $CaCl_2$ (2.2); $MgCl_2$ (2.1); glucose (5.6); $NaHCO_3$ (6.0).

2.7. Contractile Reactivity Evaluation

As described above, the uterus was assembled and after the stabilization period (40 min), a contraction with 60 mMKCl was induced to verify the organ's functionality. After 15 min, two cumulative concentration–response curves for KCl or oxytocin were obtained. The contractile reactivity was calculated from the maximum contraction of the uterus of the animals from the groups that received supplementation with S. platensis and/or were submitted to strength training, being that obtained by the average of the maximum amplitudes of the control curves. Comparisons were made between groups that received supplementation with S. platensis and/or underwent strength training, using maximum effect values (Emax) and the negative logarithm (base 10) of the concentration of KCl or oxytocin producing 50% of the Emax (pEC_{50}).

2.8. Relaxation Reactivity Evaluation

After the stabilization period, a uterine contraction was induced with oxytocin (10^{-2} IU/mL) or KCl (60 mM). After the formation of the tonic component, isoprenaline or nifedipine was added cumulatively to the organ bath of all groups, in different preparations [32]. The relaxation response was observed and expressed as the reverse percentage of the initial contraction produced by the contractile agents. Comparisons were made between groups that received supplementation with algae and/or underwent strength training, with the means of the maximum amplitudes of the control curves, based on the Emax and pEC$_{50}$ values of the relaxation substances, being calculated from the cumulative concentration–response curves that were obtained.

2.9. Evaluation of Oxidative Stress (MDA) and Antioxidant Defenses (CAT)

After the animals were euthanized, the cervical vessels were sectioned to collect blood in test tubes with anticoagulant (EDTA) and were centrifuged at 1198× g for 10 min. The supernatant was stored in Eppendorf® tubes and refrigerated at 20 °C [33,34]. To obtain the homogenates, the uterine horns were isolated and frozen at 20 °C. The tissue was weighed, macerated and homogenized with 10% KCl at a ratio of 1:1. Afterwards, the samples were centrifuged (1198× g/10 min) and the supernatant was separated for testing.

Lipid peroxidation was evaluated by quantifying the MDA production. This was performed using the method of quantification of thiobarbituric acid reactive species (TBARS) in which two TBA molecules condense with one MDA molecule through a reaction colorimetric; this product can be easily detected by spectrophotometry. After obtaining plasma and uterine homogenate, 250 μL aliquots were incubated at 37 °C in a water bath for 60 min. Afterwards, samples were precipitated with 400 μL of 35% perchloric acid and centrifuged at 16,851× g for 20 min at 4 °C. The supernatant was transferred to Eppendorf® tubes, 400 μL of thiobarbituric acid (TBA) 0.6% was added to the samples and incubated at 95–100 °C for 1 h. Then, after cooling, the samples were read in a spectrophotometer at 532 nm. The turbid samples taken after the water bath were centrifuged again at 1198× g for 10 min before reading [35].

The colorimetric method of the reduction of DPPH was used to assess the total antioxidant capacity (CAT). This method is based on the ability of the sample to reduce the DPPH radical, which has a purple color, to 1,1-diphenyl-2-picryl hydrazine, a colored transparent, which is detected by spectrophotometry. Thus, 50 μL of plasma or pulmonary homogenate and 2 mL of DPPH solution dissolved in absolute ethanol (0.012 g/L) were added to a centrifuge tube and protected from light; then, the tubes were vortexed for 10 s and kept at rest for 30 min. Next, the samples were centrifuged at 7489× g for 15 min at 20 °C. The supernatant was read in a spectrophotometer at 515 nm. [36]

Analyses was performed to compare the MDA levels (μmol/L of sample) or the CAT (%) between the CG, TG, TG50 and TG100 groups.

2.10. Statistical Analysis

The functional results obtained were expressed as mean and standard error of the mean (S.E.M.) (n = 5) and statistically analyzed for intergroup comparison using Student's t-test. The results were statistically analyzed using two-way analysis of variance (ANOVA) followed by Tukey's post-test. The differences between the means were considered significant when $p < 0.05$. The pCE$_{50}$ values were calculated using linear regression, and E_{max} was obtained by averaging the maximum percentages of contraction or relaxation. All results were analyzed using Graph Pad Prism version 5.01 (Graph Pad Software Inc., San Diego, CA, USA).

3. Results

3.1. Effects of Strength Training and Supplementation with S. platensis on the Contractile Reactivity of the Uterus to KCl and Oxytocin

In the group submitted to strength training (GT), there was a reduction in potency and an increase in contractile efficacy in response to KCl (pCE$_{50}$ = 1.0 ± 0.03; E$_{max}$ = 172.7 ± 8.1%) when compared to the CG (pCE$_{50}$ = 2.0 ± 0.07; E$_{max}$ = 100%). Supplementation with S. platensis in GT50 (pCE$_{50}$ = 1.6 ± 0.02; E$_{max}$ = 84.3 ± 8.8%) and in GT100 (pCE$_{50}$ = 2.1 ± 0.05; E$_{max}$ = 119.7 ± 9.1%) prevented the increase in efficiency and reduced the potency of KCl (Figure 1a).

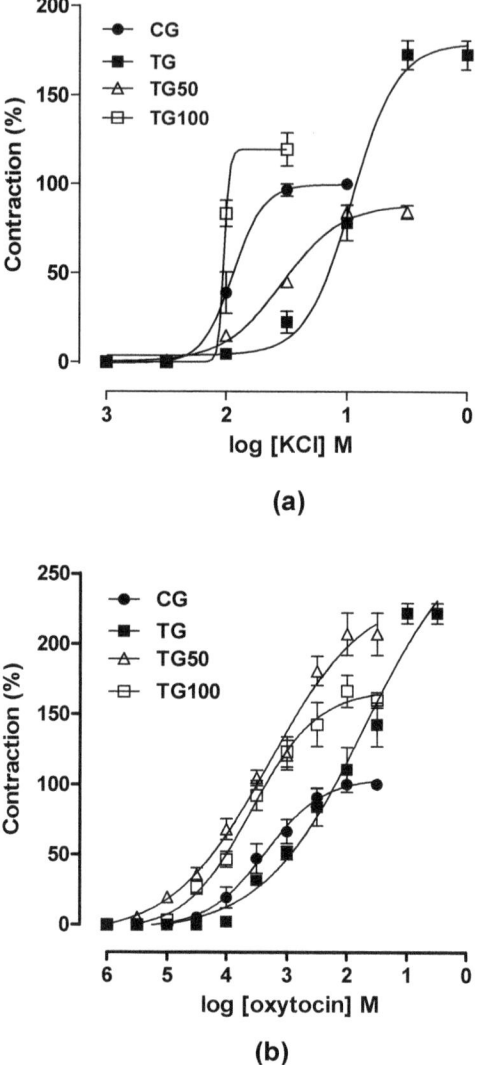

Figure 1. Effect of strength training and food supplementation with *S. platensis* on the cumulative concentration–response curves to KCl (**a**) and oxytocin (**b**) in isolated rat uterus, in CG (●), TG (■), TG50 (△) and TG100 (□). The symbols and vertical bars represent the mean and the e.p.m., respectively ($n = 5$). ANOVA one-way followed by Tukey's post-test.

In female rats submitted to strength training, there was a reduction in potency and an increase in the contractile efficacy of oxytocin ($pCE_{50} = 2.1 \pm 0.1$; $E_{max} = 222.0 \pm 7.1\%$) compared to the CG ($pCE_{50} = 3.4 \pm 0.2$; $E_{max} = 100.0\%$) and food supplementation with *S. platensis* in GT50 ($pCE50 = 3.5 \pm 0.1$; $E_{max} = 207.2 \pm 15.0\%$) and in GT100 ($pCE_{50} = 3.5 \pm 0.1$; $E_{max} = 169.1 \pm 7.7\%$) partially prevented the increase in efficiency and reduced the potency of this agonist (Figure 1b).

3.2. Effect of Strength Training and Supplementation with S. platensis on the Relaxing Response in Utero to Nifedipine and Isoprenaline

Strength training did not alter the potency or relaxing efficacy of nifedipine ($pCE_{50} = 11.0 \pm 0.2$; $E_{max} = 100\%$) compared to the CG ($pCE_{50} = 10.6 \pm 0.08$; $E_{max} = 100\%$). However, dietary supplementation with seaweed in the GT50 ($pCE_{50} = 8.8 \pm 0.2$; $E_{max} = 100\%$) and in the GT100 ($pCE_{50} = 8.6 \pm 0.2$; $E_{max} = 100.0\%$), decreased the relaxing potency of nifedipine, with no change in efficacy (Figure 2a).

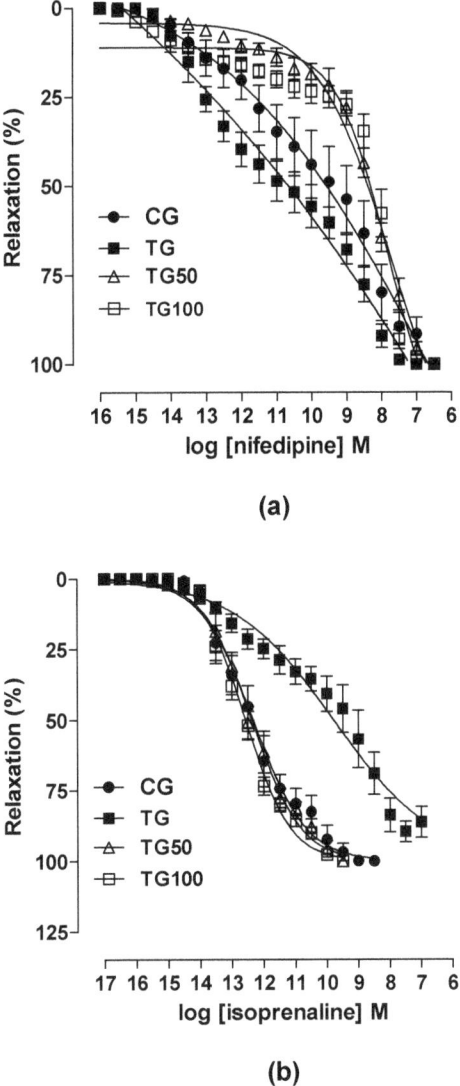

Figure 2. Effect of strength training and food supplementation with *S. platensis* on the cumulative concentration–response curves to nifedipine (**a**) and isoprenaline (**b**) in uterus of rats pre-contracted with KCl and oxytocin, respectively, in in CG (•), TG (■), TG50 (Δ) and TG100 (□). The symbols and vertical bars represent the mean and the e.p.m., respectively ($n = 5$). ANOVA one-way followed by Tukey's post-test.

Strength training (E_{max} = 89.6 ± 3.6%) decreased the relaxing efficacy of isoprenaline in relation to CG (E_{max} = 100%) and supplementation with algae in GT50 and GT100 (E_{max} = 100%) prevented the decrease in effectiveness. In relation to the potency, the GT (pCE50 = 9.8 ± 0.3) decreased the relaxing power of isoprenaline compared to the CG (pCE$_{50}$ = 12.0 ± 0.3); food supplementation with S. platensis prevented this reduction in both doses (GT50–pCE$_{50}$ = 12.0 ± 0.2; GT100–pCE$_{50}$= 12.3 ± 0.2) (Figure 2b).

3.3. Effect of Strength Training and/or Food Supplementation with S. platensis on the Concentration of MDA in the Plasma and Uterus of Rats

In female rats submitted to strength training and supplemented with S. platensis at doses of 50 and 100 mg/kg, no difference was observed in the plasma MDA concentration of the TG (3.6 ± 0.2), TG50 (3, 8 ± 0.4) and TG100 (3.1 ± 0.1) compared to the control CG (3.2 ± 0.1) (Figure 3a).

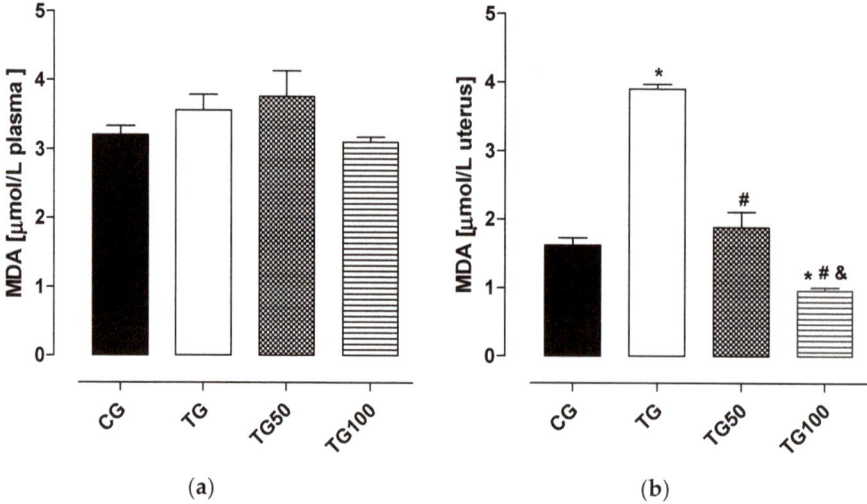

Figure 3. Effect of strength training and/or food supplementation with S. platensis on the concentration of MDA in the plasma (a) and in the uterus (b) of rats, in groups CG, TG, TG50 and TG100.The symbols and vertical bars represent the mean and the e.p.m., respectively (n = 5). ANOVA one-way followed by Tukey's post-test, * $p < 0.05$ (TG, TG50 and TG100 vs. CG); # $p < 0.05$ (TG50 and TG100 vs. TG); & $p < 0.05$ (TG100 and TG50 vs. TG). CG = control group; TG = trained group; TG50 = group trained and supplemented with algae at a dose of 50 mg/kg; TG100 = group trained and supplemented with algae at a dose of 100 mg/kg.

When analyzing the samples of uterine tissue, the concentration of MDA was increased in the TG group (3.9 ± 0.1) and this increase was prevented by supplementation with algae in the TG50 groups (1.9 ± 0.2) and more markedly in TG100 (1.0 ± 0.05) compared to the control CG (1.6 ± 0.1) (Figure 3b).

3.4. Effect of Strength Training and/or Food Supplementation with S. platensis on the Total Antioxidant Capacity in Plasma and Rat Uterus

In rats trained and supplemented with S. platensis, it was shown that strength training decreased the percentage of inhibition of oxidation in plasma (15.2 ± 0.4%) and that supplementation with seaweed in TG50 (22.4 ± 0.1%) and TG100 (24.6 ± 0.9%) attenuated this effect compared to the CG (28.4 ± 0.7%) (Figure 4a).

In the uterus, the oxidation percentage was increased by TG strength training (97.4 ± 1.3%) and by supplementation with S. platensis in TG50 (107.4 ± 1.9%), with this increase being marked in TG100 (130.8 ± 4.0%) compared to the CG (83.6 ± 3.4%) (Figure 4b).

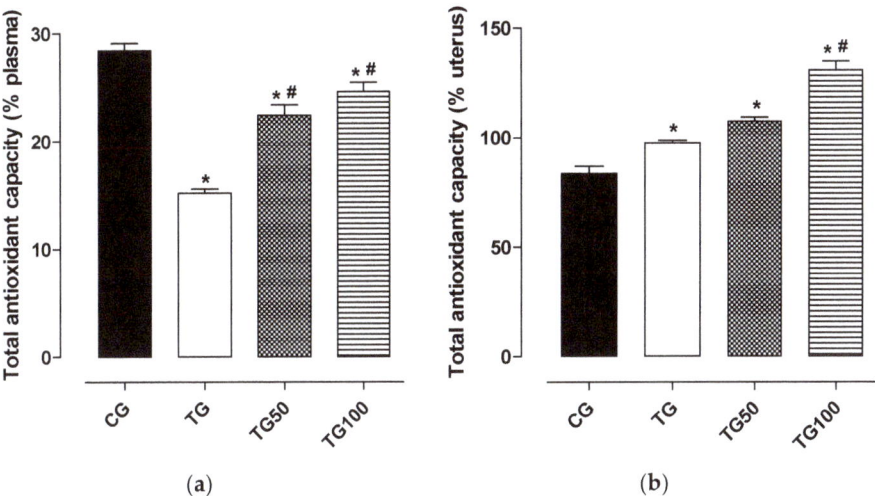

Figure 4. Effect of strength training and/or food supplementation with *S. platensis* on the percentage of antioxidant capacity in plasma (**a**) and in uterus (**b**) in rats, in CG, TG, TG50 and TG100. The symbols and vertical bars represent the mean and the e.p.m., respectively ($n = 5$). ANOVA one-way followed by Tukey's post-test, * $p < 0.05$ (TG, TG50 and TG100 vs. CG); # $p < 0.05$ (TG50 and TG100 vs. TG). CG = control group; TG = trained group; TG50 = group trained and supplemented with *S. platensis* at a dose of 50 mg/kg; TG100 = group trained and supplemented with *S. platensis* at a dose of 100 mg/kg.

4. Discussion

In this research, we investigated the modulation of contractile reactivity in the uterus of rats by strength training and in the association of dietary supplementation with training, as well as its effects on the balance of oxidative stress and antioxidant defenses. As a result, we demonstrated that strength training decreases potency and increases contractile efficacy, and decreases relaxing potency in rats' wombs, and these effects were prevented by dietary supplementation with *Spirulina platensis*. In addition, we found that supplementation with kelp prevented the increase in oxidative stress and improved uterine antioxidant defenses in trained female rats.

Several studies have shown that the pathophysiology of diseases that affect organs covered by smooth muscle, such as the intestine, vessels and uterus, may involve the deregulation of oxidative stress, as this is harmful to the contraction of smooth muscle. In addition it promotes changes in the function of various proteins from receptors to ion channels, which are responsible for triggering contractile processes [37]. The reactivity of the uterine smooth muscle plays a critical role in regulating and controlling the contractile activity of the myometrium. Many problems such as abortions, premature births, postpartum hemorrhages and uterine colic are associated with the abnormal regulation of the contractility of this muscle [38–40].

It is also important to emphasize that when women who practice physical exercise are subjected to excessive exercise, which is often accompanied by inadequate recovery, this can lead to disturbances in the body's homeostasis and hormonal dysregulation, which, in turn, can cause disorders in the reproductive system related to oxidative stress [5].

The correlation between oxidative stress and diseases involving the female reproductive system has led to an increase in the consumption of antioxidant supplements as a useful non-invasive tool, especially by women who exercise, and are seeking to decrease muscle damage, improve exercise performance and prevent or reduce oxidative stress. In addition, the concomitant use of these supplements has been shown to be promising and important for obtaining the positive results of the exercise [41]. In this scenario,

Spirulina platensis stands out, and it is used by athletes and physical activity practitioners due to its antioxidant potential and its high protein concentration [42].

From this, it was hypothesized that strength training promotes deleterious changes in uterine contractile and relaxing reactivity by increasing oxidative stress and that dietary supplementation of rats with *Spirulina platensis* would prevent the effects of exercise on the uterine reactivity of rats by decreasing oxidative stress.

Uterine contractions happen through pharmaco-mechanical and electromechanical coupling, which predominantly occurs through an increase in cytosolic calcium concentration ($[Ca^{2+}]_c$) [43], with pharmaco-mechanical coupling being induced by the release of calcium (Ca^{2+}) from intracellular cells mediated by inositol 1,4,5-triphosphate (IP3), while electromechanical contraction coupling is related to the change in resting potential, which promotes membrane depolarization, triggering the influx of Ca^{2+} through voltage-dependent calcium channels (Ca_V), and consequently, a contractile response. Thus, oxytocin, an agonist of oxytocin receptors (OT), was used as a pharmaco-mechanical contractile agent and to simulate the myogenic of this musculature [44]. KCl was used as a depolarizing agent of the cell membrane, resulting in an influx of Ca^{2+} and contraction.

Our data showed that strength training induced an increase in contractile efficacy in the two investigated couplings, demonstrating that uterine contractile reactivity is a target for exercise, and that dietary supplementation with *Spirulina platensis* prevented these effects in all tested doses. These results indicate that *Spirulina platensis* acts to prevent the formation of contractile compounds resulting from the practice of strength training, which in turn reduces the influx of Ca^{2+} and promotes a decrease in the contractile reactivity of the uterine smooth muscle.

Brito (2014) [28] demonstrated that supplementation with *S. platensis* potentiates the relaxing reactivity of the aorta (at doses of 150 and 500 mg/kg), against acetylcholine, and a decrease in contractile reactivity towards phenylephrine in the aorta of healthy rats. Similarly, Souza (2018) [45] found that supplementation with *S. platensis* potentiated the relaxing reactivity of the cavernous body of a rat. Thus, it was hypothesized that food supplementation with *S. platensis* would alter the relaxing reactivity of a rat uterus.

With regard to the relaxing response using nifedipine, an electromechanical agent Ca_V blocker, it was observed that strength training is not related to that component of the relaxing response. In the evaluation of the pharmaco-mechanical relaxation coupling, it was observed that the effect promoted by isoprenaline, a pharmaco-mechanical agonist, once again demonstrated the preventive effect of *S. platensis*, since the reduction in the relaxing potency was prevented in all doses tested. These data corroborate those observed in contractile reactivity and indicate that *Spirulina platensis* might target specific points that have been modulated by exercise.

In view of the data presented, it appears that the strength training model promoted changes in the contractile and relaxing uterine reactivity, with a resulting increase in contractile function, and that these changes were prevented by supplementation with *S. platensis*. It is known that strength exercise is strongly associated with the generation of ROS that alter tissue homeostasis, leading to different adaptations of the physiological changes induced by the deviation in cardiac output and hypoxia, which can affect the female reproductive system [5]. These adjustments are reflected by changes in contractile proteins, mitochondrial function, metabolic changes, intracellular signaling and transcriptional responses [46]. Thus, it was postulated that strength training and supplementation with *S. platensis* would modify the oxidative stress/antioxidant defense balance in plasma.

For this study, we used a methodology that determines MDA levels through a colorimetric reaction that results in the formation of a fluorescent pink chromogen that can be detected by means of a spectrophotometer reading [47], to confirm or discard the hypothesis that food supplementation with *S. platensis* reduces the formation of free radicals and prevents oxidative stress induced by strength training in the uterus of female rats Wistar.

When analyzing the rats submitted to the training protocol, an increase in MDA levels was observed, which was prevented by supplementation with seaweed in the tested doses. Although a sharp increase in the production of oxidants is necessary for myocellular adaptations to exercise, a chronic increase in protein oxidation can have serious consequences.

The chronic response to both aerobic and anaerobic training is to improve the antioxidant capacity of plasma, and the acute response relates to the production of specific antioxidants [48]. Based on this premise and that oxidative damage stimulates antioxidant defenses, we evaluated whether food supplementation with S. platensis and strength training would alter the systemic and tissue antioxidant capacity of Wistar rats [49].

When we analyzed the groups submitted to strength training, a decrease in the percentage of plasma oxidation inhibition was observed, demonstrating that strength training can decrease the systemic antioxidant capacity and that supplementation with S. platensis partially prevented this decrease. Despite this, there were no consequences related to systemic lipid peroxidation. However, when analyzing this parameter at the tissue level, there was an increase in antioxidant capacity in all groups tested, indicating that S. platensis potentiates the increase in antioxidant capacity in rats' uterus induced by strength training, strongly suggesting that a decrease in contractile free radicals resulting from the practice of strength exercise is one of the possible mechanisms to explain this preventive effect.

It is already well-established that pro-oxidant and antioxidant factors interact in a complex way to reach levels that do not damage the intracellular environment. When this balance is disturbed by an increase in free oxidizing substances, oxidative stress occurs and this event affects the whole body [19]. Such conditions are related to muscle fatigue [50], diabetes [51], arterial hypertension [52] and intermittent ischemia induced by myometrium contractions that restrict blood flow to the uterus, causing a state of reperfusion/ischemia [53,54].

Therefore, when physical exercise is not prescribed correctly, ROS can induce lipid peroxidation leading to problems such as inactivation of cell membrane enzymes, necrosis of muscle fibers, release of cellular enzymes into the blood, decreased effectiveness of immune system and alteration of mitochondrial function, leading to decreased muscle performance, overtraining and impairing important adaptations to training [55].

Thus, one can suggest that dietary supplementation with S. platensis has promising potential in pathophysiological processes that involve dysregulations in uterine contractile homeostasis such as dysmenorrhea, premature birth and abortion, as well as its preventive action for women who practice intense physical activity.

5. Conclusions

Based on the data presented and the discussion above, it was demonstrated, for the first time, a beneficial preventive effect of dietary supplementation with S. platensis, as well as its association with strength training. These preliminary data provide new insights into the mechanisms involved in this effect, and require tests in humans to confirm the possible effects, such as the reduction in uterine oxidative damage, which may contribute to better uterine functioning, especially for practitioners of progressively intense exercise during exposure to stress.

Author Contributions: P.B.F., A.S.S. and B.A.d.S. developed the hypothesis and experimental design. P.B.F., A.F.A.D. and M.d.C.C.S. analyzed the data and wrote the manuscript. P.B.F., F.F.L.J. and G.A.C. performed the experimental work. P.B.F., A.S.S., A.F.A.D. and F.F.L.J. contributed to the in vivo work. All authors have read and agreed to the published version of the manuscript.

Funding: This research received funding from the National Council for Scientific and Technological Development (CNPq), through a grant and project (protocol 433232/2016-1), and Coordination for the Improvement of Higher Education Personnel (CAPES) for supporting postgraduate activities the Academic Excellence Program (PROEX) and Periodical Publications Portal.

Institutional Review Board Statement: All work protocols were approved by the Ethics Committee on the Use of Animals of UFPB n° 0211/2014) and followed the norms for the ethical use of animals of the National Council for Experimental Control Animals (Brazil).

Acknowledgments: We thank Coordenação de Aperfeiçoamento de Pessoal de Nível Superior (CAPES), Conselho Nacional de Desenvolvimento Científico e Tecnológico (CNPq) for their financial support and Federal University of Paraíba for logistical support.

Conflicts of Interest: The authors declare that the research was conducted in the absence of any commercial or financial relationships that could be construed as a potential conflict of interest.

Abbreviations

Ach	acetylcholine
DPPH	1,1-diphenyl-2-picrylhydrazyl radical
EDTA	ethylenediamine tetra-acetic acid
E_{max}	maximum effect
MDA	malondialdehyde
SEM.	standard error of the mean
CG	control group
TG	group trained for 8 weeks
TG50	group trained and supplemented with *S. platensis* at 50 mg/kg
TG100	group trained and supplemented with *S. platensis* at 500 mg/kg
TBARS	thiobarbituric acid reactive substances

References

1. Coggan, A.R.; Williams, B.D. Metabolic adaptations to endurance training: Substrate metabolism during exercise. *Exerc. Metab.* **1995**, *183*, 177–210.
2. Garber, C.E.; Blissmer, B.; Deschenes, M.R.; Franklin, B.A.; Lamonte, M.J.; Lee, I.M.; Nieman, D.C.; Swain, D.P. American College of Sports Medicine. American College of Sports Medicine position stand. Quantity and quality of exercise for developing and maintaining cardiorespiratory, musculoskeletal, and neuromotor fitness in apparently healthy adults: Guidance for prescribing exercise. *Med. Sci. Sports Exerc.* **2011**, *43*, 1334–1359. [PubMed]
3. Marcus, B.H.; Forsyth, L.H.; Stone, E.J.; Dubbert, P.M.; Mckenzie, T.L.; Dunn, A.L.; Blair, S.N. Physical activity behavior change: Issues in adoption and maintenance. *Health Psychol.* **2000**, *19*, 32. [CrossRef]
4. Banting, L.K.; Gibson-Helm, M.; Polman, R.; Teede, H.J.; Stepto, N.K. Physical activity and mental health in women with polycystic ovary syndrome. *BMC Women's Health* **2014**, *14*, 51. [CrossRef] [PubMed]
5. Warren, M.P.; Perlroth, N.E. The effects of intense exercise on the female reproductive system. *J. Endocrinol.* **2001**, *170*, 3–11. [CrossRef]
6. De Souza, M.J.; Williams, N.I. Physiological aspects and clinical sequelae of energy deficiency and hypoestrogenism in exercising women. *Hum. Reprod. Update* **2004**, *10*, 433–448. [CrossRef]
7. Agarwal, A.; Guptaa, S.; Sikkab, S. The role of free radicals and antioxidants in reproduction. *Curr. Opin. Obstet. Gynecol.* **2006**, *18*, 325–332. [CrossRef] [PubMed]
8. Simioni, C.; Zauli, G.; Martelli, A.M.; Vitale, M.; Sacchetti, G.; Gonelli, A.; Neri, L.M.; Simioni, C.; Zauli, G.; Martelli, A.M.; et al. Oxidative stress: Role of physical exercise and antioxidant nutraceuticals in adulthood and aging. *Oncotarget* **2018**, *9*, 17181. [CrossRef]
9. Webb, R.C. Smooth muscle contraction and relaxation. *Adv. Physiol. Educ.* **2003**, *27*, 201–206. [CrossRef]
10. Wilson, G.; Dos Remedios, C.; Stephenson, D.; Williams, D. Effects of sulphydryl modification on skinned rat skeletal musclefibres using 5,5′-dithiobis (2-nitrobenzoic acid). *J. Physiol.* **1991**, *437*, 409–430. [CrossRef]
11. Aghdasi, B.; Zhang, J.-Z.; Wu, Y.; Reid, M.; Hamilton, S. Multiple classes of sulfhydryls modulate the skeletal muscle Ca^{2+} release channel. *J. Biol. Chem.* **1997**, *272*, 3739–3748. [CrossRef] [PubMed]
12. Andrade, F.H.; Reid, M.B.; Allen, D.G.; Westerblad, H. Effect of hydrogen peroxide and dithiothreitol on contractile function of single skeletal muscle fibres from the mouse. *J. Physiol.* **1998**, *509*, 565–575. [CrossRef]
13. Bentley, D.J.; Ackerman, J.; Clifford, T.; Slattery, K.S. Acute and chronic effects of antioxidant supplementation on exercise performance. In *Antioxidants in Sportnutrition*, 1st ed.; Lamprecht, M., Ed.; CRC Press: Boca Raton, FL, USA, 2015; p. 125.
14. Peternelj, T.; Coombes, J.S. Antioxidant supplementation during exercise training. *Sports Med.* **2011**, *41*, 1043–1069. [CrossRef]
15. Brisswalter, J.; Louis, J. Vitamin supplementation benefits in master athletes. *Sports Med.* **2014**, *44*, 311–318. [CrossRef]
16. Mason, S.A.; Trewin, A.J.; Parker, L.; Wadley, G.D. Antioxidant supplements and endurance exercise: Current evidence and mechanistic insights. *Redox Biol.* **2020**, *35*, 101471. [CrossRef]

17. De Almeida, C.L.; Falcão, H.S.; Lima, G.R.; Montenegro, C.A.; Lira, N.S.; Athayde-Filho, P.F.; Rodrigues, L.C.; De Souza, M.F.; Barbosa-Filho, J.M.; Batista, L.M. Bioactivities from marine algae of the genus Gracilaria. *Int. J. Mol. Sci.* **2011**, *12*, 4550–4573. [CrossRef] [PubMed]
18. Sharma, M.K.; Sharma, A.; Kumar, A.; Kumar, M. Spirulina fusiformis provides protection against mercuric chloride induced oxidative stress in Swiss albino mice. *Food Chem. Toxicol.* **2007**, *45*, 2412–2419. [CrossRef] [PubMed]
19. De Freitas Brito, A.; Silva, A.S.; de Souza, A.A.; Ferreira, P.B.; de Souza, I.L.L.; da Cunha Araujo, L.C.; da Silva Félix, G.; de Souza Sampaio, R.; da Conceição Correia Silva, M.; Tavares, R.L.; et al. Supplementation with Spirulina platensis modulates aortic vascular reactivity through nitric oxide and antioxidant activity. *Oxidative Med. Cell.* **2019**, *2019*, 7838149. [CrossRef] [PubMed]
20. Brito, A.F.; Silva, A.S.; Souza, I.L.L.; Pereira, J.C.; Silva, B.A. Intensity of swimming exercise influences aortic reactivity in rats. *Braz. J. Med. Biol. Res.* **2015**, *48*, 996–1003. [CrossRef] [PubMed]
21. Ferreira, E.S. Suplementação alimentar com *Spirulina platensis* promove efeito antiobesidade e restaura a reatividade contrátil de íleo em ratos Wistar. In *Dissertação (Mestrado em Produtos Naturais e Sintéticos Bioativos)*; Universidade Federal da Paraíba: João Pessoa, Brazil, 2017.
22. Diniz, A.F.; De Souza, I.L.L.; Dos Santos Ferreira, E.; De Lima Carvalho, M.T.; Barros, B.; Ferreira, P.B.; Da Conceição Correia Silva, M.; Lacerdam, J.; De Lima Tavares Toscano, L.; Silva, A.S.; et al. Potential Therapeutic Role of Dietary Supplementation with on the Erectile Function of Obese Rats Fed a Hypercaloric Diet. *Oxidative Med. Cell. Longev.* **2020**, *2020*, 1–14. [CrossRef] [PubMed]
23. Araujo, L.C.; Brito, A.F.; Souza, I.L.; Ferreira, P.B.; Vasconcelos, L.H.C.; Silva, A.S.; Silva, B.A. *Spirulina Platensis* Supplementation Coupled to Strength Exercise Improves Redox Balance and Reduces Intestinal Contractile Reactivity in Rat Ileum. *Mar. Drugs* **2020**, *18*, 89. [CrossRef] [PubMed]
24. Brito, A.F.; Silva, A.S.; de Oliveira, C.; de Souza, A.A.; Ferreira, P.B.; de Souza, I.; da Cunha Araujo, L.C.; da Silva Félix, G.; de Souza Sampaio, R.; Tavares, R.L.; et al. Spirulina platensis prevents oxidative stress and inflammation promoted by strength training in rats: Dose-response relation study. *Sci. Rep.* **2020**, *10*, 6382. [CrossRef] [PubMed]
25. Sherwin, C.M.; Christiansen, S.B.; Duncan, I.J.H.; Erhard, H.W.; Lay, D.C.; Mench, J.A.; O'connor, C.E.; Petherick, C.J. Guidelines for the ethical use of animals in applied animal behavior research. *Appl. Anim. Behav. Sci.* **2003**, *81*, 291–305. [CrossRef]
26. Brasil. Ministério da Ciência, Tecnologia e Inovação. Conselho Nacional de Experimentação Animal. Guia Brasileiro de Produção, Manutenção ou Utilização de Animais em Atividades de Ensino ou Pesquisa Científica: Fascículo 1: Introdução Geral. *Brasília–DF* **2016**. Available online: https://antigo.mctic.gov.br/mctic/opencms/institucional/concea/paginas/guia.html (accessed on 1 July 2021).
27. Juárez-Oropeza, M.A.; Mascher, D.; Torres-Durán, P.V.; Farias, J.M.; Paredes-Carbajal, M.C. Effects of dietary Spirulina on vascular reactivity. *J. Med. Food* **2009**, *12*, 15–20. [CrossRef]
28. Brito, A.F. Treinamento de força e suplementação alimentar com Spirulina platensis modulam a reatividade vascular de aorta de ratos wistar saudáveis dependente do óxido nítrico e da atividade antioxidante. In *Tese (Doutorado em Produtos Naturais e Sintéticos Bioativos)*; Universidade Federal da Paraíba: João Pessoa, Brazil, 2014.
29. Marqueti, R.C.; Parizotto, N.A.; Chriguer, R.S.; Perez, S.E.; Selistre-De-Araujo, H.S. Androgenic-anabolic steroids associated with mechanical loading inhibit matrix metallopeptidase activity and affect the remodeling of the achilles tendon in rats. *Am. J. Sports Med.* **2006**, *34*, 1274–1280. [CrossRef]
30. Moura, L.P.; Gurjão, A.L.; Jambassi Filho, J.C.; Mizuno, J.; Suemi, C.; Mello, M.A. Spirulina, exercise and serum glucose control in diabetic rats. *Arq. Bras. Endocrinol. Metabol.* **2012**, *1*, 25–32. [CrossRef] [PubMed]
31. Revuelta, M.P.; Cantabrana, B.; Hidalgo, A.; Revuelta, M.P.; Cantabrana, B.; Hidalgo, A. Depolarization-dependent effect of flavonoids in rat uterine smooth muscle contraction elicited by $CaCl_2$. *Gen. Pharmacol.* **1997**, *29*, 847–857. [CrossRef]
32. Heylen, E.; Guerrero, F.; Mansourati, J.; Theron, M.; Thioub, S.; Saiag, B. Effect of training frequency on endothelium-dependent vasorelaxation in rats. *Eur. J. Prev. Cardiol.* **2008**, *15*, 52–58. [CrossRef]
33. Okafor, O.; Erukainure, O.; Ajiboye, J.; Adejobi, R.; Owolabi, F.; Kosoko, S. Modulatory effect of pineapple peel extract on lipid peroxidation, catalase activity and hepatic biomarker levels in blood plasma of alcohol–induced oxidative stressed rats. *Asian Pac. J. Trop. Biomed.* **2011**, *1*, 12–14. [CrossRef]
34. Silva, A.S.; Paim, F.C.; Santos, R.C.; Sangoi, M.B.; Moresco, R.N.; Lopes, S.T.; Jaques, J.A.; Baldissarelli, J.; Morsch, V.M.; Monteiro, S.G. Nitric oxide level, protein oxidation and antioxidant enzymes in rats infected by Trypanosoma evansi. *Exp. Parasitol.* **2012**, *132*, 166–170.
35. Ohkawa, H.; Ohishi, N.; Yagi, K. Assay for lipid peroxides in animal tissues by thiobarbituric acid reaction. *Anal. Biochem.* **1979**, *95*, 351–358. [CrossRef]
36. Brand-Williams, W.; Cuvelier, M.E.; Berset, C.L.W.T. Use of a free radical method to evaluate antioxidant activity. *LWT-Food Sci. Technol.* **1995**, *28*, 25–30. [CrossRef]
37. Van Der Vliet, A. Effect of oxidative stress on receptors and signal transmission. *Chem.-Biol. Interact.* **1992**, *85*, 95–116. [CrossRef]
38. Word, R.A. Myosin phosphorylation and the control of miometrial contraction/relaxation. *Semin. Perinatol.* **1995**, *19*, 3–14. [CrossRef]
39. Wray, S.; Kupittayanant, S.; Shmigol, A.; Smith, R.D.; Burdyga, T. The physiological basis of uterine contractility: A short review. *Exp. Physiol.* **2001**, *86*, 239–246. [CrossRef]

40. Shmygol, A.; Wray, S. Functional architecture of the SR calcium store in uterine smooth muscle. *Cell Calcium* **2004**, *35*, 501–508. [CrossRef]
41. Pingitore, A.; Lima, G.P.P.; Mastorci, F.; Quinones, A.; Iervasi, G.; Vassalle, C. Exerciseandoxidative stress: Potential effects of antioxidant diet ary strategies in sports. *Nutrition* **2015**, *31*, 916–922. [CrossRef] [PubMed]
42. Carvalho, L.F.D.; Moreira, J.B.; Oliveira, M.S.; Costa, J.A.V. Novel food supplements formulated with Spirulina to meet athletes' needs. *Braz. Arch. Biol. Technol.* **2017**, *60*, 1–11.
43. Aguilar, H.N.; Mitchell, B.F. Physiological pathways and molecular mechanisms regulating uterine contractility. *Hum. Reprod. Update* **2010**, *16*, 725–744. [CrossRef]
44. Wray, S.; Jones, K.; Kupittayanant, S.; Li, Y.; Matthew, A.; MonirBishty, E.; Noble, K.; Pierce, S.J.; Quenby, S.; Shmygol, A.V. Calcium signaling and uterine contractility. *J. Gynecol.* **2003**, *10*, 252–264. [CrossRef]
45. Souza, I.L.L. Suplementação alimentar com Spirulina platensis previne o desenvolvimento da obesidade e da disfunção erétil em ratos Wistar por modular os fatores derivados do endotélio e o estresse oxidativo. In *Tese (Doutorado em Produtos Naturais e Sintéticos Bioativos)*; Universidade Federal da Paraíba: João Pessoa, Brazil, 2018.
46. Pedersen, B.K.; Ostrowski, K.; Rohde, T.; Bruunsgaard, H. The cytokine response to strenuous exercise. *Can. J. Physiol. Pharmacol.* **1998**, *76*, 505–511. [CrossRef] [PubMed]
47. Giera, M.; Lingeman, H.; Niessen, W.M. Recent advancements in the LC-and GC-based analysis of malondialdehyde (MDA): A brief overview. *Chromatographia* **2012**, *75*, 433–440. [CrossRef]
48. Atalay, M.; Laaksonen, D.E. Diabetes, oxidative stress and physical exercise. *J. Sports Sci. Med.* **2002**, *1*, 1.
49. Kinnunen, S.; Atalay, M.; Hyyppä, S.; Lehmuskero, A.; Hänninen, O.; Oksala, N. Effects of prolonged exercise on oxidative stress and antioxidant defense in endurance horse. *J. Sports Sci. Med.* **2005**, *4*, 415. [CrossRef] [PubMed]
50. Davies, K.P.; Melman, A. Markers of erectile dysfunction. *Indian J. Urol.* **2008**, *24*, 320. [CrossRef] [PubMed]
51. Karasu, C. Time course of changes in endothelium-dependent and -independent relaxation of chronically diabetic aorta: Role of reactive oxygen species. *Eur. J. Pharmacol.* **2000**, *392*, 163–173. [CrossRef]
52. Lacy, F.; O'connor, D.T. Plasma hydrogen peroxide production in hypertensives and normotensive subjects at genetic risk of hypertension. *J. Hypertens* **1998**, *16*, 291–303. [CrossRef]
53. Nakai, A.; Oya, A.; Kobe, H.; Asakura, H.; Yokota, A.; Koshino, T.; Araki, T. Changes in maternal lipid peroxidation levels and antioxidante enzymatic activities before and after delivery. *J. Nippon Med. Sch.* **2000**, *67*, 434–439. [CrossRef] [PubMed]
54. Warren, A.Y.; Matharoo-Ball, B.; Shaw, R.W.; Khan, R.N. Hydrogen peroxide and superoxide anion modulate pregnant human myometrial contractility. *Reproduction* **2005**, *130*, 539–544. [CrossRef] [PubMed]
55. Powers, S.K.; Jackson, M.J. Exercise-induce doxidative stress: Cellular mechanisms and impacton muscle force production. *Pshysiol. Rev.* **2008**, *88*, 1234–1276.

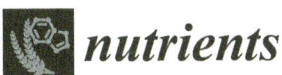

Review

Phytoprogestins: Unexplored Food Compounds with Potential Preventive and Therapeutic Effects in Female Diseases

Stefania Greco [1], Pamela Pellegrino [1], Alessandro Zannotti [1,2], Giovanni Delli Carpini [2], Andrea Ciavattini [2], Fernando M. Reis [3] and Pasquapina Ciarmela [1,*]

[1] Department of Experimental and Clinical Medicine, Università Politecnica delle Marche, 60126 Ancona, Italy; s.greco@staff.univpm.it (S.G.); p.pellegrino@pm.univpm.it (P.P.); a.zannotti@pm.univpm.it (A.Z.)

[2] Department of Specialist and Odontostomatological Clinical Sciences, Università Politecnica delle Marche, 60126 Ancona, Italy; g.dellicarpini@staff.univpm.it (G.D.C.); a.ciavattini@univpm.it (A.C.)

[3] Department of Obstetrics and Gynecology, Universidade Federal de Minas Gerais, Belo Horizonte 30130-100, Brazil; fmreis@ufmg.br

* Correspondence: p.ciarmela@univpm.it; Tel.: +39-0712206270

Abstract: In recent years, there has been an increasing interest in natural therapies to prevent or treat female diseases. In particular, many studies have focused on searching natural compounds with less side effects than standard hormonal therapies. While phytoestrogen-based therapies have been extensively studied, treatments with phytoprogestins reported in the literature are very rare. In this review, we focused on compounds of natural origin, which have progestin effects and that could be good candidates for preventing and treating female diseases. We identified the following phytoprogestins: kaempferol, apigenin, luteolin, and naringenin. In vitro studies showed promising results such as the antitumoral effects of kaempferol, apigenin and luteolin, and the anti-fibrotic effects of naringenin. Although limited data are available, it seems that phytoprogestins could be a promising tool for preventing and treating hormone-dependent diseases.

Keywords: female disease; progesterone; phytoprogestins; phytochemical compounds

1. Introduction

In recent years, there has been an increasing interest in alternative and natural methods for the prevention or treatment of female diseases. In particular, many studies have focused on searching for adequate compounds with less side effects than standard hormonal therapies. Although the etiopathogenetic mechanisms of many gynecological diseases, such as endometriosis [1] and uterine fibroids [2] are still not clear, the role of steroid hormones is undoubted. Indeed, there is an important hormonal imbalance, for example, in endometriosis [3], uterine leiomyomas [4], ovarian cancer [5], and breast cancer [6].

The father of medicine, Hippocrates, proclaimed "Let food be the medicine and medicine be the food" around 25 centuries ago. In recent studies, there is a high interest in dietary phytochemicals. Phytochemicals are chemical compounds of natural origin that can be used as therapeutic or preventive agents.

Nutraceutical compounds can exert their effects on health in different ways, including through hormonal activity. Their mechanism of action is: 1. Competition with the hormone for binding to the corresponding receptor, thanks to a structural similarity; 2. Influence on the activity of key enzymes of the biosynthetic pathway, such as in the case of isoflavones, which are moderate aromatase inhibitors, thus reducing estrogen synthesis; 3. Influence on the epigenome by affecting DNA methylation activity, histone modification, and microRNA regulation [7].

Phytoestrogens and phytoprogestins are phytochemical compounds of natural origin, which have estrogenic and progestagenic effects, respectively [8,9]. While phytoestrogen-based therapies have been extensively studied in the clinical setting, treatments with

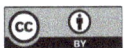

phytoprogestin are still in the preclinical stage, and their potential remains unexplored [8]. Therefore, we decided to review the current evidence supporting the preventive and therapeutic effects of phytoprogestins in female diseases.

2. Methods

In this narrative review, we performed a bibliographic search of studies evaluating the effects of dietary phytoprogestins on reproductive cells and tissues and the possible association of these nutritional compounds with gynecological diseases. The search was carried out on Pubmed using combinations of the following terms: phytochemicals [MeSH], flavonoids [MeSH], kaempferol, apigenin, naringenin, luteolin, women, uterine fibroids, endometriosis, ovarian cancer, and breast cancer. The search was narrowed to studies in humans or relevant animal models of human diseases and complemented by screening the reference lists of the selected articles. We also briefly review the pharmacological mechanisms of progesterone receptor activation and progesterone-based therapies in order to provide a background to the discussion of phytoprogestins.

3. Progesterone

Progesterone is a sex steroid hormone essential in female reproduction, including the menstrual cycle and the establishment and maintenance of pregnancy [10]. The etymology of the name derives from the Latin "pro gestationem" [11], as it allows the endometrium to pass from the proliferative to the secretory stage, facilitating the nesting of the blastocyst and is essential for maintaining pregnancy; in fact, it promotes the uterine growth and suppresses the contractility of the muscular tissue of the uterus (myometrium). In the mammary gland, it promotes the development of the gland for the secretion of milk. In addition, progesterone plays an essential role in the physiology of non-reproductive tissues, such as the cardiovascular system, the central nervous system, and bone tissue. In the brain, progesterone is neuroprotective, and its metabolite allopregnanolone is a GABAergic agonist [12,13] (Figure 1).

Steroids are ancestral molecules [11] characterized by a common base structure of cyclopentane–perhydro–phenanthrene, a polycyclic complex of 17 carbon atoms making a four-ring system. Based on the number of carbon atoms, sex steroids can be categorized into three groups: progesterone and progestins, with 21 carbon atoms, androgens, which have 19 carbon atoms, and finally estrogens, with 18 carbon atoms.

The biosynthesis of steroid hormones is the same in all organs where they are produced, such as the ovary, testis, adrenal cortex, brain, and placenta. The gonadal progesterone is mainly transported by blood to reach the target cells, while the progesterone produced by adrenal gland is mostly locally converted into glucocorticoids and androgens [14]. Progesterone circulates in the bloodstream bound to cortisol-binding globulin (approximately 10%) and serum albumin and has a relatively short half-life of only five minutes. The metabolites mainly produced in the liver are sulfates and glucuronides, which are excreted in the urine. Circulating progesterone is converted by the kidney into a mineralocorticoid, deoxycorticosterone (DOC). During the luteal phase, pregnancy, and administration of exogenous progesterone, most circulating DOC arises from this pathway and may bring unbearable side effects [14].

Progesterone exerts its physiological effect by binding to target cells via specific nuclear progesterone receptors (PR) or by binding to membrane receptors (progesterone receptor membrane component, PGRMC, or mPR). The binding with the nuclear receptors gives rise to a genomic pathway that requires a much longer response than the non-genomic one, which is triggered when progesterone binds to membrane receptors.

PRs are expressed in the human ovary [15], uterus [16], testis [17], brain [18], pancreas [19], bone tissue [20], mammary gland [21] and urinary tract [22]. PRs, together with the receptors for estradiol, mineralocorticoids, glucocorticoids, and androgens, belong to the superfamily of nuclear receptors. The nuclear progesterone receptor consists of a central binding domain for DNA (DBD) and a carboxylic terminal binding domain for the ligand

(LBD). In addition, the receptor has transcription activation function (TAF) domains that interact with coactivators and corepressors to regulate the downstream target genes [23] (Figure 2). The newly transcribed progesterone receptor is assembled into an inactive multiprotein chaperone complex in the cytoplasm [24]. The receptor at this level must be inactive [25] since its activation occurs only in the presence of a link with the hormone, which induces a conformational change of the receptor [26].

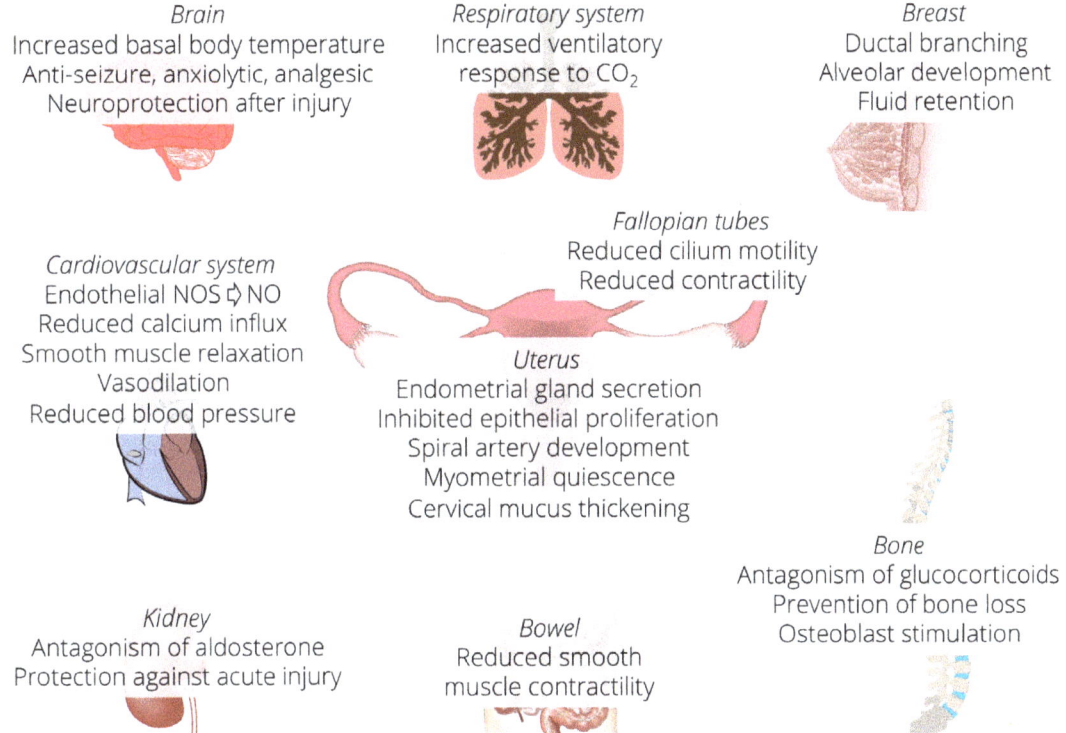

Figure 1. Schematic representation of the organs in which progesterone performs functions. Progesterone acts in reproductive as well as in non-reproductive tissues. NOS = nitric oxide synthase, NO = nitric oxide.

Two isoforms of PR are transcribed from a single gene by alternative splicing from two distinct promoters [27,28], giving rise to transcripts that encode, respectively, for the protein isoforms A (PRA) and B (PRB) (Figure 2). PRA and PRB are identical in sequence, except that PRA lacks 164 amino acids at the N-terminal, making it the shorter of the two proteins [28].

Progesterone may act through a genomic (slow process) or a non-genomic (fast process) pathway. The classical pathways of progesterone actions are mediated via nuclear receptors. Progesterone enters the cell and binds PRs, inducing their conformational change and dimerization. The complex of progesterone with PR translocates to the nucleus and interacts with DNA-binding elements in the genome, activating the transcription of progesterone-responsive genes (Figure 2). The non-genomic (also called non-classical or extranuclear) progesterone action initiates at the cell surface with the activation of the cytoplasmic PRs or membrane-bound PRs (mPRs) and determines an intracellular signaling that elicits a rapid response [29]. These proteins include the progesterone receptor membrane component 1

(PGRMC1), its counterpart PGRMC2, and the family of membrane progesterone receptors (mPR), also known as PAQR (progestin and adipoQ) receptors [30].

Studies in mice have shown that the elimination of the PRB isoform resulted in the unhealthy development of the mammary gland [31], while the elimination of PRA caused an abnormal development of the uterus and impaired its reproductive function [32]. Therefore, in animals, a dominant expression of one of the two isoforms seems to be necessary for the normal functioning and development of some organs. On the other hand, in humans, all healthy tissues, including those of the mammary gland and uterus, have epithelial cells that express PR with the co-expression of both the PRA and PRB isoforms [33,34]. This condition suggests that the colocalization and thus the cooperative activity of PRA and PRB mediate the action of PR in humans. Although the two isoforms are expressed in the same way in most human tissues, there is a different expression in the endometrium. In fact, during the secretory phase of the menstrual cycle, when there are high levels of circulating progesterone, the PRA isoform is poorly expressed, resulting in a clear predominance of PRB [33].

In breast and endometrial cancers, there are substantial differences in progesterone levels and its isoforms compared to normal tissues. In fact, in healthy tissues deriving from the mammary gland, epithelial cells equally express both PR isoforms [34], while in neoplastic biopsies, it is possible to see a significant increase in the expression, alternatively, of PRA or PRB [34,35]. Similarly, in endometrial cancer, it is common to find only one of the two isoforms expressed, either PRA or PRB, suggesting that the lack of co-expression of both isoforms is an early event of the onset of endometrial cancer [36].

A third isoform (PRC) has been identified in the human placenta [37]. PRC is an isoform with a truncated N-terminal domain, with a molecular mass of approximately 60 kDa, present in the cytoplasm. PRC lacks the first zinc finger of the DBD, but it can still bind progesterone. The actions of PRC are not clear, but it can form heterodimers with PRA and PRB and, in this way, regulate the transcriptional activity of the PR isoforms [37,38].

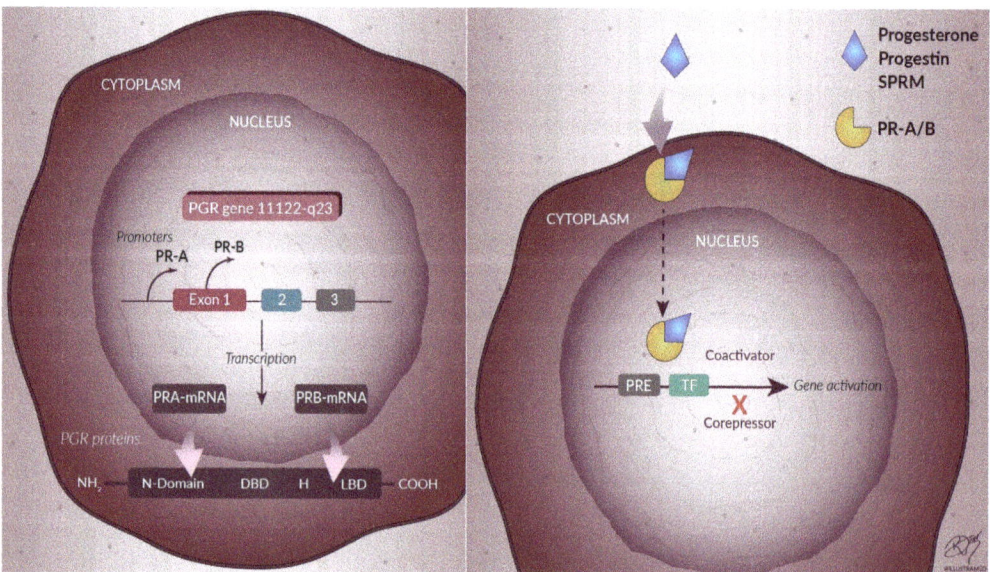

Figure 2. Progesterone receptors and their activation. The nuclear receptor is formed by two promoter regions on the PR gene, one for PRA and one for PRB, and these two promoters allow the synthesis of the two separate mRNA transcripts that code for the two different isoforms PRA and PRB. DBD = DNA-binding domain, H = hinge, LBD = ligand-binding domain, SPRM = selective progesterone receptor modulator, PRE = progesterone responsive element, TF = transcription factor.

4. Progesterone-Based Drug Therapy

Progestogens are the most common compounds used as drug therapy for the treatment of women's diseases. Many gynecological diseases are treated with synthetic progestin-based drugs. In the United States, endometrial cancer is one of the most common gynecological cancers, with 46,470 new cases and 8,120 deaths in 2011 [39]. Even if the molecular mechanisms involved in endometrial carcinogenesis are not clear, it seems that chronic exposure to estrogen and its metabolites without sufficient counterbalance of progesterone has proliferative effects [40,41] and is harmful to DNA [42,43]. Based on the antiestrogenic role of progesterone, many patients affected by endometrial cancer may have an indication to progesterone-based therapy, particularly in case of contraindications to surgery or desire for fertility maintenance. Indeed, women with endometrial hyperplasia and well-differentiated endometrial adenocarcinoma show a good response to progestogen therapy [44]. However, as the severity of the disease increases, the efficacy of progestogens decreases [45].

Other estrogen-dependent female pathologies with a high social impact, such as endometriosis, are often treated with progestin therapies [46,47], including synthetic progestins such as medroxyprogesterone acetate or dienogest [48,49]. Uterine fibroids may also be treated with progestins. Since the first reports of decades ago [50], studies have focused on the effects of different progestins on uterine fibroids, with different drug dosages and regimens. For example, medroxyprogesterone acetate [51] and dienogest [52,53] have shown a regressive effect on uterine fibroids.

Moreover, progestogens are widely used as a contraceptive method and in menopausal hormone therapy, in combination with estrogens. These therapies may also have an effect of prevention of ovarian cancer, but they increase the risk of venous thromboembolism and present side effects [54,55]. Therefore, the identification of alternative progestogens is clinically significant. Numerous studies in the literature indicate a great interest in developing phytoprogestogens, such as botanical extracts or food supplements, hoping to provide the beneficial effects of progestins while avoiding the side effects.

Selective progesterone receptor modulator (SPRM) is a class of synthetic ligands that act on the PR and tend to be more tissue-specific than progestins. The mechanism of action of SPRMs occurs through binding to PR, resulting in a conformational change of the receptor. The action can be agonistic, antagonistic, or mixed. The agonist action of SPRMs involves the recruitment of different coactivators to induce transcriptional activity and occurs in tissues where high levels of coactivators are present, while antagonist activity occurs where corepressors are in excess (Figure 2).

When the PR is inactive, SPRMs bind to the receptor and activate it. The binding involves nuclear import, which gives the receptor the property of dimerization. In the nucleus, the dimer interacts with the response element in the DNA, causing the up-regulation or down-regulation of the gene [56,57]. The action of SPRMs also depends on the ratio of PR-A and PR-B in the tissue and on the specific binding affinity of the SPRMs for each receptor isoform [58]. SPRMs have been developed for clinical applications, considering their tissue selectivity and low rate of side effects [59]. Their application is principally for the treatment of uterine fibroids [60], endometriosis [61], and breast cancer [62].

Despite having beneficial effects, for example, in the treatment of uterine fibroids, the prolonged use of SPRMs may lead to endometrial hyperplasia and other side effects. Indeed, it has been shown that long-term use of the SPRM asoprisnil results in long-term damage to the endometrium. Ulipristal acetate has been approved in Canada and Europe as a presurgical therapy for patients with uterine fibroids to control bleeding, and in the United States for emergency contraception. However, it has raised concerns due to liver toxicity [63], as well as telapristone acetate, which was stopped in 2009. Vilaprisan is still under study, and its possible collateral effects are not yet known [64].

5. Phytoprogestins

Phytoprogestins are chemical compounds of vegetal origin that have progesterone-like activity and can function as non-steroidal SPRMs. Unlike estrogenic counterparts, which have been extensively studied, the literature reports much fewer studies on phytoprogestins. The following phytoprogestins have been identified: kaempferol, apigenin, luteolin, and naringenin (Figure 3).

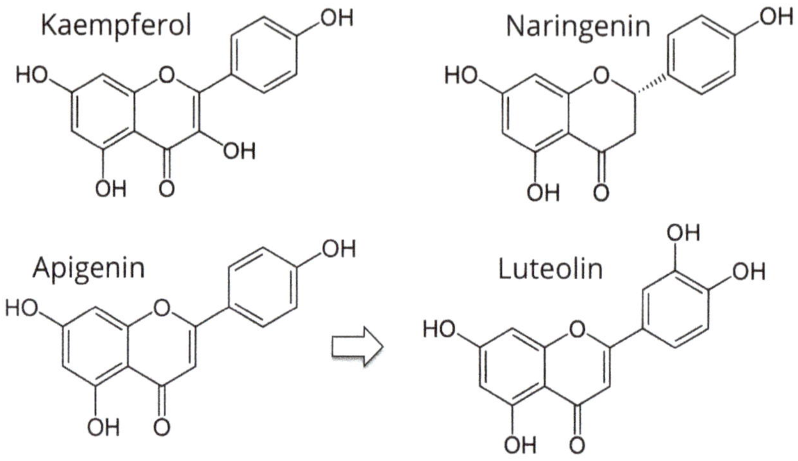

Figure 3. Chemical structure of phytoprogestins.

5.1. Kaempferol

Kaempferol (KP: 3,5,7-trihydroxy-2-(4-hydroxyphenyl)-4H-1-benzopyran-4-one) is a flavonoid found in several botanical families, including Pteridophyta, Pinophyta, and Magnoliophyta (Figure 3). Flavonoids are a group of secondary metabolites widespread in nature. These substances are known for the benefits of their consumption, which seems to reduce the risk of cancer and cardiovascular diseases [65]. A case–control study showed a 40% reduction (adjusted odds ratio 0.60) in breast cancer risk in Chinese women in the upper quartile of serum KP levels [66]. The risk of epithelial ovarian cancer was also decreased by 40% among women in the highest quintile of KP dietary intake of a large prospective cohort in the USA, the Nurses' Health Study [67]. Several studies have shown that KP has excellent antioxidant properties. In fact, it is able to decrease, even at low concentrations, the levels of the hydroxyl radical and peroxynitrite, highly reactive species capable of causing severe damage to DNA, proteins, and lipids [68]. In addition, KP has anti-inflammatory properties not only in vitro but also in vivo [69,70].

KP inhibits estrogen receptor-α, causing antiestrogenic effects, depending on the concentration of endogenous estrogens. The antiestrogenic activity of KP results in the inhibition of the growth of hormone-dependent tumors; this activity has been demonstrated in numerous in vitro studies, for example, in endometrial carcinoma cells [71] and two lines of breast cancer cells [72].

In uterine fibroids, despite being hormone-dependent tumors with severe symptoms, the effects of KP have not been extensively studied. KP treatment reduces the expression of the estrogen receptor, thus inhibiting the cell proliferation of human uterine leiomyoma cells in vitro [73], although its therapeutic effect in vivo remains unknown (Table 1).

Table 1. Effects of phytoprogestins that suggest their potential to treat women's diseases.

Substance	Study Design	Effects	Significance	References
Kaempferol	Experiments in mice and rats	Anti-inflammatory	Could be useful to treat chronic pelvic pain and its causes	[69,70]
	In vitro culture of human neutrophils	Antioxidant	Another potential therapeutic mechanism to treat endometriosis	[68]
	In vitro culture of endometrial cancer cells	Growth inhibition and apoptosis	Could be effective against endometrial hyperplasia and cancer	[71]
Apigenin	In vitro culture of human cancer cell lines	Growth inhibition and apoptosis VEGF inhibition	Could be effective against endometrial hyperplasia and cancer	[74,75]
Luteolin	Human breast tumor xenografts in nude mice	Inhibition of tumor growth and angiogenesis	Could be an adjuvant therapy of breast cancer	[76,77]
Naringenin	Mouse model in vivo	Analgesic, anti-inflammatory and antioxidant	Could be useful to treat chronic pelvic pain and its causes	[78]
	Rat model of hepatic injury in vivo	Antifibrotic	Could be effective to treat uterine fibroids	[79]

5.2. Apigenin and Luteolin

Apigenin (4',5,7-trihydroxyflavone) is found in a wide range of plants, including chamomile (*Matricaria recutita*). The traditional use of chamomile as a treatment for insomnia and anxiety has led to investigations of its active constituents, including apigenin. Apigenin is mainly present as a glycosylated compound in significant quantities in vegetables (parsley, celery, onions), fruit (oranges), herbs (chamomile, thyme, oregano, basil), and vegetable drinks (tea, beer, and wine) [80]. Apigenin is considered a phytoestrogen, although it has a much lower potency than other phytoestrogens such as genistein [81]. However, in recent studies, it has emerged that apigenin is also a phytoprogestin. A study found that apigenin reduces the risk of breast tumors in women exposed to prolonged treatment with medroxyprogesterone acetate [82,83]. A study by Horwitz and Sartorius showed that prolonged progestogen therapy could lead to the development of breast cancer through the activation of stem cells that differentiate into cancer cells [84]. In animals subjected to medroxyprogesterone therapy, apigenin administration decreased the incidence of tumors by 50% [82].

Apigenin has an antitumor effect by acting through a variety of mechanisms, including the induction of cell cycle arrest and apoptosis [74], attenuation of phosphorylation of MAP kinase [85] and inhibition of the proinflammatory cytokine interleukin-6 [86]. In vitro studies have shown that treating human breast cancer cell lines [75] with apigenin significantly reduced the expression of vascular endothelial growth factor (VEGF) and its receptor VEGFR-2 [87]. The significant reduction in VEGF disadvantages the tumor growth and development in breast tissue.

Apigenin taken orally is detectable in peripheral blood at concentrations sufficient to be biologically effective [88]. Immediately after ingestion, its concentration increases, and it remains in circulation for a long time, suggesting that it can accumulate within tissues to levels sufficient to exert chemo-preventive effects [89]. Furthermore, apigenin increased the endometrial expression of Hand2, which is a transcription factor stimulated by progesterone. The activation of Hand2 by progesterone allows an antiproliferative action in the endometrium, further suggesting that apigenin is a phytoprogestin. Apigenin appears to be non-toxic even at high doses, as suggested by a study in which it was repeatedly administered to animals up to 50 mg/kg per 10–13 days, and no signs of toxicity were observed. Apigenin seems to reduce endometrial (Ishikawa) cell proliferation regardless of progesterone [90]. In vivo, apigenin is rapidly metabolized to luteolin.

Luteolin, a flavonoid found in more than 300 plant species, many of which are readily available in the human diet, has been demonstrated to be an excellent progesterone antagonist [91] (Figure 3). A study showed that luteolin effectively inhibits the growth of progestogen-dependent human xenograft tumors, inhibiting angiogenesis and limiting the conversion of breast cancer cells to stem cell-like cells [76,77]. Interestingly, preliminary results suggest that luteolin may inhibit the growth of endometriotic lesions in a mouse model [92].

5.3. Naringenin

Naringenin (4,5,7-dihydroxy-2-(4-hydroxyphenyl)-2,3-dihydrochromen- 4-one) belongs to the subclass of flavanones (Figure 3). It is a colorless compound that gives the typical bitter taste in citrus, including grapefruit, orange, and lemon [93].

Naringenin has antioxidant, immunomodulatory, anti-inflammatory, nephroprotective, hepatoprotective, neuroprotective, antidiabetic, antitumor, and anti-atherosclerotic properties. In addition, naringenin has a high bioavailability [94,95].

Naringenin is able to inhibit the recruitment and generation of reactive oxygen species (ROS), thereby reducing oxidative stress [78,96]. Moreover, it acts directly on the NF-KB pathway in vitro and in vivo [97]. This signaling pathway is known to be activated by external agents such as pathogens. In the presence of external agents, pro-inflammatory cytokines such as IL-1 and TNF-α are recalled [98]. This stimulation and this recall involve the activation of the IKB kinase complex (IKK), which eventually phosphorylates IKK β. The phosphorylated IKB allows NF-KB to translocate into the nucleus, causing inflammatory responses [99]. Naringenin can prevent the degradation of IKB, inhibiting the transcription activity of NF-KB [98].

In numerous studies, it has emerged that naringenin is also an excellent anti-fibrotic agent [79]. In fact, naringenin was able to decrease the expression of collagen, fibronectin, and Smad3 induced by TGF-β and to inhibit Plasminogen Activator-1 (PAI-1) in hepatic cells [100]. Some of these mechanisms are similar to those fueled by progesterone in uterine fibroids [4].

In a study by Rosenberg et al. [101] it emerged that naringenin may also have progestin-like activity. More specifically, the study showed that the progestin activity of naringenin is weak and acts at concentrations around 10^{-5}–10^{-6} M. These concentration levels are similar to those deemed necessary for the action of resveratrol as a weak estrogen [102], but not for the activity of synthetic progestins such as norgestrel and norgestimate. In fact, the biological activity of naringenin compared to norgestimate is about 104-fold lower.

The effects that naringenin as a phytoprogestin could have on diseases such as endometriosis and uterine fibroids remain to be investigated. An in vitro study found that naringenin induced apoptosis and inhibited the proliferation of immortalized cell lines derived from the endocervical epithelium of a premenopausal woman undergoing hysterectomy for endometriosis [103].

6. Conclusions

There is large unexplored potential in using plant-derived substances to treat human diseases. Some of these phytochemicals have been characterized as phytoprogestins, based on their similarity with progesterone and their pharmacological interaction with PR, functioning as agonists, partial agonists, or antagonists. At least four phytoprogestins have been studied in vitro with promising results such as the antitumoral effects of KP, apigenin, and luteolin, and the anti-fibrotic effects of naringenin. Although there are limited data in the literature, it appears that phytoprogestins could be a good tool for preventing and treating hormone-dependent diseases such as endometriosis, uterine fibroids, ovarian cancer, and breast cancer, with potential reduction in the side effects of currently available hormone treatments. The next step is to proceed with tests in well-characterized animal models to define the therapeutic mechanisms and safety of these substances, along with observational human studies correlating the dietary ingestion of phytoprogestins with the prevalence and incidence of gynecologic diseases.

Author Contributions: Writing, S.G., P.P., A.Z., G.D.C., A.C., F.M.R., P.C. All authors have read and agreed to the published version of the manuscript.

Funding: This research received no external funding.

Institutional Review Board Statement: Not applicable.

Informed Consent Statement: Not applicable.

Data Availability Statement: Not applicable.

Conflicts of Interest: The authors declare no conflict of interest.

References

1. Bulletti, C.; Coccia, M.E.; Battistoni, S.; Borini, A. Endometriosis and infertility. *J. Assist. Reprod. Genet.* **2010**, *27*, 441–447. [CrossRef]
2. Islam, M.S.; Greco, S.; Janjusevic, M.; Ciavattini, A.; Giannubilo, S.R.; D'Adderio, A.; Biagini, A.; Fiorini, R.; Castellucci, M.; Ciarmela, P. Growth factors and pathogenesis. *Best Pract. Res. Clin. Obstet. Gynaecol.* **2016**, *34*, 25–36. [CrossRef]
3. Marquardt, R.M.; Kim, T.H.; Shin, J.H.; Jeong, J.W. Progesterone and Estrogen Signaling in the Endometrium: What Goes Wrong in Endometriosis? *Int. J. Mol. Sci.* **2019**, *20*, 3822. [CrossRef] [PubMed]
4. Reis, F.M.; Bloise, E.; Ortiga-Carvalho, T.M. Hormones and pathogenesis of uterine fibroids. *Best Pract. Res. Clin. Obstet. Gynaecol.* **2016**, *34*, 13–24. [CrossRef] [PubMed]
5. Momenimovahed, Z.; Tiznobaik, A.; Taheri, S.; Salehiniya, H. Ovarian cancer in the world: Epidemiology and risk factors. *Int. J. Womens Health* **2019**, *11*, 287–299. [CrossRef]
6. Group, E.C.W. Hormones and breast cancer. *Hum. Reprod. Update* **2004**, *10*, 281–293. [CrossRef] [PubMed]
7. Dietz, B.M.; Hajirahimkhan, A.; Dunlap, T.L.; Bolton, J.L. Botanicals and Their Bioactive Phytochemicals for Women's Health. *Pharmacol. Rev.* **2016**, *68*, 1026–1073. [CrossRef]
8. Hajirahimkhan, A.; Dietz, B.M.; Bolton, J.L. Botanical modulation of menopausal symptoms: Mechanisms of action? *Planta Med.* **2013**, *79*, 538–553. [CrossRef]
9. Zava, D.T.; Dollbaum, C.M.; Blen, M. Estrogen and progestin bioactivity of foods, herbs, and spices. *Proc. Soc. Exp. Biol. Med.* **1998**, *217*, 369–378. [CrossRef]
10. Scarpin, K.M.; Graham, J.D.; Mote, P.A.; Clarke, C.L. Progesterone action in human tissues: Regulation by progesterone receptor (PR) isoform expression, nuclear positioning and coregulator expression. *Nucl. Recept. Signal* **2009**, *7*, e009. [CrossRef]
11. Taraborrelli, S. Physiology, production and action of progesterone. *Acta Obstet. Gynecol. Scand.* **2015**, *94*, 8–16. [CrossRef] [PubMed]
12. Guennoun, R. Progesterone in the Brain: Hormone, Neurosteroid and Neuroprotectant. *Int. J. Mol. Sci.* **2020**, *21*, 5271. [CrossRef] [PubMed]
13. Piette, P.C.M. The pharmacodynamics and safety of progesterone. *Best Pract. Res. Clin. Obstet. Gynaecol.* **2020**, *69*, 13–29. [CrossRef]
14. Amadori, A.; Cavallari, C.; Giacomucci, E.; Macrelli, S.; Mastronuzzi, G.; Ucci, N. *Fisiologia Della Riproduzione*; CLUEB: Bologna, Italy, 1994; pp. 1–92.
15. Horie, K.; Takakura, K.; Fujiwara, H.; Suginami, H.; Liao, S.; Mori, T. Immunohistochemical localization of androgen receptor in the human ovary throughout the menstrual cycle in relation to oestrogen and progesterone receptor expression. *Hum. Reprod.* **1992**, *7*, 184–190. [CrossRef] [PubMed]
16. Thijssen, J.H. Progesterone receptors in the human uterus and their possible role in parturition. *J. Steroid Biochem. Mol. Biol.* **2005**, *97*, 397–400. [CrossRef] [PubMed]
17. Abid, S.; Gokral, J.; Maitra, A.; Meherji, P.; Kadam, S.; Pires, E.; Modi, D. Altered expression of progesterone receptors in testis of infertile men. *Reprod. Biomed. Online* **2008**, *17*, 175–184. [CrossRef]
18. Brinton, R.D.; Thompson, R.F.; Foy, M.R.; Baudry, M.; Wang, J.; Finch, C.E.; Morgan, T.E.; Pike, C.J.; Mack, W.J.; Stanczyk, F.Z.; et al. Progesterone receptors: Form and function in brain. *Front. Neuroendocrinol.* **2008**, *29*, 313–339. [CrossRef]
19. Doglioni, C.; Gambacorta, M.; Zamboni, G.; Coggi, G.; Viale, G. Immunocytochemical localization of progesterone receptors in endocrine cells of the human pancreas. *Am. J. Pathol.* **1990**, *137*, 999–1005.
20. Bland, R. Steroid hormone receptor expression and action in bone. *Clin. Sci.* **2000**, *98*, 217–240. [CrossRef]
21. Branchini, G.; Schneider, L.; Cericatto, R.; Capp, E.; Brum, I.S. Progesterone receptors A and B and estrogen receptor alpha expression in normal breast tissue and fibroadenomas. *Endocrine* **2009**, *35*, 459–466. [CrossRef]
22. Batra, S.C.; Iosif, C.S. Progesterone receptors in the female lower urinary tract. *J. Urol.* **1987**, *138*, 1301–1304. [CrossRef]

23. Lonard, D.M.; Lanz, R.B.; O'Malley, B.W. Nuclear receptor coregulators and human disease. *Endocr. Rev.* **2007**, *28*, 575–587. [CrossRef] [PubMed]
24. Smith, D.F.; Faber, L.E.; Toft, D.O. Purification of unactivated progesterone receptor and identification of novel receptor-associated proteins. *J. Biol. Chem.* **1990**, *265*, 3996–4003. [CrossRef]
25. Pratt, W.B.; Galigniana, M.D.; Morishima, Y.; Murphy, P.J. Role of molecular chaperones in steroid receptor action. *Essays Biochem.* **2004**, *40*, 41–58. [CrossRef] [PubMed]
26. Tata, J.R. Signalling through nuclear receptors. *Nat. Rev. Mol. Cell Biol.* **2002**, *3*, 702–710. [CrossRef] [PubMed]
27. Gronemeyer, H.; Meyer, M.E.; Bocquel, M.T.; Kastner, P.; Turcotte, B.; Chambon, P. Progestin receptors: Isoforms and antihormone action. *J. Steroid. Biochem. Mol. Biol.* **1991**, *40*, 271–278. [CrossRef]
28. Kastner, P.; Krust, A.; Turcotte, B.; Stropp, U.; Tora, L.; Gronemeyer, H.; Chambon, P. Two distinct estrogen-regulated promoters generate transcripts encoding the two functionally different human progesterone receptor forms A and B. *EMBO J.* **1990**, *9*, 1603–1614. [CrossRef]
29. Losel, R.M.; Besong, D.; Peluso, J.J.; Wehling, M. Progesterone receptor membrane component 1–many tasks for a versatile protein. *Steroids* **2008**, *73*, 929–934. [CrossRef]
30. Kowalik, M.K.; Rekawiecki, R.; Kotwica, J. The putative roles of nuclear and membrane-bound progesterone receptors in the female reproductive tract. *Reprod. Biol.* **2013**, *13*, 279–289. [CrossRef] [PubMed]
31. Mulac-Jericevic, B.; Lydon, J.P.; DeMayo, F.J.; Conneely, O.M. Defective mammary gland morphogenesis in mice lacking the progesterone receptor B isoform. *Proc. Natl. Acad. Sci. USA* **2003**, *100*, 9744–9749. [CrossRef]
32. Mulac-Jericevic, B.; Mullinax, R.A.; De Mayo, F.J.; Lydon, J.P.; Conneely, O.M. Subgroup of reproductive functions of progesterone mediated by progesterone receptor-B isoform. *Science* **2000**, *289*, 1751–1754. [CrossRef] [PubMed]
33. Mote, P.A.; Balleine, R.L.; McGowan, E.M.; Clarke, C.L. Colocalization of progesterone receptors A and B by dual immunofluorescent histochemistry in human endometrium during the menstrual cycle. *J. Clin. Endocrinol. Metab.* **1999**, *84*, 2963–2971. [CrossRef] [PubMed]
34. Mote, P.A.; Bartow, S.; Tran, N.; Clarke, C.L. Loss of co-ordinate expression of progesterone receptors A and B is an early event in breast carcinogenesis. *Breast Cancer Res. Treat.* **2002**, *72*, 163–172. [CrossRef]
35. Graham, J.D.; Yeates, C.; Balleine, R.L.; Harvey, S.S.; Milliken, J.S.; Bilous, A.M.; Clarke, C.L. Characterization of progesterone receptor A and B expression in human breast cancer. *Cancer Res.* **1995**, *55*, 5063–5068. [PubMed]
36. Arnett-Mansfield, R.L.; deFazio, A.; Wain, G.V.; Jaworski, R.C.; Byth, K.; Mote, P.A.; Clarke, C.L. Relative expression of progesterone receptors A and B in endometrioid cancers of the endometrium. *Cancer Res.* **2001**, *61*, 4576–4582.
37. Taylor, A.H.; McParland, P.C.; Taylor, D.J.; Bell, S.C. The cytoplasmic 60 kDa progesterone receptor isoform predominates in the human amniochorion and placenta at term. *Reprod. Biol. Endocrinol.* **2009**, *7*, 22. [CrossRef] [PubMed]
38. Wei, L.L.; Hawkins, P.; Baker, C.; Norris, B.; Sheridan, P.L.; Quinn, P.G. An amino-terminal truncated progesterone receptor isoform, PRc, enhances progestin-induced transcriptional activity. *Mol. Endocrinol.* **1996**, *10*, 1379–1387. [CrossRef]
39. Siegel, R.; Ward, E.; Brawley, O.; Jemal, A. Cancer statistics, 2011: The impact of eliminating socioeconomic and racial disparities on premature cancer deaths. *CA Cancer J. Clin.* **2011**, *61*, 212–236. [CrossRef]
40. Key, T.J.; Pike, M.C. The dose-effect relationship between 'unopposed' oestrogens and endometrial mitotic rate: Its central role in explaining and predicting endometrial cancer risk. *Br. J. Cancer* **1988**, *57*, 205–212. [CrossRef]
41. Siiteri, P.K. Steroid hormones and endometrial cancer. *Cancer Res.* **1978**, *38*, 4360–4366.
42. Doherty, J.A.; Weiss, N.S.; Fish, S.; Fan, W.; Loomis, M.M.; Sakoda, L.C.; Rossing, M.A.; Zhao, L.P.; Chen, C. Polymorphisms in nucleotide excision repair genes and endometrial cancer risk. *Cancer Epidemiol. Biomarkers Prev.* **2011**, *20*, 1873–1882. [CrossRef] [PubMed]
43. Shibutani, S.; Ravindernath, A.; Suzuki, N.; Terashima, I.; Sugarman, S.M.; Grollman, A.P.; Pearl, M.L. Identification of tamoxifen-DNA adducts in the endometrium of women treated with tamoxifen. *Carcinogenesis* **2000**, *21*, 1461–1467. [CrossRef]
44. Gompel, A. Progesterone and endometrial cancer. *Best Pract. Res. Clin. Obstet. Gynaecol.* **2020**, *69*, 95–107. [CrossRef] [PubMed]
45. Ethier, J.L.; Desautels, D.N.; Amir, E.; MacKay, H. Is hormonal therapy effective in advanced endometrial cancer? A systematic review and meta-analysis. *Gynecol. Oncol.* **2017**, *147*, 158–166. [CrossRef] [PubMed]
46. Vierikko, P.; Kauppila, A.; Ronnberg, L.; Vihko, R. Steroidal regulation of endometriosis tissue: Lack of induction of 17 beta-hydroxysteroid dehydrogenase activity by progesterone, medroxyprogesterone acetate, or danazol. *Fertil. Steril.* **1985**, *43*, 218–224. [CrossRef]
47. Brandon, D.D.; Erickson, T.E.; Keenan, E.J.; Strawn, E.Y.; Novy, M.J.; Burry, K.A.; Warner, C.; Clinton, G.M. Estrogen receptor gene expression in human uterine leiomyomata. *J. Clin. Endocrinol. Metab.* **1995**, *80*, 1876–1881. [CrossRef]
48. Soper, J.T.; McCarty, K.S., Jr.; Creasman, W.T.; Clarke-Pearson, D.L. Induction of cytoplasmic progesterone receptor in human endometrial carcinoma transplanted into nude mice. *Am. J. Obstet. Gynecol.* **1984**, *150*, 437–439. [CrossRef]
49. Murji, A.; Biberoglu, K.; Leng, J.; Mueller, M.D.; Romer, T.; Vignali, M.; Yarmolinskaya, M. Use of dienogest in endometriosis: A narrative literature review and expert commentary. *Curr. Med. Res. Opin.* **2020**, *36*, 895–907. [CrossRef]
50. Goodman, A.L. Progesterone therapy in uterine fibromyoma. *J. Clin. Endocrinol. Metab.* **1946**, *6*, 402–408. [CrossRef]
51. Lumbiganon, P.; Rugpao, S.; Phandhu-fung, S.; Laopaiboon, M.; Vudhikamraksa, N.; Werawatakul, Y. Protective effect of depot-medroxyprogesterone acetate on surgically treated uterine leiomyomas: A multicentre case-control study. *BJOG Int. J. Obstet. Gynaecol.* **1996**, *103*, 909–914. [CrossRef]

52. Schindler, A.E.; Campagnoli, C.; Druckmann, R.; Huber, J.; Pasqualini, J.R.; Schweppe, K.W.; Thijssen, J.H. Classification and pharmacology of progestins. *Maturitas* **2008**, *61*, 171–180. [CrossRef] [PubMed]
53. Ichigo, S.; Takagi, H.; Matsunami, K.; Suzuki, N.; Imai, A. Beneficial effects of dienogest on uterine myoma volume: A retrospective controlled study comparing with gonadotropin-releasing hormone agonist. *Arch. Gynecol. Obstet.* **2011**, *284*, 667–670. [CrossRef] [PubMed]
54. Rott, H. Thrombotic risks of oral contraceptives. *Curr. Opin. Obstet. Gynecol.* **2012**, *24*, 235–240. [CrossRef] [PubMed]
55. Practice Committee of the American Society for Reproductive Medicine. Combined hormonal contraception and the risk of venous thromboembolism: A guideline. *Fertil. Steril.* **2017**, *107*, 43–51. [CrossRef]
56. DeMarzo, A.M.; Beck, C.A.; Onate, S.A.; Edwards, D.P. Dimerization of mammalian progesterone receptors occurs in the absence of DNA and is related to the release of the 90-kDa heat shock protein. *Proc. Natl. Acad. Sci. USA* **1991**, *88*, 72–76. [CrossRef]
57. Smith, C.L.; O'Malley, B.W. Coregulator function: A key to understanding tissue specificity of selective receptor modulators. *Endocr. Rev.* **2004**, *25*, 45–71. [CrossRef]
58. Bouchard, P.; Chabbert-Buffet, N.; Fauser, B.C. Selective progesterone receptor modulators in reproductive medicine: Pharmacology, clinical efficacy and safety. *Fertil. Steril.* **2011**, *96*, 1175–1189. [CrossRef]
59. Wilkens, J.; Male, V.; Ghazal, P.; Forster, T.; Gibson, D.A.; Williams, A.R.; Brito-Mutunayagam, S.L.; Craigon, M.; Lourenco, P.; Cameron, I.T.; et al. Uterine NK cells regulate endometrial bleeding in women and are suppressed by the progesterone receptor modulator asoprisnil. *J. Immunol.* **2013**, *191*, 2226–2235. [CrossRef]
60. Donnez, J. Uterine Fibroids and Progestogen Treatment: Lack of Evidence of Its Efficacy: A Review. *J. Clin. Med.* **2020**, *9*, 3948. [CrossRef]
61. Bressler, L.H.; Bernardi, L.A.; Snyder, M.A.; Wei, J.J.; Bulun, S. Treatment of endometriosis-related chronic pelvic pain with Ulipristal Acetate and associated endometrial changes. *HSOA J. Reprod. Med. Gynaecol. Obstet.* **2017**, *2*. [CrossRef]
62. Lee, O.; Sullivan, M.E.; Xu, Y.; Rogers, C.; Muzzio, M.; Helenowski, I.; Shidfar, A.; Zeng, Z.; Singhal, H.; Jovanovic, B.; et al. Selective Progesterone Receptor Modulators in Early-Stage Breast Cancer: A Randomized, Placebo-Controlled Phase II Window-of-Opportunity Trial Using Telapristone Acetate. *Clin. Cancer Res.* **2020**, *26*, 25–34. [CrossRef]
63. Dinis-Oliveira, R.J. Pharmacokinetics, toxicological and clinical aspects of ulipristal acetate: Insights into the mechanisms implicated in the hepatic toxicity. *Drug Metab. Rev.* **2021**, 1–9. [CrossRef]
64. Islam, M.S.; Afrin, S.; Jones, S.I.; Segars, J. Selective Progesterone Receptor Modulators-Mechanisms and Therapeutic Utility. *Endocr. Rev.* **2020**, *41*, 643–694. [CrossRef]
65. Middleton, E., Jr.; Kandaswami, C.; Theoharides, T.C. The effects of plant flavonoids on mammalian cells: Implications for inflammation, heart disease, and cancer. *Pharmacol. Rev.* **2000**, *52*, 673–751. [PubMed]
66. Feng, X.L.; Zhan, X.X.; Zuo, L.S.; Mo, X.F.; Zhang, X.; Liu, K.Y.; Li, L.; Zhang, C.X. Associations between serum concentration of flavonoids and breast cancer risk among Chinese women. *Eur. J. Nutr.* **2021**, *60*, 1347–1362. [CrossRef] [PubMed]
67. Gates, M.A.; Tworoger, S.S.; Hecht, J.L.; De Vivo, I.; Rosner, B.; Hankinson, S.E. A prospective study of dietary flavonoid intake and incidence of epithelial ovarian cancer. *Int. J. Cancer* **2007**, *121*, 2225–2232. [CrossRef] [PubMed]
68. Wang, L.; Tu, Y.C.; Lian, T.W.; Hung, J.T.; Yen, J.H.; Wu, M.J. Distinctive antioxidant and antiinflammatory effects of flavonols. *J. Agric. Food Chem.* **2006**, *54*, 9798–9804. [CrossRef] [PubMed]
69. Orhan, I.; Kupeli, E.; Terzioglu, S.; Yesilada, E. Bioassay-guided isolation of kaempferol-3-O-beta-D-galactoside with anti-inflammatory and antinociceptive activity from the aerial part of Calluna vulgaris L. *J. Ethnopharmacol.* **2007**, *114*, 32–37. [CrossRef]
70. Park, M.J.; Lee, E.K.; Heo, H.S.; Kim, M.S.; Sung, B.; Kim, M.K.; Lee, J.; Kim, N.D.; Anton, S.; Choi, J.S.; et al. The anti-inflammatory effect of kaempferol in aged kidney tissues: The involvement of nuclear factor-kappaB via nuclear factor-inducing kinase/IkappaB kinase and mitogen-activated protein kinase pathways. *J. Med. Food* **2009**, *12*, 351–358. [CrossRef]
71. Chuwa, A.H.; Sone, K.; Oda, K.; Tanikawa, M.; Kukita, A.; Kojima, M.; Oki, S.; Fukuda, T.; Takeuchi, M.; Miyasaka, A.; et al. Kaempferol, a natural dietary flavonoid, suppresses 17beta-estradiol-induced survivin expression and causes apoptotic cell death in endometrial cancer. *Oncol. Lett.* **2018**, *16*, 6195–6201. [CrossRef]
72. Hu, G.; Liu, H.; Wang, M.; Peng, W. IQ Motif Containing GTPase-Activating Protein 3 (IQGAP3) Inhibits Kaempferol-Induced Apoptosis in Breast Cancer Cells by Extracellular Signal-Regulated Kinases 1/2 (ERK1/2) Signaling Activation. *Med. Sci. Monit.* **2019**, *25*, 7666–7674. [CrossRef]
73. Li, Y.; Ding, Z.; Wu, C. Mechanistic Study of the Inhibitory Effect of Kaempferol on Uterine Fibroids In Vitro. *Med. Sci. Monit.* **2016**, *22*, 4803–4808. [CrossRef]
74. Horinaka, M.; Yoshida, T.; Shiraishi, T.; Nakata, S.; Wakada, M.; Sakai, T. The dietary flavonoid apigenin sensitizes malignant tumor cells to tumor necrosis factor-related apoptosis-inducing ligand. *Mol. Cancer Ther.* **2006**, *5*, 945–951. [CrossRef]
75. Mafuvadze, B.; Benakanakere, I.; Hyder, S.M. Apigenin blocks induction of vascular endothelial growth factor mRNA and protein in progestin-treated human breast cancer cells. *Menopause* **2010**, *17*, 1055–1063. [CrossRef] [PubMed]
76. Cook, M.T.; Liang, Y.; Besch-Williford, C.; Goyette, S.; Mafuvadze, B.; Hyder, S.M. Luteolin inhibits progestin-dependent angiogenesis, stem cell-like characteristics, and growth of human breast cancer xenografts. *Springerplus* **2015**, *4*, 444. [CrossRef] [PubMed]
77. Cook, M.T.; Liang, Y.; Besch-Williford, C.; Hyder, S.M. Luteolin inhibits lung metastasis, cell migration, and viability of triple-negative breast cancer cells. *Breast Cancer* **2017**, *9*, 9–19. [CrossRef] [PubMed]

78. Manchope, M.F.; Calixto-Campos, C.; Coelho-Silva, L.; Zarpelon, A.C.; Pinho-Ribeiro, F.A.; Georgetti, S.R.; Baracat, M.M.; Casagrande, R.; Verri, W.A., Jr. Naringenin Inhibits Superoxide Anion-Induced Inflammatory Pain: Role of Oxidative Stress, Cytokines, Nrf-2 and the NO-cGMP-PKG-KATP Channel Signaling Pathway. *PLoS ONE* **2016**, *11*, e0153015. [CrossRef] [PubMed]
79. Lee, M.H.; Yoon, S.; Moon, J.O. The flavonoid naringenin inhibits dimethylnitrosamine-induced liver damage in rats. *Biol. Pharm. Bull.* **2004**, *27*, 72–76. [CrossRef] [PubMed]
80. Hostetler, G.L.; Ralston, R.A.; Schwartz, S.J. Flavones: Food Sources, Bioavailability, Metabolism, and Bioactivity. *Adv. Nutr.* **2017**, *8*, 423–435. [CrossRef]
81. Mabry, T.; Markham, K.R.; Thomas, M.B. *The Systematic Identification of Flavonoids*; Springer: Berlin/Heidelberg, Germany, 2012.
82. Mafuvadze, B.; Benakanakere, I.; Lopez Perez, F.R.; Besch-Williford, C.; Ellersieck, M.R.; Hyder, S.M. Apigenin prevents development of medroxyprogesterone acetate-accelerated 7,12-dimethylbenz(a)anthracene-induced mammary tumors in Sprague-Dawley rats. *Cancer Prev. Res.* **2011**, *4*, 1316–1324. [CrossRef]
83. Mafuvadze, B.; Liang, Y.; Besch-Williford, C.; Zhang, X.; Hyder, S.M. Apigenin induces apoptosis and blocks growth of medroxyprogesterone acetate-dependent BT-474 xenograft tumors. *Horm. Cancer* **2012**, *3*, 160–171. [CrossRef] [PubMed]
84. Horwitz, K.B.; Sartorius, C.A. Progestins in hormone replacement therapies reactivate cancer stem cells in women with preexisting breast cancers: A hypothesis. *J. Clin. Endocrinol. Metab.* **2008**, *93*, 3295–3298. [CrossRef]
85. Yin, F.; Giuliano, A.E.; Law, R.E.; Van Herle, A.J. Apigenin inhibits growth and induces G2/M arrest by modulating cyclin-CDK regulators and ERK MAP kinase activation in breast carcinoma cells. *Anticancer Res.* **2001**, *21*, 413–420. [PubMed]
86. Lee, H.H.; Jung, J.; Moon, A.; Kang, H.; Cho, H. Antitumor and Anti-Invasive Effect of Apigenin on Human Breast Carcinoma through Suppression of IL-6 Expression. *Int. J. Mol. Sci.* **2019**, *20*, 3143. [CrossRef] [PubMed]
87. Hyder, S.M. Sex-steroid regulation of vascular endothelial growth factor in breast cancer. *Endocr. Relat. Cancer* **2006**, *13*, 667–687. [CrossRef]
88. Meyer, H.; Bolarinwa, A.; Wolfram, G.; Linseisen, J. Bioavailability of apigenin from apiin-rich parsley in humans. *Ann. Nutr. Metab.* **2006**, *50*, 167–172. [CrossRef]
89. Chen, D.; Landis-Piwowar, K.R.; Chen, M.S.; Dou, Q.P. Inhibition of proteasome activity by the dietary flavonoid apigenin is associated with growth inhibition in cultured breast cancer cells and xenografts. *Breast Cancer Res.* **2007**, *9*, R80. [CrossRef]
90. Dean, M.; Austin, J.; Jinhong, R.; Johnson, M.E.; Lantvit, D.D.; Burdette, J.E. The Flavonoid Apigenin Is a Progesterone Receptor Modulator with In Vivo Activity in the Uterus. *Horm. Cancer* **2018**, *9*, 265–277. [CrossRef]
91. Fidelis, Q.C.; Faraone, I.; Russo, D.; Aragao Catunda, F.E., Jr.; Vignola, L.; de Carvalho, M.G.; de Tommasi, N.; Milella, L. Chemical and Biological insights of *Ouratea hexasperma* (A. St.-Hil.) Baill.: A source of bioactive compounds with multifunctional properties. *Nat. Prod. Res.* **2019**, *33*, 1500–1503. [CrossRef]
92. Park, S.; Lim, W.; You, S.; Song, G. Ameliorative effects of luteolin against endometriosis progression in vitro and in vivo. *J. Nutr. Biochem.* **2019**, *67*, 161–172. [CrossRef]
93. Zaidun, N.H.; Thent, Z.C.; Latiff, A.A. Combating oxidative stress disorders with citrus flavonoid: Naringenin. *Life Sci.* **2018**, *208*, 111–122. [CrossRef]
94. Pereira-Caro, G.; Borges, G.; van der Hooft, J.; Clifford, M.N.; Del Rio, D.; Lean, M.E.; Roberts, S.A.; Kellerhals, M.B.; Crozier, A. Orange juice (poly)phenols are highly bioavailable in humans. *Am. J. Clin. Nutr.* **2014**, *100*, 1378–1384. [CrossRef]
95. Kanaze, F.I.; Bounartzi, M.I.; Georgarakis, M.; Niopas, I. Pharmacokinetics of the citrus flavanone aglycones hesperetin and naringenin after single oral administration in human subjects. *Eur. J. Clin. Nutr.* **2007**, *61*, 472–477. [CrossRef] [PubMed]
96. Martinez, R.M.; Pinho-Ribeiro, F.A.; Steffen, V.S.; Caviglione, C.V.; Vignoli, J.A.; Barbosa, D.S.; Baracat, M.M.; Georgetti, S.R.; Verri, W.A., Jr.; Casagrande, R. Naringenin Inhibits UVB Irradiation-Induced Inflammation and Oxidative Stress in the Skin of Hairless Mice. *J. Nat. Prod.* **2015**, *78*, 1647–1655. [CrossRef] [PubMed]
97. Pinho-Ribeiro, F.A.; Zarpelon, A.C.; Fattori, V.; Manchope, M.F.; Mizokami, S.S.; Casagrande, R.; Verri, W.A., Jr. Naringenin reduces inflammatory pain in mice. *Neuropharmacology* **2016**, *105*, 508–519. [CrossRef] [PubMed]
98. Lawrence, T. The nuclear factor NF-kappaB pathway in inflammation. *Cold Spring Harb. Perspect. Biol.* **2009**, *1*, a001651. [CrossRef]
99. Ghosh, S.; Karin, M. Missing pieces in the NF-kappaB puzzle. *Cell* **2002**, *109*, S81–S96. [CrossRef]
100. Liu, X.; Wang, W.; Hu, H.; Tang, N.; Zhang, C.; Liang, W.; Wang, M. Smad3 specific inhibitor, naringenin, decreases the expression of extracellular matrix induced by TGF-beta1 in cultured rat hepatic stellate cells. *Pharm. Res.* **2006**, *23*, 82–89. [CrossRef]
101. Rosenberg, R.S.; Grass, L.; Jenkins, D.J.; Kendall, C.W.; Diamandis, E.P. Modulation of androgen and progesterone receptors by phytochemicals in breast cancer cell lines. *Biochem. Biophys. Res. Commun.* **1998**, *248*, 935–939. [CrossRef]
102. Gehm, B.D.; McAndrews, J.M.; Chien, P.Y.; Jameson, J.L. Resveratrol, a polyphenolic compound found in grapes and wine, is an agonist for the estrogen receptor. *Proc. Natl. Acad. Sci. USA* **1997**, *94*, 14138–14143. [CrossRef]
103. Park, S.; Lim, W.; Bazer, F.W.; Song, G. Naringenin induces mitochondria-mediated apoptosis and endoplasmic reticulum stress by regulating MAPK and AKT signal transduction pathways in endometriosis cells. *Mol. Hum. Reprod.* **2017**, *23*, 842–854. [CrossRef] [PubMed]

MDPI
St. Alban-Anlage 66
4052 Basel
Switzerland
Tel. +41 61 683 77 34
Fax +41 61 302 89 18
www.mdpi.com

Nutrients Editorial Office
E-mail: nutrients@mdpi.com
www.mdpi.com/journal/nutrients